MW01181580

2005
YEAR BOOK OF
PATHOLOGY
AND LABORATORY
MEDICINE®

The 2005 Year Book Series

Year Book of Allergy, Asthma, and Clinical Immunology™: Drs Rosenwasser, Boguniewicz, Milgrom, Routes, and Spahn

Year Book of Anesthesiology and Pain Management™: Drs Chestnut, Abram, Black, Gravlee, Mathru, Lee, and Roizen

Year Book of Cardiology®: Drs Gersh, Cheitlin, Graham, Kaplan, Sundt, and Waldo

Year Book of Critical Care Medicine®: Drs Dellinger, Parrillo, Balk, Bekes, Dries, and Dorman

Year Book of Dentistry®: Drs Zakariasen, Hatcher, Horswell, McIntyre, Scott, Victoroff, and Zakariasen

Year Book of Dermatology and Dermatologic Surgery™: Drs Thiers and Lang

Year Book of Diagnostic Radiology®: Drs Osborn, Birdwell, Dalinka, Gardiner, Levy, Maynard, and Oestreich

Year Book of Emergency Medicine®: Drs Burdick, Cydulka, Hamilton, Handly, Werner, and Quintana

Year Book of Endocrinology®: Drs Mazzaferri, Rubin, Molitch, Leahy, Kennedy, Kannan, Bessesen, Rogol, and Meikle

Year Book of Family Practice®: Drs Bowman, Apgar, Dexter, Miser, Neill, and Scherger

Year Book of Gastroenterology™: Drs Lichtenstein, Dempsey, Drebin, Faust, Ginsberg, Katzka, Kochman, Morris, Reddy, and Stein

Year Book of Hand and Upper Limb Surgery®: Drs Berger and Ladd

Year Book of Medicine®: Drs Barkin, Frishman, Klahr, Loehrer, Mazzaferri, Phillips, Pillinger, and Snydman

Year Book of Neonatal and Perinatal Medicine®: Drs Fanaroff, Maisels, and Stevenson

Year Book of Neurology and Neurosurgery®: Drs Gibbs and Verma

Year Book of Nuclear Medicine®: Drs Coleman, Blaufox, Royal, Strauss, and Zubal

Year Book of Obstetrics, Gynecology, and Women's Health®: Dr Shulman

Year Book of Oncology®: Drs Loehrer, Arceci, Glatstein, Gordon, Hanna, Morrow, and Thigpen

Year Book of Ophthalmology®: Drs Rapuano, Cohen, Eagle, Grossman, Hammersmith, Myers, Nelson, Penne, Sergott, Shields, Tipperman, and Vander

Year Book of Orthopedics®: Drs Morrey, Beauchamp, Peterson, Swiontkowski, Trigg, and Yaszemski

Year Book of Otolaryngology-Head and Neck Surgery®: Drs Paparella, Otto, and Keefe

2005

The Year Book of PATHOLOGY AND LABORATORY MEDICINE®

Editors-in-Chief

Stephen S. Raab, MD

Director of Cytology and Director of Pathology Quality and Healthcare Research, University of Pittsburgh Medical Center; and Professor of Pathology, University of Pittsburgh School of Medicine, Pittsburgh, Pennsylvania

Dana Marie Grzybicki, MD, PhD

Assistant Professor, Department of Pathology, University of Pittsburgh School of Medicine; University of Pittsburgh Medical Center, Pittsburgh, Pennsylvania

Editors

Pablo A. Bejarano, MD

Associate Professor, University of Miami School of Medicine; and Pathologist, Jackson Memorial Hospital, Miami, Florida

Michael G. Bissell, MD, PhD, MPH

Professor of Pathology, Ohio State University; and Director of Clinical Chemistry and Toxicology, Ohio State University Medical Center, Columbus, Ohio

Michael W. Stanley, MD

Professor of Pathology, University of Minnesota; Pathologist, Hospital Pathology Associates, Minneapolis, Minnesota

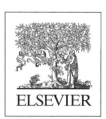

ELSEVIER

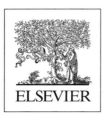

Vice President, Continuity Publishing: Timothy M. Griswold
Managing Editor, Continuity Production: David Orzechowski
Associate Developmental Editor: Tim Maxwell
Senior Manager, Continuity Production: Idelle L. Winer
Issue Manager: Jason Gonulsen
Illustrations and Permissions Coordinator: Kimberly E. Denando

2005 EDITION

Printed in the United States of America
Composition by Thomas Technology Solutions, Inc.
Printing/binding by Sheridan Books, Inc.

Editorial Office:
Elsevier
300 East
170 South Independence Mall West
Philadelphia, PA 19106-3399

International Standard Serial Number: 1077-9108
International Standard Book Number: 0-323-02115-8

Contributing Editors

Marta E. Couce, MD, PhD
Assistant Professor of Pathology, Division of Neuropathology, University of Pittsburgh, Pittsburgh, Pennsylvania

Fiona Craig, MD
Associate Professor, Medical Director, Clinical Flow Cytometry Lab, Presbyterian University Hospital, Pathology Department, Pittsburgh, Pennsylvania

Rajiv Dhir, MD
Division Director, Genitourinary Pathology, UPMC Shadyside, Department of Pathology, Pittsburgh, Pennsylvania

Ronald Jaffe, MB, BCh
Chief of Pathology, Children's Hospital of Pittsburgh; and Professor of Pathology and Pediatrics, University of Pittsburgh School of Medicine, Pittsburgh, Pennsylvania

Drazen M. Jukic, MD, PhD
Assistant Professor, Departments of Dermatology and Pathology; and Director, Dermatopathology, University of Pittsburgh School of Medicine, Pittsburgh, Pennsylvania

Frederico Monzon-Bordonaba, MD
Assistant Professor of Pathology, Medical Director, Cancer Biomarkers Laboratory, Pathology Informatics, Pittsburgh, Pennsylvania

Table of Contents

Journals Represented

Journals represented in this YEAR BOOK are listed below.

American Journal of Clinical Pathology
American Journal of Dermatopathology
American Journal of Gastroenterology
American Journal of Human Genetics
American Journal of Kidney Diseases
American Journal of Medicine
American Journal of Pathology
American Journal of Surgery
American Journal of Surgical Pathology
American Surgeon
Annals of Diagnostic Pathology
Annals of Internal Medicine
Annals of Surgical Oncology
Annals of Thoracic Surgery
Archives of Dermatology
Archives of Pathology and Laboratory Medicine
Archives of Surgery
Blood
Brain Research
Breast Journal
British Journal of Cancer
British Journal of Haematology
British Journal of Surgery
British Journal of Urology International
CA: A Cancer Journal for Clinicians
Cancer
Cancer Epidemiology, Biomarkers and Prevention
Cardiovascular Pathology
Chest
Clinical Cancer Research
Clinical Chemistry
Clinical Infectious Diseases
Diabetes Care
European Journal of Cancer
European Journal of Surgical Oncology (London)
European Respiratory Journal
Forensic Science International
Gastrointestinal Endoscopy
Gut
Gynecologic Oncology
Head and Neck
Hepatology
Histopathology
Human Pathology
International Journal of Cancer
International Journal of Gynecological Pathology
International Journal of Oral and Maxillofacial Surgery
Journal of Clinical Endocrinology and Metabolism
Journal of Clinical Investigation

Journal of Clinical Microbiology
Journal of Clinical Oncology
Journal of Clinical Pathology
Journal of Cutaneous Pathology
Journal of Diabetes and Its Complications
Journal of Experimental Medicine
Journal of Investigative Dermatology
Journal of Laryngology and Otology
Journal of Molecular Diagnostics
Journal of Pathology
Journal of Pediatric Gastroenterology and Nutrition
Journal of Pediatric Hematology/Oncology
Journal of Thoracic and Cardiovascular Surgery
Journal of Urology
Journal of the American College of Surgeons
Journal of the American Medical Association
Journal of the National Cancer Institute
Leukemia
Metabolism: Clinical and Experimental
Modern Pathology
Neurology
New England Journal of Medicine
Oral Surgery, Oral Medicine, Oral Pathology, Oral Radiology Endodontics
Otolaryngology-Head and Neck Surgery
Pediatric and Developmental Pathology
Proceedings of the National Academy of Sciences
Public Health Reports
Science
Stroke
Surgery
Thrombosis Research
Transfusion
Transplantation
Urology

STANDARD ABBREVIATIONS

The following terms are abbreviated in this edition: acquired immunodeficiency syndrome (AIDS), cardiopulmonary resuscitation (CPR), central nervous system (CNS), cerebrospinal fluid (CSF), computed tomography (CT), deoxyribonucleic acid (DNA), electrocardiography (ECG), health maintenance organization (HMO), human immunodeficiency virus (HIV), intensive care unit (ICU), intramuscular (IM), intravenous (IV), magnetic resonance (MR) imaging (MRI), ribonucleic acid (RNA), ultrasound (US), and ultraviolet (UV).

NOTE

The YEAR BOOK OF PATHOLOGY AND LABORATORY MEDICINE is a literature survey service providing abstracts of articles published in the professional literature. Every effort is made to assure the accuracy of the information presented in these pages. Neither the editors nor the publisher of the YEAR BOOK OF PATHOLOGY AND LABORATORY MEDICINE can be responsible for errors in the original materials. The editors' comments are their own opinions. Mention of specific products within this publication does not constitute endorsement.

To facilitate the use of the YEAR BOOK OF PATHOLOGY AND LABORATORY MEDICINE as a reference tool, all illustrations and tables included in this publication are now identified as they appear in the original article. This change is meant to help the reader recognize that any illustration or table appearing in the YEAR BOOK OF PATHOLOGY AND LABORATORY MEDICINE may be only one of many in the original article. For this reason, figure and table numbers will often appear to be out of sequence within the YEAR BOOK OF PATHOLOGY AND LABORATORY MEDICINE.

Introduction

Welcome to the 2005 YEAR BOOK OF PATHOLOGY AND LABORATORY MEDICINE! We believe that this year's YEAR BOOK contains a number of abstracted articles that bring us up to date on the important areas in anatomic and clinical pathology. These articles include current data on practice management issues, new uses of immunohistochemistry and other technologies, and state of the art in diagnoses.

As usual, the contributing editors provide insightful, humorous, and concise views of most of these articles. For many of these articles, the editors provide a list of suggested readings, which, in their opinion, are important reviews or the major sources of information for the current topics. The editors include Drs Michael Stanley (Hennepin County Medical Center), Michael Bissell (Ohio State University), and Pablo Bejarano (University of Miami). Other contributors include Drs Fiona Craig, Frederico Monzon-Bordonaba, Marta Couce, Drazen Jukic, Rajiv Dhir, and Ronald Jaffe.

We hope you enjoy the abstracts and commentary. Please feel free to provide either of us feedback: (raabss@msx.upmc.edu or grzybickidm@msx.upmc.edu). Thank you and good reading!!

Stephen S. Raab, MD
Dana M. Grzybicki, MD, PhD
Editors-in-Chief

PART I

ANATOMIC PATHOLOGY

1 Outcome Analysis

Interinstitutional Pathology Consultations: A Reassessment
Weir MM, Jan E, Colgan TJ (Univ of Western Ontario, London, Canada; Univ of Toronto)
Am J Clin Pathol 120:405-412, 2003   1–1

Introduction.—The Association of Directors of Anatomic and Surgical Pathology recommended about 1 decade ago the adoption of interinstitutional pathology consultations (IPCs). Despite the call for mandatory IPCs, there is no consensus regarding the adoption of this practice. The value of IPCs was evaluated in a publicly funded (single-payer) Canadian health care system.

Methods.—The clinical impact of 1000 randomly chosen IPCs was retrospectively examined. All specimens from each patient were reviewed during the IPC. The IPCs were classified as either concordant or discordant with the original diagnosis. Discordant IPCs were further classified as having clinical impact or no clinical impact. Discordant IPCs involved in interpretation differences were further subclassified.

Results.—A total of 1522 IPC specimens were reviewed (1204 histology; 318 cytology). Of these, 923 (92.3%) were concordant, 9 (0.9%) were indeterminate, and 68 (6.8%) were discordant (clinical impact, 37; no impact, 31). Reasons for discordant IPCs included interpretation differences in 45 cases, additional sectioning in 7, ancillary testing in 1, clerical errors in 5, and a combination of reasons in 10 cases. Reasons for 26 discordant IPCs with clinical impact because of interpretation differences were overdiagnosis in 11 cases, tumor subtype change in 4, stage change in 4, underdiagnosis in 3, resection margin status change in 2, undergrading in 1, and understaging with resection margin status change in 1 case.

Conclusion.—An IPC may identify diagnostic discrepancies that affect the management of some patients. The prevalence of a clinical impact of IPC on management differs according to body site. Mandatory IPCs ensure the identification of clinically important discrepancies.

▶ This fine study by a group of Canadian pathologists in Toronto illustrates the utility of IPCs for improving patient outcomes by preinterventional detection of diagnostic discrepancies that impact patient clinical management. The general findings of these authors are not unique, but the detailed examination they perform regarding the underlying reasons for discrepancies is new information, and their comprehensive and thoughtful discussion is highly worthwhile reading. These authors find an overall diagnostic discrepancy rate of 6.8%, with a little over half of the detected discrepancies (3.7%) resulting in significant clinical management changes. Detailed stratification of their discrepancies revealed a majority that were caused by discrepancies in pathologist interpretations, although other reasons, such as lack of original ancillary testing, were also identified.

This article is highly timely in light of the current emphasis on improving patient safety in all areas of health care. The authors point out in their discussion the relatively low level of compliance in the general pathology community with adoption of IPCs for all cases referred for surgical management, citing consultation remuneration issues, labor intensity issues, and pathologist and clinician need for more effective evidence as major reasons for noncompliance. Similar to implementation of many, if not all, quality improvement interventions, resistance based on fears of revenue loss and change, as well as unwavering perceptions of lack of time and adequate convincing data, appears to hamper the widespread implementation of this quality improvement process. In the face of continuing undeniable evidence supporting the usefulness of this procedure, pathologists should do the right thing for patients and create changes in their departments allowing for the general adoption of this safety improvement process.

D. M. Grzybicki, MD, PhD

Slide Review in Gynecologic Oncology Ensures Completeness of Reporting and Diagnostic Accuracy
Khalifa MA, Dodge J, Covens A, et al (Sunnybrook and Women's College Health Sciences Ctr, Toronto)
Gynecol Oncol 90:425-430, 2003   1–2

Introduction.—Despite the nearly universal application of routine pathology review in clinical practice, few publications have concentrated on the value of interinstitutional pathology review for gynecologic oncology patients referred to tertiary care medical centers for either primary surgery or adjuvant therapy. Medical records were reviewed in a tertiary care teaching hospital to investigate the value of the mandatory slide review policy in gynecologic oncology, with emphasis on completeness of reports.

Methods.—Cases reviewed between October 2001 through September 2002 were evaluated. Clinical data were obtained from discussions at the weekly tumor board and from medical record review. The standardized reporting guidelines in benchmark surgical pathology textbooks were used to examine the completeness of original pathology reports of excisional specimens (Table 1). Diagnostic discrepancies were classified as major if the resultant change altered patient management and minor if patient management was unaffected.

Results.—Of 351 cases reviewed, 173 were biopsies and 178 were excisional specimens. One hundred forty (78.8%) of the original pathology re-

TABLE 1.—The Database Scheme Used for Entering Results of Each Pathology Review

Patient's demographic information section

Case review by another academic gynecologic pathologist   ☐ Yes   ☐ No

Nature of specimen   ☐ Biopsy   ☐ Excision

Result of the review

I. Accuracy of original diagnosis

☐ Agree with original diagnosis   ☐ Disagree with original diagnosis

     Nature of the change in diagnosis

       ☐ Increase the stage
       ☐ Lower the stage
       ☐ Increase the grade
       ☐ Lower the grade
       ☐ Cell type change
       ☐ Benign versus malignant
       ☐ Other

     Clinical-pathologic correlation
     Does discrepancy change management?

       ☐ Yes   ☐ No

II. Completeness of original report (for excisional specimens only)

☐ Original report is complete   ☐ Original report is incomplete

     Missing information ————————

     Clinical-pathologic correlation
     Is the missing information essential?

       ☐ Yes   ☐ No

(Courtesy of Khalifa MA, Dodge J, Covens A, et al: Slide review in gynecologic oncology ensures completeness of reporting and diagnostic accuracy. *Gynecol Oncol* 90:425-430, 2003. Copyright 2003 by Elsevier Science.)

ports of excisional specimens conformed to standardized reporting guidelines. Of 38 incomplete reports, 18 were missing crucial information needed for planning further therapy; this represented 10.1% of reports of all excisional specimens. There was agreement with the original diagnosis in 252 cases (71.8%). Minor discrepancies were recorded in 70 (19.9%) and major discrepancies in 29 cases (8.3%). No major discrepancies resulted from reviewing any of the vulvar specimens or cases already reviewed by gynecologic pathologists from other academic institutes.

Conclusion.—Mandatory slide review in gynecologic oncology is important in the management of gynecologic cancer since it completes reporting on missing parameters necessary for planning subsequent therapy in 10.1% of cases and identifies discrepancies that alter management in 8.3% of patients.

▶ At the risk of seeming repetitive in my selection of articles this year, I decided to go ahead and include this article as recommended reading for all pathologists for 3 major reasons. First, these authors show, in their single study, the usefulness of mandatory slide review for all gynecologic cancer cases referred for treatment for detecting both reporting and diagnostic interpretation errors that may significantly impact patient management and outcomes. Second, they provide a very concise but highly useful quality assurance/quality improvement data collection sheet for case review that could be easily and quickly completed by pathologists in all practice types for cancer cases from any anatomic site. Finally, a current major health policy and health services research question is, "How do we effectively incorporate the best practice information we are generating into daily medical practice?" As a result of the findings of this study, the authors received funding to host an active education and dissemination workshop where synoptic reporting will be reviewed and practiced, and where attendees will receive CD-ROMs with digital files of report templates that may be inserted into current pathology reports. Pathology reports of referred cases will then be monitored for the subsequent year to assess the effectiveness of this workshop method.

D. M. Grzybicki, MD, PhD

Concordance With Breast Cancer Pathology Reporting Practice Guidelines
Wilkinson NW, Shahryarinejad A, Winston JS, et al (Roswell Park Cancer Inst, Buffalo, NY; State Univ of New York, Buffalo)
J Am Coll Surg 196:38-43, 2003   1–3

Background.—Accurate pathology reporting is an essential aspect of proper medical and surgical treatment of breast cancer. In 1998, the College of American Pathologists (CAP) distributed guidelines for reporting pathologic findings from cancer specimens. The purpose of this study was to determine community-wide concordance with CAP breast cancer reporting guidelines.

Methods.—The pathology reporting of stage I and II breast cancers was examined for adherence to CAP guidelines. Pathology reports were reviewed from 100 consecutive patients with invasive breast cancer referred to Roswell Park Cancer Institute in 1998 or 1999 after excisional breast biopsy. Also reviewed were 20 consecutive patients who underwent excisional biopsy at the Institute. Adherence to CAP guidelines on clinically relevant items was determined from the original pathology report for each patient.

Results.—A total of 101 cases met the inclusion criteria. Reports for most of these patients did not include at least 1 of the elements required by the CAP guidelines. Surgical margins were inked in only 77% of cases, and the margins were oriented in only 25% of cases, with many specimens not being oriented by the surgeon. Grade was reported in most cases, but use of the Bloom Scarf Richardson scale for grade was reported in only 6% of cases. The presence or absence of lymphovascular invasion was reported in 57% of cases, and the presence or absence of coexisting in situ disease was reported in 71% of cases.

Conclusions.—This study found wide variations in breast cancer pathology reporting. In many cases, key elements affecting treatment were omitted, including description of gross specimen and tumor size, orientation and involvement of surgical margins, and histologic features. The passive distribution of CAP practice guidelines may be insufficient to accomplish community-wide quality improvement in breast pathology reporting.

▶ This study provides evidence supporting the fact that CAP reporting guidelines for breast cancer surgical pathology diagnostic specimens are poorly adhered to in daily practice. Since appropriate treatment requires complete and accurate pathologic information at the time of original diagnosis, these findings are clearly highly clinically relevant and suggest that in some cases, optimal care may not be given or may not be given in a timely manner as a consequence of omissions in pathology reports. A major limitation of the study is the lack of outcome information for the patients whose reports contained serious omissions. A complete understanding of the impact of reporting omissions may provide information useful for prioritizing elements of the current recommendations, for more effective dissemination of the current guidelines, or both. Previous studies examining effective methods for practice guideline dissemination and acceptance have shown that passive methods are, by and large, inadequate, and that some form of audit after implementation is necessary to ensure ongoing compliance. Therefore, for the current CAP guidelines to be adopted in everyday practice, active methods involving the CAP leadership and other pathology leaders will need to be utilized, and a method for auditing compliance by a body willing to insist on accountability will need to be instituted.

D. M. Grzybicki, MD, PhD

Risk of Cervical Cancer Associated With Extending the Interval Between Cervical-Cancer Screenings

Sawaya GF, McConnell KJ, Kulasingam SL, et al (Univ of California, San Francisco; Oregon Health and Science Univ, Portland; Duke Univ, Durham, NC; et al)
N Engl J Med 349:1501-1509, 2003   1–4

Background.—Guidelines from the US Preventive Services Task Force and other groups recommend screening for cervical cancer be performed "at least every 3 years," rather than every year, for women more than 30 years old who have had 3 or more consecutive negative cervical cytologic exams. Still, many practitioners continue to recommend annual cervical exams, perhaps in part because they believe less frequent screening may increase the risk of cervical cancer. These authors created a Markov model to examine the excess risk of cervical cancer associated with triennial cervical cytologic exams in low-risk women.

Methods.—Data from the Centers for Disease Control and Prevention's National Breast and Cervical Cancer Early Detection Program were examined to determine the incidence of biopsy-proven cervical neoplasia among 938,576 women aged 30 to 64 years. Subjects were stratified according to their number of previous consecutive negative Papanicolaou tests. Then the authors used a Markov model to estimate the risk of cervical cancer within 3 years after a given number of negative Papanicolaou tests. They also estimated the number of additional exams that would be required to prevent 1 case of cervical cancer with triennial versus annual screening.

Results.—In all, there were 31,728 women aged 30 to 64 years who had 3 or more consecutive negative cervical cytologic exam results. Among this group, 9 women (0.028%) had biopsy-proven cervical intraepithelial neoplasia (CIN) grade 2, and 6 women (0.019%) had CIN grade 3; none had invasive cervical cancer. According to the Markov model, the estimated risk of cervical cancer with annual screening for 3 years was 2 per 100,000 in women aged 30 to 44 years, 1 per 100,000 in women aged 45 to 59 years, and 1 per 100,000 in women aged 60 to 64 years. If screening were performed only once 3 years after the last negative exam, the corresponding estimates would be 5, 2, and 1 per 100,000, respectively. To prevent 1 additional case of cervical cancer by screening 100,000 women annually for 3 years rather than once 3 years after the last negative test, women aged 30 to 44 years would need 69,665 additional Papanicolaou tests and 3861 colposcopic exams; women aged 45 to 59 years would need 209,342 additional Papanicolaou tests and 11,502 colposcopic exams.

Conclusion.—Screening women aged 30 to 64 years with 3 or more consecutive negative cervical cancer screening results every 3 years is associated with only a small excess risk of cervical cancer compared with annual screening (on average, approximately 3 per 100,000 women). These findings support the recommendations for triennial cervical cancer screening in low-risk women.

▶ This article provides, for those pathologists interested in clinical outcomes research, a well-designed, well-performed, and well-reported study exquisitely relevant to cytology and surgical pathology practice. With Markov modeling, this study provides the confirmatory evidence supporting extension of the cervical cancer screening interval in women aged 30 to 64 years who have had 3 previous consecutive negative Papanicolaou tests, a recommendation that has been adopted by the American Cancer Society, the Centers for Disease Control and Prevention, and the U.S. Preventive Services Task Force. Importantly, the authors stress that these recommendations should be considered in the context of the level of dysplasia risk in the particular patient population.

D. M. Grzybicki, MD, PhD

Eight False Negative Sentinel Node Procedures in Breast Cancer: What Went Wrong?

Estourgie SH, Nieweg OE, Valdés Olmos RA, et al (The Netherlands Cancer Inst, Amsterdam)
Eur J Surg Oncol 29:336-340, 2003   1–5

Background.—Even though sentinel lymph node (SLN) biopsy has become popular for staging breast cancer, false-negative cases do occur. These authors review their experience with false-negative SLN cases to determine what went wrong in these procedures and what could be done to prevent such failures in the future.

Methods.—The subjects were 599 women with clinically node-negative breast cancer who underwent 606 SLN biopsy procedures between January 1997 and November 2001. During the learning phase (ie, until January 1999), 81 patients underwent routine axillary clearance. Beginning in November 1999, all patients underwent preoperative axillary US to confirm nodal status. SLN procedures were performed over a 2-day period, with intratumoral injection of radiotracer and lymphoscintigraphy on day 1, followed the next day by intratumoral blue dye injection and excision of the SLNs. SLNs were formalin fixed, bisected, paraffin embedded, and cut through at least 6 levels at 50- to 150-µm intervals. Cases in which the SLN was negative but another non-SLN was positive, as determined during axillary clearance or by clinical follow-up, were examined in detail.

Results.—SLNs were identified in 565 (93.2%) of the 606 procedures. Of these, 204 SLNs (36.1%) revealed metastasis. There were 8 false-negative findings. Two of these false-negative cases were discovered by axillary clearance during the learning phase. In 2 other cases, the axillary tail of the simple mastectomy specimen was found to harbor diseased lymph nodes. In 3 cases, a non-SLN that was negative for both blue dye and radiotracer, but which nevertheless was positive for tumor, was present. In 1 case, axillary recurrence developed 22 months after surgery. After careful analysis, the presumptive causes of these false-negative findings were determined to be surgical delay in 1 case, sampling error of the pathologic specimen in 3 cases, obstruction of lymphatic flow by the tumor in 2 cases, and indeterminable in 2 cases.

Conclusion.—Based on their analyses of what went wrong in these 8 false-negative cases, the authors make the following suggestions for SLN biopsy in breast cancer. First, preoperative US of the axilla can help ensure nodes are negative. The procedure should include both radioactive tracer and blue dye injections, and if performed as a 2-day procedure, surgery should take place first thing in the morning on day 2 to ensure the radiotracer has not dissipated. Intraoperative palpation of the biopsy wound should be performed to identify any suspicious lymph nodes. A target of 7 specimen slices at 50- to

150-µm intervals seems to strike an acceptable balance between sensitivity and pathologist workload.

▶ This extremely interesting study describes application of root cause analysis to a particular anatomic pathology diagnostic error, specifically, false-negative SLN diagnoses in breast cancer patients. I think this study is important for pathologists to read because this kind of analysis uncommonly takes place in anatomic pathology practice, and it is rarely reported in the pathology literature. As a consequence of the authors' willingness to investigate causes underlying rare negative events in an effort to improve quality of care, they discovered causative factors on both the laboratory and the clinical sides of the care equation that they felt contributed to these errors. Most importantly, they were able to formulate process change recommendations that may prevent these errors from happening in the future.

D. M. Grzybicki, MD, PhD

Interobserver and Intraobserver Reproducibility in the Histopathology of Follicular Thyroid Carcinoma
Franc B, de la Salmonière P, Lange F, et al (Ambroise Paré Hosp, Boulogne, France; Univ of Versailles, St Quentin en Yvelines, France; Univ of Paris VI; et al)
Hum Pathol 34:1092-1100, 2003   1–6

Background.—Follicular thyroid carcinoma (FTC) is difficult to diagnose, in part because these tumors contain many nuclear features also seen in papillary thyroid carcinoma. The reproducibility of histopathologic diagnosis in FTC was examined, and areas of interobserver and intraobserver disagreements were explored.
Methods.—Formalin-fixed, paraffin-embedded specimens from 41 cases of FTC were retrieved and stained with hematoxylin and eosin for review. Five pathologists independently reviewed each case and completed a standardized questionnaire regarding, among other features, the presence of capsular invasion and the presence and number of vascular invasions. Pathologists also reviewed 31 of the same specimens twice. FTCs were diagnosed as minimally invasive FTC (MIFTC) or non-MIFTC according to World Health Organization classification criteria. At the end of the study, the 5 pathologists met around a multiheaded microscope to review each case until a final consensus diagnosis (FCD) was reached. Intraobserver and interobserver reproducibility was evaluated by the kappa statistic (for qualitative data) and the intraclass correlation coefficient (for quantitative data).
Results.—The FCD classified 30 cases as malignant, including 24 cases of FTC (17 non-MIFTC and 7 MIFTC), 2 follicular variants of papillary carcinoma, 1 well-differentiated carcinoma not otherwise specified, 1 medullary thyroid carcinoma, 1 lymphoma, and 1 undifferentiated carcinoma with small areas of FTC. FCD excluded malignancy in 11 cases, including 6 atypical adenomas, 3 follicular adenomas, and 2 oxyphilic cell-type follicular ad-

enomas. The levels of agreement between each pathologist's initial diagnosis and the FCD were 0.69, 0.41, 0.35, 0.28, and 0.11. All 5 pathologists were in agreement in 10 of the non-MIFTC cases (59%), and diagnostic reproducibility was acceptable for non-MIFTC. However, in only 3 (43%) of the 7 cases of MIFTC were all 5 pathologists in unanimous agreement, and the diagnosis of MIFTC was poorly reproducible. Interobserver agreement for a diagnosis of FTC was 0.23, and the intraobserver agreement was 0.68. Interobserver agreement about the presence of vascular and capsular invasion was low (0.20 and 0.27, respectively), but the corresponding intraobserver agreement was higher (0.51 and 0.70). Interobserver and intraobserver agreement about the number of vascular invasions was moderate (0.42 and 0.65).

Conclusion.—The diagnostic reproducibility of MIFTC is rather low, which has implications both for clinical practice and for research. The agreement between the initial diagnosis and the FCD varied widely, which suggests 1 of the pathologists was regarded as a leader and the other pathologists tended to defer to him at the consensus conference.

▶ This study, reported by a large group of French pathologists, is an excellent examination of diagnostic variability among pathologists. I think it is an excellent study because the authors' intent was not only to document the low level of agreement among pathologists for the diagnosis of FTC but also to explore the reasons underlying the diagnostic difficulty with these lesions. They describe findings of a consensus conference, which was part of the study, during which the 5 pathologist observers sat down together at a multiheaded microscope to discuss the cases. Their description of some of the difficulties encountered at the consensus conference, including the occurrence of psychosocial phenomena such as the "leadership phenomenon," provides the reader with a richer view of the diagnostic process than is usually found in the pathology literature.

D. M. Grzybicki, MD, PhD

Cost-effectiveness of Laboratory Testing
Hernandez JS (Mayo Clinic, Rochester, Minn)
Arch Pathol Lab Med 127:440-445, 2003   1–7

Introduction.—It is no longer enough for laboratories to provide efficient testing. With increasing frequency, payers are demanding to know the value of tests, with value equaling quality per unit cost. Payers request that laboratories prove that tests are cost-effective. Clinicians are asked to eliminate overuse and misuse of laboratory tests. An in-depth review of the literature on cost-effectiveness of laboratory testing was performed, and an expository model for analyzing the value of newer laboratory tests was created.

Findings.—Documents in the National Library of Medicine were searched to identify literature concerning the cost-effectiveness of laboratory testing. Relatively few investigations address this issue. There are similarities between evidence-based medicine and cost-effectiveness, but important differences exist. Advocates of evidence-based medicine allude to the *individual* clinical ethic of doing everything possible (where efficacious) for the patient, whereas advocates of cost-effectiveness support the *social* ethic of obtaining the maximum gains in population health, recognizing the restraints of a finite budget. With budget restraints forcing a broader, more global view, medical directors have to look beyond the walls of the laboratory and analyze how the laboratory affects the hospital and the integrated health care system. In examining the efficacy of their operations, laboratories need to address 3 major factors: (1) assay performance (sensitivity, specificity, reproducibility, supplemental testing, quality assurance, and turnaround time); (2) epidemiology (prevalence, clinical setting, and risk indicators [demographic, behavioral, and clinical variables]); and (3) cost (testing and nontesting costs). The overlap of these 3 factors encompass cost-effectiveness, cost benefit, and cost utility.

Discussion/Conclusion.—The demand for providing the value of newer and more expensive medical technologies, including newer medical tests, will rise markedly. Payers, including Medicare, commercial insurers, and employers, will require accountability and eradication of the abuse and misuse of ineffective testing strategies. Pathologists and laboratorians have an important role in guiding the most cost-effective use of testing strategies, including the judicious use of algorithms.

Cost-effectiveness of Immediate Specimen Adequacy Assessment of Thyroid Fine-Needle Aspirations

Eedes CR, Wang HH (Harvard Med School, Boston)
Am J Clin Pathol 121:64-69, 2004   1–8

Introduction.—Pathologists and cytotechnologists commonly provide immediate specimen adequacy assessment of thyroid fine-needle aspirations to ensure that diagnostic material is obtained. The cost-effectiveness of this practice was examined in 311 patients.

Methods.—The mean age of 261 women and 50 men was 49.4 years. Patients were divided into 2 groups: those with (group 1) and those without (group 2) immediate adequacy assessment. Specimen adequacy was compared between groups. The time spent to conduct the adequacy evaluation was documented.

Results.—Of 311 patients, 291 underwent a single procedure, and 20 underwent 2 procedures (total, 331 specimens). Compared with group 2, group 1 had more specimens with diagnostic cellular material (67.2% vs 47.0%) and fewer specimens with suboptimal (23.3% vs 38.1%) or nondiagnostic cellular material (9.5% vs 14.9%) ($P = .002$). At the time of adequacy evaluation, 98% (60/61) of the adequate specimens were obtained with 3 or fewer passes. The improved rate of diagnostic material was accomplished at a cost of 220 minutes of cytologists' time per additional diagnostic specimen, compared with group 2.

Conclusion.—It may be cost-effective to routinely obtain immediate adequacy evaluation during special circumstances, such as repeated procedures. The increase was accomplished at the cost of 220 minutes of cytologists' time per additional adequate case. The cost would be lower (177 minutes) if all adequacy evaluations could be performed in a designated location and at a designated time, such as in the thyroid nodule clinic.

▶ Cost is a critically important outcome measure in the current health care environment, with organizations and payers utilizing information from cost analyses for decision making regarding provision of services and reimbursement. The majority of recent published studies formally examining cost outcomes utilize cost-effectiveness analyses, although other formal measures of cost include cost-utility and cost-benefit analyses.

The recommended article by Dr Hernandez (Abstract 1–7) is highly worthwhile reading because he provides an excellent, concise review of the literature on the cost-effectiveness of laboratory testing, placing it in the context of efficacy and effectiveness measurement in clinical patient care settings. He makes the point up front that pathologists have traditionally focused on measurement of diagnostic performance in laboratory testing, rarely addressing broader outcomes like cost-effectiveness.

The second article by Eedes and Wang (Abstract 1–8) is a good example of this general lack of pathologist understanding of clinical outcomes measurement. Although the authors state in their title that a cost-effectiveness analysis was performed, they did not perform one. Unfortunately, the editor of the journal in which this article appeared chose to publish this highly unscientific article, confirming for interested health services researchers who might read it that pathologists don't know how to do outcomes research. Instead of performing the rigorous economic analysis that a true cost-effectiveness study requires, the authors provide a description of their current practice for performing fine-needle aspirations, perform some invalid pathologist compensation calculations, and state their opinion that cytologists shouldn't be wasting their time performing immediate interpretations on thyroid fine-needle aspirations. The authors of this article and any other interested readers are urged to read a recent, scientifically sound cost-effectiveness analysis examining this same question.[1]

D. M. Grzybicki, MD, PhD

Reference

1. Nasuti JF, Gupta PK, Baloch ZW: Diagnostic value and cost-effectiveness of on-site evaluation of fine-needle aspiration specimens: Review of 5,688 cases. *Diagn Cytopathol* 27:1-4, 2002.

Value of Fetal Autopsy After Medical Termination of Pregnancy

Piercecchi-Marti MD, Liprandi A, Sigaudy S, et al (CHU Timone, Marseille Cedex, France)
Forensic Sci Int 144:7-10, 2004   1–9

Introduction.—The liberalization of the law allowing abortion for medical reasons in France has resulted in an increasing number of medical terminations of pregnancy (MTP) for fetal indications. In 1997, prenatal diagnosis centers with specialists in obstetrics, ultrasonography, fetal medicine, legal medicine, and pathology were established to assess and validate the management strategy of fetal abnormalities and to improve the quality of the information provided to couples. The indications for MTP were examined. Prenatal US findings were compared with fetal autopsy results to demonstrate the contribution of the pathologic examination of the fetus to prenatal diagnosis and to genetic counseling, as well as the need to verify by autopsy the quality of US screening.

Findings.—A total of 352 MTPs performed in a large French administrative region over 2 consecutive years were retrospectively reviewed. Preliminary analysis of the indications for MTP revealed that in 69.9%, US screening had been performed and showed primarily brain abnormalities and heart defects generally linked with chromosomal abnormalities (22.2% and 32.1%, respectively). Prenatal findings were in agreement with autopsy results. There were no false-positive prenatal diagnoses. Verification was not possible at autopsy in 7.9% of cases in which brain abnormalities were identified because of tissue autolysis, demonstrating the need for optimal conditions of expulsion. Verification of diagnosis by autopsy was not helpful for patient management in 35.8% of cases, yet still added medical knowledge and demonstrated to the mother the reality of the defects. The autopsy findings were decisive for genetic counseling in 50.9% of cases.

Conclusion.—Fetal autopsy findings and karyotyping in a large number of MTPs demonstrate the value of autopsy in the overall management of couples and in genetic counseling. The obstetrician or ultrasonographer benefits from a comparison of pathologic findings with abnormalities identified prenatally.

Infectious Diseases Detected at Autopsy at an Urban Public Hospital, 1996-2001

Bonds LA, Gaido L, Woods JE, et al (Univ of Colorado, Denver)
Am J Clin Pathol 119:866-872, 2003   1–10

Introduction.—Earlier reports have revealed significant discrepancy rates between clinical and autopsy diagnoses. Infectious diseases have not been emphasized in these trials. The discrepancy rate for infectious diseases at an urban public hospital was examined during a 6-year period. Findings were categorized in terms of their clinical importance by using an established classification system.

Methods.—A retrospective review was performed of clinical (premortem) and autopsy records of 276 patients (182 adults; 94 fetuses and neonates) who died and underwent autopsy between 1996 and 2001. The Goldman classification scheme was used to compare clinical and autopsy diagnoses.

Results.—A total of 137 adults (75.3%) had an infectious disease at autopsy. In 59 of these patients (43.1%), the infectious disease diagnoses were not known clinically. Forty-five fetuses and neonates (48%) had an infectious disease at autopsy; in 26 (58%), the infectious disease diagnoses were not known before death.

Conclusion.—There are marked discrepancies between clinical and autopsy diagnoses of infectious diseases. In adults, acute bronchopneumonia is the infectious disease most commonly missed clinically; in fetuses and neonates, it is acute chorioamnionitis.

▶ Despite continually low autopsy rates, several articles are published each year reconfirming not only the usefulness of the autopsy for multiple purposes, including quality assurance and education, but also the maintenance of overall clinical-pathologic diagnostic discrepancy rates in the range of 10% to 20%, with discrepancy rates even higher for particular diseases. The first of these 2 articles (Abstract 1–9) also demonstrates the effectiveness of fetal autopsy findings after medical termination of pregnancy for providing parents with important information that they would otherwise not receive: confirmation of prenatal radiologic diagnoses and genetic information decisive for genetic counseling. It would be interesting to actually measure the value parents place on this information and, therefore, on the value of the autopsy in this clinical context, using survey methods.

The second article (Abstract 1–10) confirms continuing substantial numbers of discrepancies between clinical and autopsy diagnoses of infectious diseases, with 2 very common diseases, acute bronchopneumonia in adults and acute chorioamnionitis in fetuses and neonates, the diseases most often missed clinically in this study sample. Hypothetically, this autopsy information, if provided in a timely manner to the appropriate clinical staff in a nonpunitive and clinically significant manner, could result in increased rates of premortem pneumonia and chorioamnionitis diagnostic rates and improved patient care. Definitive demonstration of this positive effect on patient outcomes would require collection of prospective autopsy data, which is highly limited by currently low autopsy rates.

Both of these articles clearly demonstrate the continuing value of the autopsy in current medical practice; they also demonstrate the lack of definitive information demonstrating the positive impact of autopsy information on defined outcome measures. In order to effect change regarding financial compensation for medical autopsy performance (currently received exclusively by individual private practice pathologists with autopsy businesses from patients paying out-of-pocket) and to increase autopsy rates, such formal outcomes studies are needed.

D. M. Grzybicki, MD, PhD

An Evidence-Based Staging System for Cutaneous Melanoma

Balch CM, Soong S-J, Atkins MB, et al (Johns Hopkins Med Ctr, Baltimore, Md; Univ of Alabama, Birmingham; Beth Israel Deaconess Med Ctr, Boston; et al)
CA Cancer J Clin 54:131-149, 2004   1–11

Introduction.—Melanoma is estimated to be the fifth and seventh most frequent cancer in men and women, respectively. It is responsible for 1% to 2% of all cancer deaths in the United States. Physicians involved in diagnosing and treating cancer need to know about the staging of this common malignancy. In 2003, a totally revised staging system for cutaneous melanoma was implemented. The changes were validated with a prognostic factors analysis that involved 17,600 patients with melanoma from prospective databases. The resultant collaborative project is the largest prognostic factors analysis of melanoma ever performed. These data were used by the American Joint Committee on Cancer to develop criteria for an evidence-based staging system.

Findings.—Important findings that shaped staging criteria involved both the tumor-node-metastases criteria and stage grouping for all 4 stages of melanoma. Important changes in the staging system include the following: (1) melanoma thickness and ulceration are the dominant predictors of survival in patients with localized melanoma (stages I and II); a deeper level of invasion (stages IV and V) is independently correlated with reduced survival only in patients with thin or T1 melanomas. (2) The number of metastatic lymph nodes and the tumor burden are the most dominant predictors of survival in persons with stage III melanoma; patients with metastatic nodes identified by palpation have a shorter survival than those whose nodal metastases are initially detected by sentinel node excision of clinically occult or "microscopic" metastases. (3) The site of distant metastases (nonvisceral vs lung vs all other visceral metastatic sites) and the presence of elevated serum lactate dehydrogenase levels are the strongest predictors of outcome in patients with stage IV or distant metastases. (4) An upstaging was initiated for all patients who had stage I, II, and III disease when a primary melanoma was ulcerated by histopathologic criteria. (5) Satellite metastases around a primary melanoma and in-transit metastases were merged into a single staging entity that was categorized into stage III disease. (6) A new convention was begun for defining clinical and pathologic staging to include the new staging information gained for lymphatic mapping and sentinel node biopsy.

Conclusion.—The prognostic factors identified by this analysis should be the primary stratification criteria and end-results reporting criteria of melanoma clinical trials.

▶ This important article describes the recently revised staging system for cutaneous melanoma that was implemented in 2003. The authors describe this system as an evidence-based staging system because it is based on information collected in large clinical outcomes databases. Development and validation of this revised system involved prognostic factor analysis from the largest to date prospective collaborative study of melanoma patients. Although the article is lengthy, it is worthwhile reading for both practicing pathologists and pathology residents interested in detailed information about how the commonly referenced American Joint Committee on Cancer Staging Manual guidelines are developed.

D. M. Grzybicki, MD, PhD

2 Breast

Does Core Needle Breast Biopsy Accurately Reflect Breast Pathology?

Crowe JP Jr, Rim A, Patrick RJ, et al (Cleveland Clinic Found, Ohio)
Surgery 134:523-528, 2003   2–1

Background.—In many cases of suspicious breast lesions, core needle breast biopsy (CB) has replaced excisional biopsy as the initial diagnostic biopsy procedure. However, CB is still a sampling procedure. The extent of agreement between histology obtained at CB and that obtained at a subsequent excisional procedure (EP) was determined.

Methods.—Data on 3035 CBs were collected prospectively between January 1995 and July 2002. Breast radiologists performed the procedures with US or stereotactic guidance. Subsequent EP was done within 1 year in 1410 cases (46%). Histologic categories were invasive breast cancer, ductal carcinoma in situ (DCIS), atypia/lobular carcinoma in situ, and benign. The principal histology of CB and EP was compared.

Findings.—Overall, agreement was moderate between CB and EP histology. Complete agreement was documented in 83% of the procedures. Of the remaining procedures, principal histology was detected only at CB in 5% and only after EP in 12% (Table 1).

TABLE 1.—Principal Histology Finding at CB Relative to EP

CB	Invasive	DCIS	Atypia/LCIS	Benign	Total
Invasive	858	27	1	10	896
DCIS	62	140	3	9	214
Atypia/LCIS	17	22	15	28	82
Benign	32	14	17	155	218
Total	969	203	36	202	1410

κ = 0.669; *P* < .001.

Abbreviations: DCIS, Ductal carcinoma in situ; *LCIS,* lobular carcinoma in situ.

(Courtesy of Crowe JP Jr, Rim A, Patrick RJ, et al: Does core needle breast biopsy accurately reflect breast pathology? *Surgery* 134:523-528, 2003. Copyright 2003 by Elsevier.)

Conclusions.—In this series, histologic agreement was exact in 83% of CB and EP cases. CB was diagnostic in 88% of the procedures.

▶ Much like the authors of this paper, most of us hypothesize a very high degree of agreement between CB of the breast and the pathology ultimately identified in excision specimens. I think many of us will be surprised at the relatively poor degree of correlation as shown by the overall kappa statistic (0.669) and by the somewhat more detailed description of results offered in Table 1. Most alarming for the pathologist on the day of sign-out will be those cases in which invasive carcinoma was identified on a CB without evidence of malignancy in the subsequent excision specimen. This represented only 1% of all cases with subsequent excision specimens but would certainly necessitate careful review of the CB. Of greater clinical importance, however, are those cases in which a benign CB was followed by an excision procedure showing either invasive or in situ carcinoma. I was very surprised to turn the crank and realize that this happened in approximately 20% of benign CBs followed by EP. I suspect that most of us do our daily work without any idea that the false-negative rate of radiographically guided CB can be this high. A more careful look at the methods suggest that these numbers may be misleading, however. There is a mix of stereotactic and US guided procedures as well as variation in needle size (11 or 14 gauge) and a limited number of cores (3-5 per case). Furthermore, the time period over which the biopsies were obtained is 7 years in length and almost surely involves a large number of individuals performing the biopsies. In most clinical practice, a smaller number of radiologists will be obtaining samples, and current trends seem to be toward larger needles and a greater number of cores. Thus, the degree to which the data in this paper can be generalized to our current practices remains to be seen. Another factor discussed by these authors but also difficult to generalize is the patient selection criteria and the referral nature of the author's practice. Other factors that make these data difficult to generalize include the fact that we are not privy to discussions among colleagues of the type that lead clinicians to conclude that a given breast abnormality has not been adequately explained by a single CB. Furthermore, some EPs are instigated on the basis of follow-up considerations, including interval changes in breast radiographs or persistence of abnormalities previously regarded as equivocal.

M. W. Stanley, MD

Core Needle Biopsy as a Diagnostic Tool to Differentiate Phyllodes Tumor From Fibroadenoma
Komenaka IK, El-Tamer M, Pile-Spellman E, et al (Columbia Univ, New York)
Arch Surg 138:987-990, 2003   2–2

Background.—Core needle biopsy may be useful for differentiating phyllodes from fibroadenoma. A patient database was reviewed to determine the efficacy of large-core needle biopsy for this purpose.

Methods.—Data on 57 core needle biopsies performed between August 1998 and December 2001 and yielding the possibility of phyllodes tumor were obtained. Patient age ranged from 16 to 77 years. Core needle biopsy diagnoses were compared with postoperative pathologic diagnoses.

Findings.—Twenty-five of the 57 specimens had core biopsies in which pathologic findings favored the diagnosis of fibroadenoma over phyllodes tumor. In 23 cases, initial core biopsies favored phyllodes tumor. Nine core biopsies were equivocal. Excisional biopsy confirmed the diagnosis of fibroadenoma in 23 of 25 patients with specimens that favored fibroadenoma. Phyllodes tumor was identified in the remaining 2. Thus, the negative predictive value of core needle biopsy was 93%. Nineteen of the 23 core biopsies favoring phyllodes tumor were confirmed on excisional biopsy. The remaining 4 were fibroadenoma. The positive predictive value of core needle biopsy was 83%. Five of the equivocal core biopsies were fibroadenoma on final pathologic analysis, and 4 were phyllodes tumor. None of the lesions was found to be malignant on final examination.

Conclusions.—Core needle biopsy can significantly decrease the need for surgical management of fibroepithelial tumors. A core needle biopsy result favoring fibroadenoma should prompt treatment as a fibroadenoma, with observation and close follow-up or enucleation. Core needle histologic examination of phyllodes tumor enables preoperative planning for definitive management at one surgical procedure, decreasing the need for additional surgery.

▶ The main conclusion of this article is that one can at least strongly suspect phyllodes tumors at the time of core needle biopsy. Furthermore, in most instances the authors suggest that this sometimes aggressive tumor can be readily distinguished from fibroadenomas in most patients. This is certainly a clinically useful conclusion. The problems I have in reading this report virtually all stem from the fact that it gives no hint that anybody with pathology expertise was involved in the study. I find it very difficult to understand why a series of only 57 cases was not submitted for coordinated review by an individual with expertise in breast pathology. At some point, the distinction between fibroadenomas, especially those with hypercellular stroma, and phyllodes tumor can be subjective. We are left to wonder about things like phyllodes tumors in patients younger than 20 years and instances in which this diagnosis was applied to very small lesions. Especially telling is the comment that "None of the lesions studied was determined to be malignant on final pathologic analysis." The terms "benign" and "malignant" to describe phyllodes tumors is of course an oversimplification that would have been avoided by central pathology review. Thus, while this paper tells an interesting story, I find its conclusion somewhat suspect and would like to see the same type of study done from a large institution with careful pathology review.

M. W. Stanley, MD

Malignant Phyllodes Tumours Show Stromal Overexpression of c-myc and c-kit

Sawyer EJ, Poulsom R, Hunt FT, et al (Cancer Research UK, London; City Hosp, Nottingham; Guy's Hosp, London; et al)

J Pathol 200:59-64, 2003   2–3

Background.—The stroma of phyllodes tumors, fibroepithelial breast neoplasms, can undergo malignant progression to sarcoma. The frequency of malignant tumors ranges from 5% to 30% in different series. Potential molecular mechanisms in the progression to malignancy in phyllodes tumors were defined.

Methods and Findings.—Expression of c-myc and c-kit was assessed in 30 phyllodes tumors by in situ hybridization and immunohistochemistry. Nine of 10 malignant tumors and only 7 of 20 benign tumors demonstrated c-myc expression in the stroma. Stromal c-kit expression was detected in half of 10

TABLE 2.—Summary of Immunohistochemistry Data

Specimen	Histology	c-kit Stromal Staining	c-myc Stromal Staining	c-myc Epithelial Staining
1	Malignant	Strong	Moderate	Weak†
2	Malignant	Strong	Strong	Weak
3	Malignant	Strong	Weak	Weak
4	Malignant	Negative	Moderate	Weak
5	Malignant	Moderate	Strong	Weak
6	Malignant	Negative	Strong	Weak
7	Malignant	Negative	Strong	Weak
8	Malignant	Strong	Moderate	Weak
9	Borderline	Negative	Moderate	Moderate
10	Borderline	Negative	Strong	Moderate
11	Benign	Moderate	Strong	Strong
12	Benign	Negative	Negative	Weak
13	Benign	Negative	Weak	Moderate
14	Benign	Negative	nw*	Weak
15	Benign	Negative	Weak	Moderate
16	Benign	Negative	nw	Weak
17	Benign	Negative	Moderate	Weak
18	Benign	Negative	Negative	Weak
19	Benign	Negative	Strong	Strong
20	Benign	Negative	Weak	Weak
21	Benign	Negative	Negative	Weak
22	Benign	Negative	Strong	Moderate
23	Benign	Negative	Negative	Moderate
24	Benign	Negative	Moderate	Moderate
25	Benign	Negative	Weak	Weak
26	Benign	Weak	Strong	Weak
27	Benign	Negative	Moderate	Weak
28	Benign	Negative	Negative	Weak
29	Benign	Weak	Weak	Weak
30	Benign	Negative	Weak	Weak

*Not worked (nw).
†Weak epithelial staining was present in normal epithelium.
(Courtesy of Sawyer EJ, Poulsom R, Hunt FT, et al: Malignant phyllodes tumors show stromal overexpression of c-myc and c-kit. *J Pathol* 200:59-64, 2003. Reprinted by permission of John Wiley & Sons, Ltd.)

Benign Plyllodes Tumours

Malignant Phyllodes Tumours

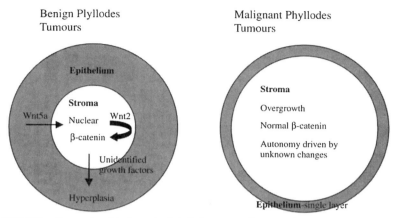

FIGURE 1.—Proposed model of growth of phyllodes tumors. (Courtesy of Sawyer EJ, Poulsom R, Hunt FT, et al: Malignant phyllodes tumors show stromal overexpression of c-myc and c-kit. *J Pathol* 200:59-64, 2003. Reprinted by permission of John Wiley & Sons, Ltd.)

malignant tumors and in only 1 of 20 benign tumors (Table 2). Although 1 tumor had high-level amplification of c-myc, no evidence of c-kit mutations was found (Fig 1).

Conclusions.—Overexpression of c-myc may drive stromal proliferation in malignant phyllodes tumors. Overexpression of c-kit contributes to the growth of these tumors. In addition, c-kit may be a new therapeutic target in these lesions.

▶ One of the themes that emerges from this year's series of commentaries is the ever-expanding role of c-kit analysis in a wide variety of neoplasms. While this paper presents other information and attempts to postulate molecular mechanisms for stromal expansion in more aggressive examples of phyllodes tumor, the description of immunohistochemically demonstrable c-kit expression will emerge as the most interesting finding for those of us who do diagnostic pathology. However, some potentially useful information is missing from this article. When faced with a phyllodes tumor and asked to predict its biologic potential, we struggle with imperfect but well-recognized criteria. These include stromal cellularity, stromal overgrowth of epithelial elements, stromal cell atypia, mitotic rates, in periductal stroma cells, and the presence or absence of heterologous elements. It would have been interesting to see the molecular data in this report correlated with these histopathologic findings and with the clinical characteristics of patients. Thus, it would have been useful if the authors had expanded Table 2 to include this information. We can hope that this type of clinical, pathologic, and molecular correlative study will be the subject of a subsequent publication by this group. Identification of abnormalities by c-kit (CD117) immunostaining opens up the possibility of chemical treatment of phyllodes tumor in a manner analogous to that used for gastrointestinal stromal tumors at this time. While only 10% of phyllodes tumors exhibit metastatic behavior—involving mostly the brain, lungs, or bones—any improvement of treatment for the more common and frequently very aggressive chest wall local recurrences would be welcome.

M. W. Stanley, MD

Epithelial Lesions in Prophylactic Mastectomy Specimens From Women With *BRCA* Mutations

Kauff ND, Brogi E, Scheuer L, et al (Mem Sloan-Kettering Cancer Ctr, New York; Michigan State Univ, East Lansing)

Cancer 97:1601-1608, 2003   2–4

Background.—Women with germline mutations in *BRCA1* or *BRCA2* are at a significantly increased risk of developing breast carcinoma. In recent prospective cohort studies, women with these mutations in specialized surveillance programs developed invasive breast carcinoma at an annual rate of 33-41 per 1,000 women. About half of the invasive tumors in these studies were diagnosed in the intervals between radiographic screening evaluations, despite careful monitoring with clinical examination and frequent radiographic evaluation. *BRCA*-associated breast carcinomas are thought to lack a detectable preinvasive phase. The present study investigated this hypothesis by comparing the prevalence of histopathologic lesions in prophylactic

TABLE 3.—Pathologic Findings in Risk-Reducing Mastectomy Specimens of Women With *BRCA* Mutations

Characteristics	Cases (*n* = 24) (%)	Comparison Group (*n* = 48) (%)	*P* Value*
Mean age (years)	41.5 (range, 29-58)	41.6 (range, 30-58)	0.965
Atypical ductal hyperplasia	38	4	0.001
Atypical lobular hyperplasia	13	0	0.034
Ductal carcinoma in situ	13	0	0.034
Columnar changes†	33	4	0.002
Sclerosing adenosis	38	17	0.076
Radial scar	8	6	NS
Adenosis	25	19	NS
Apocrine metaplasia	63	67	NS
Cyst formation	83	83	NS
Fibroadenoma	17	27	NS
Fibroadenoid changes	46	31	NS
Papillomas	4	6	NS
Papillomatous changes	4	4	NS
Duct ectasia	23	21	NS
Secretory changes	13	15	NS
Calcifications	71	71	NS
Ductal hyperplasia atypia	46	40	NS
Blunt duct adenosis	13	8	NS
Lobular carcinoma in situ	4	2	NS

*Comparison of all mutation carriers vs comparison group. *P* values were determined by the Fisher exact test.

†Columnar change was noted if the change involved the epithelium of the lobules, and no nuclear or architectural atypia was noted. Secretory changes were not included.

Abbreviation: NS, Not significant.

(Courtesy of Kauff ND, Brogi E, Scheuer L, et al: Epithelial lesions in prophylactic mastectomy specimens from women with *BRCA* mutations. *Cancer* 97[7]:1601-1608, 2003. Copyright 2003, American Cancer Society. Reprinted by permission of Wiley-Liss, Inc, a subsidiary of John Wiley & Sons, Inc.)

TABLE 4.—OR for Neoplastic Findings in PM Specimens of Women With *BRCA* Mutations Compared With Women Without a Known Cancer Predisposition*

Characteristics	Cases (%)	Comparison Group (%)	P Value	OR (95% CI)
High-risk ductal lesions (DCIS, ADH)	42	4	< 0.001	16.4 (3.2-84.0)
High-risk lobular lesions (LCIS, ALH)	13	2	0.105	6.7 (0.7-68.4)
LCIS, ADH, or ALH	42	6	0.001	10.7 (2.6-44.5)
DCIS, LCIS, ADH, or ALH	46	6	< 0.001	12.7 (3.1-52.4)

*Odds ratios, 95% confidence intervals, and P values were calculated using the method of Altman. (From Altman F: *Differences in Proportions: Practical Statistics for Medical Research*. London, Chapman Hall, 1994, p 268.)

Abbreviations: OR, Odds ratio; PM, prophylactic mastectomy; CI, confidence interval; DCIS, ductal carcinoma in situ; ADH, atypical ductal hyperplasia; LCIS, lobular carcinoma in situ; ALH, atypical lobular hyperplasia.

(Courtesy of Kauff ND, Brogi E, Scheuer L, et al: Epithelial lesions in prophylactic mastectomy specimens from women with *BRCA* mutations. *Cancer* 97[7]:1601-1608, 2003. Copyright 2003, American Cancer Society. Reprinted by permission of Wiley-Liss, Inc, a subsidiary of John Wiley & Sons, Inc.)

mastectomy (PM) specimens from women with *BRCA* mutations and in mastectomy specimens obtained at autopsy from an age- and race-matched comparison group without a known predisposition for cancer.

Methods.—Specimens obtained from women with a deleterious *BRCA1* or *BRCA2* mutation enrolled in an ongoing follow-up study and who underwent PM between November 1, 1987, and May 31, 2001, at 1 institution were reviewed. For each case, breast tissue from 2 age- and race-matched women with no known predispositions for cancer was also reviewed. The prevalence of benign, premalignant, and cancerous lesions was compared.

Findings.—Mastectomy specimens from 24 cases and 48 comparison subjects were included in this review. Ductal carcinoma in situ (DCIS), atypical ductal hyperplasia, and atypical lobular hyperplasia were all more common in PM specimens from women with *BRCA* mutations than in those from women in the comparison group (Table 3). The odds ratio for the detection of any high-risk lesion was 12.7 (95% confidence interval, 3.1 to 52.4; *P* < 0.001) (Table 4).

Conclusions.—This review found that lesions associated with an increased risk of subsequent malignancy are more common in PM specimens from women with *BRCA* mutations than in breast tissue obtained at autopsy from unaffected comparison subjects with no known predispositions to cancer. These findings suggest that a preinvasive phase for hereditary breast carcinoma may be detectable with aggressive surveillance.

▶ The results of this study are not surprising. However, the careful documentation of various histopathologic findings in breast tissue from patients with *BRCA* mutations is interesting and useful. Several of the changes that are more frequent in these patients than in controls represent lesions known to be associated with an increased risk for subsequent development of invasive breast carcinoma. In this regard, it is interesting to speculate that perhaps the lack of an increase in lobular carcinoma in situ can be attributed to the small number of such lesions identified in both groups. These findings are interesting in the light of previous speculations that a preinvasive phase for breast carcinoma may not exist in many patients. In fact, this suggestion has been used for an explanation of rapid tumor development among these women. The current study suggests that not only do these lesions exist, but that they progress much more rapidly in this group of patients. The clinical consequences of these suggestions include increased use of MRI for breast surveillance as well as a shortened interval of screening.

As an aside that has little to do with the major message of this article, this author finds it disheartening that literature describing preoperative detection of proliferative breast disease by fine-needle aspiration cytology is still being cited. Most of us with extensive expertise in breast cytology have long since given up efforts to identify premalignant lesions in cytologic samples. This is even reflected in the somewhat vague language used in the diagnoses recommended in the National Cancer Institute consensus statement on breast cytology. The latter includes such terms as indeterminate probably benign and indeterminate probably malignant.

The authors of this article do an excellent job of examining potentially limiting factors in their study. Chief among these may be errors in sampling for histology. The potential utility of these observations for chemoprevention trials is interesting, but clinical results to date have been unclear at best.

M. W. Stanley, MD

Pleomorphic Adenoma of the Breast: A Case Report and Distinction From Mucinous Carcinoma
Reid-Nicholson M, Bleiweiss I, Pace B, et al (Mount Sinai Med Ctr, New York; Queens Hosp Ctr, NY)
Arch Pathol Lab Med 127:474-477, 2003   2–5

Background.—Pleomorphic adenoma of the breast, a benign tumor, occurs most commonly in postmenopausal women. This rare lesion is characterized by an admixture of epithelial and myoepithelial cells embedded in abundant myxomatous stroma. Because its appearance clinically and histologically is difficult to interpret, it may be misdiagnosed as invasive carcinoma. One case was reported.

Case Report.—A 59-year-old woman, gravida 7, para 5, with a history of hypertension, obesity, peptic ulcer, and gastroesophageal disease had discovered a mass in her right breast 10 years earlier. The mass was firm and measured 2 cm in maximum dimension. Follow-up with serial mammography showed no significant change until a recent scan showed a slight increase in the size of the lesion. The mass was excised completely, and the patient is currently well. Histologic examination of the excised specimen demonstrated a circumscribed neoplasm consisting of epithelial, stellate, and spindle cells in pale blue myxoid stroma. In the epithelial component, tubules and cords of cuboidal cells were seen with pink cytoplasm and small oval nuclei. The stroma showed stellate and spindle-shaped myoepithelial-type cells. Adjacent to the neoplasm was an intraductal papilloma with areas of florid duct hyperplasia. The papilloma consisted of a mixture of proliferating ductal cells and darker staining, spindle-shaped, myoepithelial cells. There was no evident chondroid metaplasia. Staining of the myxoid areas was positive with mucicarmine and alcian blue. Hyaluronidase pretreatment obliterated alcian blue staining. Myoepithelial-type cells stained positively with S100 protein, vimentin, muscle-specific actin, and cytokeratin. These cells were negative for desmin and glial fibrillary acidic protein. Epithelial cell staining was strong only with cytokeratin. The histologic appearance and immunohistochemical results were consistent with pleomorphic adenoma of the breast.

Conclusions.—This report describes a mammary pleomorphic adenoma in an asymptomatic, 59-year-old woman. The use of special stains can help distinguish this entity from mucinous carcinoma.

▶ As noted by the authors, it is not surprising that pleomorphic adenomas as well as other salivary gland-type tumors occur in the breast. When presented with this tumor in this site or in a tracheobronchial location, the major diagnostic problem is usually to consider it in the differential diagnosis. This is especially true if only limited sampling or needle aspiration material are available. It is reasonable to suggest that clinical findings will be confusing when one is confronted with a postmenopausal patient whose extremely firm breast mass is well circumscribed radiographically. The occurrence of calcification within such lesions may also lead to indeterminate clinicoradiologic impressions. The authors of this paper are helpful to us when they warn that epithelial predominance or capsule penetration in pleomorphic adenomas may simulate a breast malignancy. In such settings, one would be likely to describe the otherwise helpful cartilaginous material as a heterologous element of metaplastic carcinoma. The other major potentially confusing train of thought would be mistaking the cartilaginous matrix of a mixed tumor for the extracellular material of a mucinous carcinoma. Ultimately, the greatest value of this and similar reports is that it broadens our differential diagnostic thinking and reminds us that uncommon lesions occur in various sites.

M. W. Stanley, MD

E-Cadherin Expression in Pleomorphic Lobular Carcinoma: An Aid to Differentiation From Ductal Carcinoma
Wahed A, Connelly J, Reese T (Univ of Texas, Houston; St Luke's Episcopal Hosp, Houston)
Ann Diagn Pathol 6:349-351, 2002   2–6

Background.—Pleomorphic lobular carcinoma, recently described, can be distinguished from classic lobular carcinoma by cytologic pleomorphism. The course of pleomorphic lobular carcinoma can be aggressive, and its frequency of recurrence high. Distinguishing this entity from ductal carcinoma

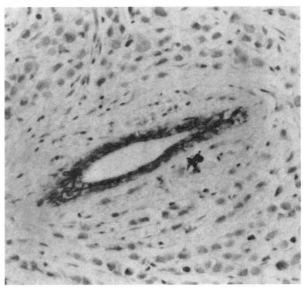

FIGURE 1.—Negative staining for pleomorphic lobular carcinoma (E-cadherin stain; magnification ×200). (Courtesy of Wahed A, Connelly J, Reese T: E-cadherin expression in pleomorphic lobular carcinoma: An aid to differentiation from ductal carcinoma. *Ann Diagn Pathol* 6:349-351, 2002.)

histologically may be difficult but is important. The pattern of E-cadherin (a transmembrane glycoprotein) expression was studied in a series of pleomorphic lobular carcinomas.

Methods.—Fourteen cases of pleomorphic lobular carcinoma were assessed by immunohistochemistry. Invasive lobular carcinoma and lobular carcinoma in situ show a complete loss of E-cadherin expression, whereas ductal carcinoma retains some E-cadherin expression.

Findings.—No staining was observed in 86% of the 14 pleomorphic lobular carcinomas (Fig 1). The remaining 2 cases displayed 10% to 25% positive cells.

Conclusions.—Detecting E-cadherin by immunohistochemistry can be useful for differentiating between ductal and lobular and also pleomorphic lobular and ductal carcinomas. This useful diagnostic aid can help clinicians interpret cases with histologically equivocal features.

▶ As I have written these commentaries over the last several years, 2 themes in our literature have been the emergence of pleomorphic lobular carcinoma and tubulolobular carcinoma as well-established diagnostic entities. The impetus for the current study stems from the fact that pleomorphic lobular carcinoma appears to be a more aggressive tumor than classic infiltrating lobular carcinoma. These authors postulate that the loss of E-cadherin expression typical of classic lobular carcinoma as well as its in situ counterpart will also characterize the pleomorphic variant of infiltrating lobular carcinoma. This concept seems to be borne out by their results. The degree to which this will improve the consistency with which we in the laboratory reach this diagnosis remains to be seen. For the moment, it appears this may provide the beginning of a molecular explanation for this tumor's aggressive behavior and for the fact that although it is morphologically distinctive, it more closely resembles ductal carcinoma than lobular carcinoma in its clinical manifestations.

M. W. Stanley, MD

Metaplastic Spindle Cell Breast Tumors Arising Within Papillomas, Complex Sclerosing Lesions, and Nipple Adenomas

Gobbi H, Simpson JF, Jensen RA, et al (Vanderbilt Univ Med Ctr, Nashville, Tenn; Federal Univ of Minas Gerais, Belo Horizonte, Brazil)
Mod Pathol 16:893-901, 2003   2–7

Background.—A slightly increased risk for subsequent carcinoma has been associated with micropapillomas/papillomas and complex sclerosing lesions of the breast, even though benign squamous metaplasia and reactive hypercellular stroma are observed in these tumors. The literature contains few reports of fibrosclerotic lesions associated with metaplastic tumors. A series of metaplastic lesions arising in fibrosclerotic breast tumors was described.

Methods.—Thirty-three metaplastic tumors associated with fibrosclerotic lesions were examined immunohistochemically for expression of cytokeratins, vimentin, and smooth muscle and muscle-specific actins. The metaplastic tumors arose within papillomas in 20 cases, complex sclerosing lesions in 7, papilloma and complex sclerosing lesions in 3, and nipple adenoma in 3.

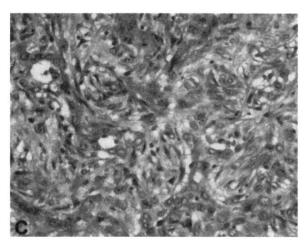

FIGURE 1.—Low-grade spindle cell metaplastic carcinoma arising within papilloma. C, Detail showing clusters of epithelioid cells (hematoxylin and eosin; magnification, 200×). (Courtesy of Gobbi H, Simpson JF, Jensen RA, et al: Metaplastic spindle cell breast tumors arising within papillomas, complex sclerosing lesions, and nipple adenomas. *Mod Pathol* 16[9]:893-901, 2003.)

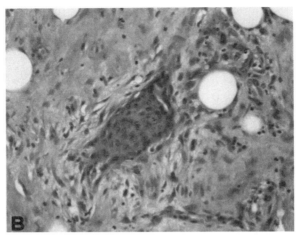

FIGURE 2.—B, Detail of **Figure 1, A**, showing bland spindle cell proliferation and tiny islands of squamous metaplasia (hematoxylin and eosin; magnification, 200×). (Courtesy of Gobbi H, Simpson JF, Jensen RA, et al: Metaplastic spindle cell breast tumors arising within papillomas, complex sclerosing lesions, and nipple adenomas. *Mod Pathol* 16[9]:893-901, 2003.)

Findings.—Most metaplastic tumors displayed a dominant spindle cell component with various degrees of atypia. These ranged from fibromatosis-like to low-grade, intermediate-grade, and high-grade fibrosarcoma phenotypes (Figs 1, C and 2, B). In 25 cases, squamous metaplasia was evident. Twenty-one cases had low-grade glandular elements. A low-grade adenosquamous growth pattern was observed in 11 tumors. Ductal carcinoma in situ was documented in 7 cases. In 5, invasive mammary carcinoma was detected. Very low grade tumors were comparable histologically to limited regions of stromal reaction and myofibroblastic proliferation, observed in partially sclerotic micropapillomas/papillomas and complex sclerosing lesions, although they were usually more cellular. Cytokeratin positivity underscored the metaplastic nature of the plumper spindled cells, which were also positive for vimentin and smooth muscle and muscle-specific actins.

Conclusions.—The study found that spindle cell metaplastic tumors, ranging from fibromatosis-like to fibrosarcoma, may arise in a variety of fibrosclerotic breast tumors. The behavior and prognosis of metaplastic lesions arising in fibrosclerotic breast tumors depend on type, extent, and grade of the metaplastic components.

▶ The authors of this study are successful in uniting a diverse group of histologic patterns and possible precursor lesions under the term metaplastic spindle cell breast tumors. The referral nature of this study makes it difficult to determine the extent of which these uncommon lesions may invariably take their origin from within one of these parent precursors. Perhaps this detailed study with access to a very wide range of material will help unify a long-term low-

TABLE 4.—Epithelial and Myoepithelial Marker Expression in Epithelial Areas in Metaplastic Spindle Cell Carcinomas

Case Number	SMA	S100	34βE12	CK5	CK14	AE1/AE3	Cam5.2	CK7	CK19	EMA
1	—	—	—	—	—	—	—	—	—	—
2	0	0	2	4	3	4	4	2	2	0
3	0	4	4	2	4	4	4	4	4	4
4	4	3	3	4	4	4	4	4	3	4
5	0	2	4	4	4	4	4	3	0	2
6	4	0	2	4	4	4	4	4	1	4
7	0	2	4	4	4	4	2	2	3	3
8	0	1	4	1	1	4	4	4	4	4
9	0	0	2	4	4	0	1	2	0	2
10	4	0	3	3	4	4	4	4	2	4
11	0	2	4	0	1	1	1	4	0	0
12	2	1	1	0	1	1	0	0	0	0
13	0	2	0	0	0	4	4	1	4	1
14	0	0	2	1	1	4	4	0	4	4
15	0	2	2	2	4	4	4	4	4	4
16	0	1	4	2	4	4	4	4	4	4
17	0	1	4	4	4	4	4	4	4	12
Total positive ≥ +2	4	7	14	11	10	13	13	13	11	12

Note: +1 staining = <10% positive cells, +2 = >10% and <50% positive cells, +3 = >50% and <90% positive cells, +4 = >90% positive cells.
(Courtesy of Dunne B, Lee AHS, Pinder SE, et al: An immunohistochemical study of metaplastic spindle cell carcinoma, phyllodes tumor and fibromatosis of the breast. *Hum Pathol* 34:1009-1015, 2003.)

for small biopsies. The CK expressed most frequently in sarcomatoid areas in this series of MSCs was 34βE12.

▶ These authors address the very difficult problem of properly classifying spindle cell breast tumors. They begin with an excellent review of this subject and its complexities. The problems are most difficult when one is faced with a spindle cell lesion showing little if any epithelial component. While its classification and prognosis depend to a very great extent on cytologic grade, distinguishing a truly mesenchymal process from a sarcomatoid carcinoma remains a difficult problem not only in this area but in other body sites as well. The results seem to indicate that a range of CK-reactive immunoreagents may be required to maximize the chance of identifying carcinomatous elements with a sarcomatoid growth pattern. However, the finding that 34βE12 is especially useful in this regard is welcome. Also, the finding that bcl-2 and CD34 may be useful in distinguishing PTs from other breast tumors with prominent spindle cells is intriguing and warrants further investigation.

M. W. Stanley, MD

The Need for Vigilance in the Pathologic Evaluation of Sentinel Lymph Nodes: A Report of Two Illustrative Cases
Scognamiglio T, Hoda RS, Edgar MA, et al (New York Presbyterian Hosp; Med Univ of South Carolina, Charleston)
Breast J 9:420-422, 2003   2–9

Background.—Sentinel lymph node (SLN) biopsy is widely performed, but major clinical issues about this procedure remain unresolved. Significant pitfalls have been reported in the pathologic handling of SLNs. Two cases were described that demonstrate the need for the utmost vigilance in the macroscopic and microscopic examination of SLN specimens.

Case 1.—Woman, 45, underwent a core needle biopsy for a left breast mass. Invasive ductal carcinoma was diagnosed, and a lumpectomy and sentinel lymphadenectomy were done. Intraoperative consultation was sought for the excised lump and SLN. Adipose tissue surrounding the SLN was trimmed. The node was then "entirely" submitted for frozen-section evaluation. The frozen-section slide demonstrated no evidence of metastatic disease, and no further axillary nodal dissection was done. However, the trimmed adipose tissue from the SLN dissection, submitted for permanent section histologic examination, showed micrometastatic carcinoma in nodal tissue. Metastatic carcinoma had been missed at frozen-section analysis because of improper sampling.
Case 2.—Woman, 70, underwent mastectomy and axillary lymphadenectomy for multicentric in situ and invasive ductal carcinoma of the left breast. Examination of 16 axillary lymph nodes showed only an intracapsular nodular aggregate of cells in one node. The dif-

ferential diagnosis of this abnormality included metastatic carcinoma and nevus cell aggregate (NCA). Metastatic lobular carcinoma in the lymph node may closely resemble NCA. However, in the former, the cells are positive for mucin and cytokeratin stains, and negative for S-100. Rare intranuclear inclusions were observed. The final diagnosis for this patient, based on histologic findings and immunohistochemical examination, was NCA in the lymph node.

Conclusions.—Two uncommon cases were reported to demonstrate possible pitfalls in the handling of SLNs. The utmost vigilance is needed both in the macroscopic and microscopic evaluation of SLN specimens.

▶ SLN biopsy has been one of the main themes recurring through the last several years of these commentaries. These authors begin this brief study with a pointed review of questions that remain regarding the relevance of SLN procedures. They then go on to report 2 practical experiences that have caused difficulty in SLN interpretation. Various benign lymph node inclusions present well-known but uncommon problems that must go through the mind of any pathologist doing frozen sections where small metastases are to be identified. The problem described in the authors' case 1 in which a trimmed lymph node is negative by frozen section but is positive in more complete permanent sections is one that has probably troubled many of us. In my experience, this also occurs when one portion of a node is not present on a frozen-section slide because adjacent adipose tissue has disrupted sectioning. The authors are correct and helpful in pointing out that a very high degree of vigilance is required of those performing intraoperative SLN examinations.

M. W. Stanley, MD

There Is More Than One Kind of Myofibroblast: Analysis of CD34 Expression in Benign, In Situ, and Invasive Breast Lesions
Chauhan H, Abraham A, Phillips JRA, et al (Univ of Leicester, England)
J Clin Pathol 56:271-276, 2003   2–10

Introduction.—Smooth muscle actin (SMA) positive myofibroblasts may be involved in tumor invasion. Acquisition of SMA is not restricted to peritumorous fibroblasts. Other changes in fibroblasts may be more specifically associated with the malignant environment. CD34 is a sialomucin that is expressed by normal breast fibroblasts; it is lost in invasive carcinomas. The association between CD34 and SMA expression in breast fibroblasts was evaluated, along with whether the loss of CD34 is specific for invasive disease.

Methods.—Immunohistochemistry for CD34 and SMA was conducted in 135 cases: 10 normal, 10 fibroadenomas, 40 infiltrating ductal carcinomas, 55 cases of ductal carcinoma in situ (DCIS), and 20 radial scar/complex sclerosing lesions. The association between staining pattern and histopathologic characteristics was documented as positive, negative, or decreased.

TABLE 1.—Summary of the Pattern of Expression of CD34 and α Smooth Muscle Antigen (αSMA) in Fibroblasts in Relation to Histopathologic Features

Histology	CD34			αSMA			Total No. Duct/Lobular Units
	+	−	+/−	+	−	+/−	
Normal	301	0	0	0	278	23	301
HUT	88	0	0	0	79	9	88
DCIS: low	28	21	11	33	16	11	60
DCIS: intermediate	22	29	26	52	3	22	77
DCIS: high	48	311	39	362	0	36	398
LCIS	12	0	0	0	12	0	12
Invasive carcinoma	0	40	0	40	0	0	40
Microinvasion	0	6	0	6	0	0	6
Radial scar	0	21	3	5	4	15	24
Fibroadenoma	10	0	0	10	0	0	10
ADH	3	0	3	0	6	0	6
Apocrine cyst	11	0	0	0	11	0	11
Postbiopsy fibrosis	0	4	0	4	0	0	4

For normal breast, ductal carcinoma in situ (DCIS), lobular carcinoma in situ (LCIS), atypical ductal hyperplasia (ADH), and hyperplasia of usual type (HUT), figures relate to individual duct-lobular units. For fibroadenomas, radial scars, postbiopsy fibrosis, and invasive carcinomas, figures relate to case numbers.

(Reprinted with permission of BMJ Publishing Group from Chauhan H, Abraham A, Phillips JRA, et al: There is more than one kind of myofibroblast: Analysis of CD34 expression in benign, in situ, and invasive breast lesions. *J Clin Pathol* 56:271-276, 2003. With permission from the BMJ Publishing Group.)

Results.—Fibroblasts around all normal duct-lobule units and those demonstrating epithelial hyperplasia were CD34 positive and primarily SMA negative. In fibroadenomas, fibroblasts retained CD34 and also acquired SMA expression. Fibroblasts around invasive carcinoma were both CD34 positive and SMA negative. In DCIS, CD34 loss was significantly more common in high-grade tumors versus low- or intermediate-grade tumors ($P <$ .001). The acquisition of SMA was observed more often than the loss of CD34, especially in non-high-grade DCIS. In all radial scars, the fibroblasts were SMA positive and CD34 negative; a similar pattern was observed in stromal cells in areas of fibrosis after core biopsy (Table 1).

Conclusion.—It appears that SMA positive myofibroblasts exhibit variable expression of CD34. This suggests that these markers are not coordinately controlled. The loss of CD34 is strongly associated with the malignant phenotype in both invasive and preinvasive disease. It is not entirely specific because radial scar fibroblasts and fibroblasts in reactive fibrosis have a similar phenotype. The functional relevance of altered CD34 expression is not clear. The focal changes implicate local signaling mechanisms that may be of epithelial origin.

3 Gastrointestinal System

Colorectal Carcinoma Nodal Staging: Frequency and Nature of Cytokeratin-Positive Cells in Sentinel and Nonsentinel Lymph Nodes
Turner RR, Nora DT, Trocha SD, et al (Saint John's Health Ctr, Santa Monica, Calif)
Arch Pathol Lab Med 127:673-679, 2003   3–1

Introduction.—Nodal staging accuracy is important in both the prognosis and selection of patients for chemotherapy. Sentinel lymph node (SLN) mapping improves staging accuracy in breast cancer and melanoma. The pathologic aspects of SLN staging for colon cancer were examined, along with the number of histologic levels necessary to identify cytokeratin-positive (CK+) tumor cells for a practical approach to accurate staging.

Methods.—SLNs were detected with a dual surgeon-pathologist technique in 51 colorectal carcinomas and 12 adenomas. The incidence of CK+ cells in mesenteric lymph nodes, both SLN and non-SLN, was determined, along with their immunohistochemical characteristics.

Results.—The median number of SLNs was 3, and the median number of total nodes was 14. The CK+ cell clusters were identified in the SLNs of 10 (29%) of 34 SLN-negative patients. Adjusted per patient, the SLNs were significantly more likely to have CK+ cells than were non-SLNs ($P < .001$). Cell clusters, cytologic atypia, and coexpression of tumor and epithelial markers p53 and E-cadherin were supportive of carcinoma cells. Single CK+ cells only were not able to be definitively characterized as isolated tumor cells. These cells usually lacked malignant cytologic characteristics and coexpression of tumor and epithelial markers; in 2 cases, they represented mesothelial cells with calretinin immunoreactivity. Colorectal adenomas were associated with a rare CK+ cell in 1 of 12 cases (8%).

Conclusion.—SLN staging with CK immunohistochemical analysis for colorectal carcinomas is highly sensitive in the identification of nodal tumor cells. Cohesive cell clusters can be reliably described as isolated tumor cells.

Single CK+ cells should be interpreted with caution since they may occasionally represent benign epithelial or mesothelial cells.

▶ If individual CK+ cells are seen in a lymph node, the pathologist has to match the immunohistochemical finding with the corresponding hematoxylin and eosin section to ensure that the cell of interest is indeed cytologically malignant before issuing a diagnosis of metastasis. These cells may represent benign epithelial or mesothelial cells. If the latter are considered, a stain for calretinin may be performed for confirmation. Apart from this exercise, the clinical significance of finding isolated CK+ cells in mesenteric lymph nodes in patients with colorectal carcinoma is still unclear. Some studies have shown worse prognosis for these patients,[1] but others[2] have demonstrated no survival differences with patients whose lymph nodes are negative in the hematoxylin and eosin section and immunohistochemical stains. Isolated CK cells in lymph nodes may be dormant cells incapable of proliferating. Long-term follow-up studies are needed to determine the significance of the finding before using the stain in every single case.

P. A. Bejarano, MD

References

1. Yasuda K, Adachi Y, Shiraishi N, et al: Pattern of lymph node micrometastasis and prognosis of patients with colorectal cancer. *Ann Surg Oncol* 8:300-304, 2001.
2. Noura S, Yamamoto H, Miyake Y, et al: Immunohistochemical assessment of localization and frequency of micrometastases in lymph nodes of colorectal cancer. *Clin Cancer Res* 8:759-767, 2002.

Histopathological and Clinical Evaluation of Serrated Adenomas of the Colon and Rectum
Bariol C, Hawkins NJ, Turner JJ, et al (St Vincent's Hosp, Sydney, Australia; Univ of New South Wales, Sydney, Australia)
Mod Pathol 16:417-423, 2003   3–2

Introduction.—Much of the uncertainty concerning the epidemiology of serrated adenomas reflects the fact that the lesions have been incompletely defined and are therefore probably underdiagnosed. The diagnostic utility of the histologic features ascribed in the literature to serrated adenomas was examined and a practical working model was created to allow their reliable identification. The incidence and location of serrated adenomas identified in an unselected series of persons undergoing colonoscopic assessment were documented, along with the clinical characteristics of those persons.

Methods.—One hundred forty consecutive persons (prospective polyp data set; 97 male, 43 females; mean age, 63.3 years [range, 29-98 years]) with 255 polyps were identified from 919 persons undergoing colonoscopy. Additional polyps previously removed from these persons were added for the purpose of histologic evaluation (extended polyp data set, 380). All polyps were examined by 2 independent examiners for 8 selected architectural and cytologic characteristics of serrated adenomas.

Results.—In the prospective polyp data set, 56 persons had 72 hyperplastic polyps, 7 had 9 serrated adenomas, 3 had 4 admixed polyps, and 98 had 170 conventional adenomas. There were no between-group differences in age, gender, or cancer association of the 7 patients with serrated adenomas, compared with other persons with polyps. The prevalence of serrated adenomas was 9 of 919 (1%) in this series. Their mean size was 5.8 mm. When examining serrated adenomas histologically, the combination of nuclear dysplasia and serration of at least 20% of crypts offered the most accurate model for identification of these lesions (sensitivity 100%, specificity 97%). Other criteria offered supportive evidence, yet did not enhance the diagnostic yield.

Conclusion.—The optimum model for the histologic identification of serrated adenomas includes the presence of a serrated architecture in at least 20% of crypts in association with surface epithelial dysplasia.

▶ Serration in a polyp is characterized by infolding of the epithelium in a sawtooth fashion within the crypt lumen. However, there is difficulty among pathologists in distinguishing a serrated hyperplastic polyp from a serrated adenoma. Previous studies on this subject have included numerous histologic criteria with complex qualitative ranking systems and, thus, they become impractical or poorly reproducible in the daily practice of a surgical pathologist. This article attempts to facilitate the approach toward making the diagnosis. The authors evaluated 5 architectural and 3 cytologic features: serration, architectural atypia, horizontal crypt orientation, basal crypt dilatation, surface tufting, surface epithelial dysplasia, increased surface mitosis, and mucin depletion. Among these criteria, 2 are the cornerstone for an accurate diagnosis. They are serrated architecture and dysplasia. The latter is characterized by the presence in surface epithelial cells of pleomorphic, hyperchromatic nuclei, nuclear elongation and pseudostratifaction, and prominent and/or irregular nucleoli. Thus, surface epithelial dysplasia is the key feature differentiating serrated adenoma from hyperplastic polyps. The area of serration must occupy at least 20% of the polyp. Although surface tufting and mitosis add little to the sensitivity and specificity, they are supporting evidence of dysplasia. I wish more pictures of better quality were presented in this article.

In a related article, O'Brien et al[1] studied the frequency of promoter region CpG island methylation phenotypes (CIMP) in 79 hyperplastic (serrated) polyps in relation to their location in the large intestine and size. CIMP was much more frequently seen in those polyps with morphologic abnormal proliferation and located more proximally than distally. Other studies are needed to confirm the criteria used in these articles for serrated polyps and correlate them with the biologic behavior and their relation to colorectal carcinoma.

P. A. Bejarano, MD

Reference

1. O'Brien MJ, Yang S, Clebanoff JL, et al: Hyperplastic (serrated) polyps of the colorectum. Relationship of CpG island methylator phenotype and K-ras mutation to location and histologic subtype. *Am J Surg Pathol* 28:423-434, 2004.

Benign Fibroblastic Polyps of the Colon: A Histologic, Immunohisto-chemical, and Ultrastructural Study

Eslami-Varzaneh F, Washington K, Robert ME, et al (Yale Univ, New Haven, Conn; Vanderbilt Univ, Nashville, Tenn; Cleveland Clinic Found, Ohio)
Am J Surg Pathol 28:374-378, 2004   3–3

Background.—Gastrointestinal polyps are commonly encountered lesions in any surgical pathology practice. These polyps may represent epithelial proliferations, lymphocytic infiltrates (benign or neoplastic), inflammation, or various types of mesenchymal/spindle cell proliferations. Most gastrointestinal polyps are epithelial and composed of hyperplastic, adenomatous, or hamartomatous polyps. In children most polyps occur in the context of a genetic polyposis syndrome, but in adults most polyps are sporadic. Mesenchymal or spindle cell proliferations presenting as mucosal lesions are much less common and may represent gastrointestinal stromal tumors, smooth muscle and neural tumors, and inflammatory fibroid polyps. Described are the clinicopathologic features of a distinctive type of mucosal polyp composed of cytologically bland spindled cells with fibroblastic features.

Methods.—Fourteen cases of mucosal polyps diagnosed with features of fibroblastic polyps from 2 centers were included in this study. Clinical and endoscopic findings were reviewed. Immunohistochemistry was performed in all cases with a panel of antibodies, and electron microscopy was performed in 2 cases.

Results.—All the lesions were solitary, and none was associated with an identifiable polyposis syndrome. Associated adenomata or hyperplastic polyps at different sites were present in 10 cases, and hyperplastic polyps were observed in close association in 3 cases. These polyps were characterized by a monomorphic spindle cell proliferation in the lamina propria without necrosis or mitotic activity (Fig 1). The lesions were observed to be intimately associated with the muscularis mucosae and resulted in wide separation and disorganization of the colonic crypts. On immunohistochemical analysis, strong and diffuse reactivity was only observed for vimentin. In 2 cases there was weak and focal reactivity for CD34 and smooth muscle actin, whereas staining for other antibodies was negative. Sparse cytoplasmic organelles and many intermediate filaments were observed on electron microscopy. These findings were suggestive of fibroblastic differentiation of these spindle cells.

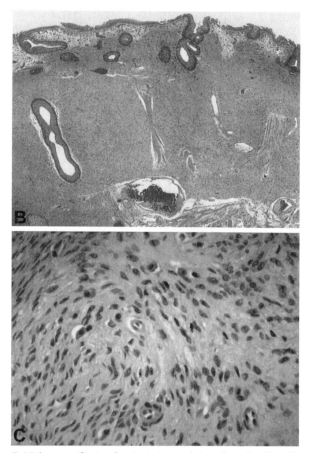

FIGURE 1.—B, Higher magnification showing intimate relation of spindle cell proliferation with muscularis mucosa seen at bottom of photograph. Longitudinal bands of smooth muscle emanating from muscularis mucosa and extending between crypts can also be noted (hematoxylin and eosin stain). **C,** Higher magnification showing monomorphic cells with oval to spindle nuclei and indistinct pale eosinophilic cytoplasm. Interspersed mast cells can be easily identified at this magnification (hematoxylin and eosin stain). (Courtesy of Eslami-Varzaneh F, Washington K, Robert ME, et al: Benign fibroblastic polyps of the colon: A histologic, immunohistochemical, and ultrastructural study. *Am J Surg Pathol* 28:374-378, 2004.)

Conclusions.—Benign fibroblastic polyps of the colon represent a distinctive type of colonic mucosal polyp that should be distinguished from other stromal polyps of the gastrointestinal tract.

▶ Most gastrointestinal polyps are of epithelial origin and are classified as hyperplastic, adenomatous, and hamartomatous polyps. Among the mesenchymal proliferations, the better known are gastrointestinal stromal tumors, smooth muscle, schwannoma neuromas, solitary fibrous tumor, ganglioneuroma, fibroepithelial polyp, and inflammatory fibrous tumor. The authors add a new kind that they named benign fibroblastic polyp of the colon, which corresponds to about 0.2% of all colonic polyps in their archival material. The mean age of the patients was 61.5 years and the median size of the polyps was 0.45 cm. Microscopically there is expansion of the lamina propria by a monomorphic and bland spindle cell proliferation without necrosis or mitotic activity. The overlying epithelium is intact, but the crypts are widely separated by the spindle cells. Stains for S100, c-Kit (CD117), epithelial membrane antigen, CD31, Bcl-2, and desmin are negative. Staining for CD34 was focal in 2 cases, not enough to classify them as solitary fibrous tumors. In addition, stain for Bcl-2 described in solitary fibrous tumor was negative. Thus, it appears that their lesions are fibroblastic in nature that stain for vimentin. Additional studies are needed to characterize them with certainty.

P. A. Bejarano, MD

Duodenal Histology in Patients With Celiac Disease After Treatment With a Gluten-Free Diet
Lee SK, Lo W, Memeo L, et al (Columbia Univ, New York)
Gastrointest Endosc 57:187-191, 2003   3–4

Background.—To diagnose celiac disease, it is necessary to show that characteristic changes have occurred in an intestinal biopsy and to show clinical improvement after the patient is given a gluten-free diet (GFD). Biopsy specimen analysis while the patient is on the GFD has been recommended. While many children exhibit a normalization of the biopsy results, whether the endoscopic appearance of the duodenal mucosa changes in adult patients on a GFD is not clear. The histopathologic and endoscopic appearance of the duodenum was systematically evaluated in patients with celiac disease who were following a GFD.

Methods.—The 39 adults (age range, 20-74 years; mean age, 52 years) had biopsy-proved celiac disease and had responded clinically to the GFD they had followed for 1 to 45 years (mean, 8.5 years). A retrospective review of the endoscopic and histopathologic appearance of their duodenal mucosa was undertaken. A blinded review of their diagnostic and posttreatment biopsy results was also conducted to assess the response of the individual patients to the dietary approach.

Results.—Only 9 patients had a normal endoscopic appearance, with the remaining patients showing at least 1 abnormality and 18 patients having multiple abnormalities. The disorders seen most often were reduced folds (46%), reduced mucosal fissures (44%), scalloping of folds (33%), and nodularity of the mucosa (33%). Histologic results were normal in 8 patients; partial villous atrophy was present in 69% of the patients and total villous atrophy in 10%. On blind review of 12 patients who had followed the GFD for 1 to 14 years (mean, 4 years), the mean intraepithelial lymphocyte (IEL) count was 61 per 100 epithelial cells before treatment and 38 after treatment; normal is less than 30 per 100 epithelial cells. The IEL count fell in all but 1 patient, and the crypt-to-villous ratio improved in all but 1 patient.

Even after 14 years on the GFD and good clinical response, none of the biopsy specimens had a normal crypt-to-villous ratio. Of the 31 patients for whom serologic results were available, 77% had negative results. Seven patients had a positive response for antigliadin antibodies, 3 for IgA and IgG, 4 for IgG only, and 1 for antiendomyseal antibody.

Conclusion.—Even though these patients had faithfully adhered to their special diet for a prolonged period of time and had demonstrated favorable clinical responses, endoscopic and histopathologic abnormalities in the duodenum persisted. While the crypt-to-villous ratio improved and the IEL count was reduced, none of the specimens examined were normal.

▶ The primary treatment of celiac disease is the institution of a GFD. While patients respond clinically to this diet, the endoscopic appearance improves only in a few patients. This study found that the small intestine is endoscopically normal in 23% of patients. However, other studies have found no normality after prolonged GFD. Although normal histologic architecture can be seen in about 20% of the biopsies, a significant number of IELs still can be seen even after 14 years of gluten restriction. As diarrhea and other symptoms improve, it appears that the histology of the distal small intestine returns to normal sooner than the proximal small intestine. This finding supports the view that the clinical manifestations of the disease depend on the extent of the intestinal involvement rather than the severity of the proximal intestinal damage. Likewise, serologies for antiendomysial and antigliadin antibodies become negative despite the persistent presence of villous atrophy. Therefore, the only way to document mucosal recovery is by examining a biopsy.

Gastroenterologists and pathologists should expect some residual atrophy and epithelial lymphocytosis in the biopsies of patients with celiac disease who are treated with GFD.

P. A. Bejarano, MD

Human Cytomegalovirus Infection of the Gastrointestinal Tract in Apparently Immunocompetent Patients

Maiorana A, Baccarini P, Foroni M, et al (Univ of Modena, Italy)
Hum Pathol 34:1331-1336, 2003   3–5

Introduction.—Human cytomegalovirus (HCMV) usually causes significant infections in immunocompromised patients, whereas active infection appears to be rare in immunocompetent individuals. The 11 cases of HCMV infection of the gastrointestinal (GI) tract reported were diagnosed in apparently immunocompetent patients, 4 of whom were found to have a malignancy.

Methods.—Cases were retrieved from the study institution files for 1999 to 2001. Diagnosis was based on identification of HCMV inclusion bodies in routine histologic sections and confirmed by immunoperoxidase staining with HCMV antiserum. None of the patients had a known cause of immunodeficiency; 2 had a history of treatment for ulcerative colitis. Biopsy specimens from the stomach (4 cases), lower third of the esophagus (1 case), and different areas of the large intestine (6 cases) were obtained for analysis.

Results.—Patients were 9 men and 2 women with a median age of 76 years. All had sought medical advice because of gastrointestinal symptoms. Findings of esophagogastroduodenoscopy or colonoscopy included ulcers, thickened mucosal folds, and mucosal erosions. Light microscopy showed chronic inflammatory infiltrate in the lamina propria in all cases. Follow-up was available for 9 patients. Subsequent to the investigation of gastrointestinal symptoms and within 2 to 5 months of the diagnosis of HCMV, 4 patients had malignancies diagnosed: a well-differentiated adenocarcinoma of the common hepatic duct, an inoperable mass in the left lung, pancreatic carcinoma with widespread peritoneal metastases, and an infiltrating adenocarcinoma of Vater's ampulla. Only the first of these 4 patients survived, and an additional patient died of a brain infarct 1 year after diagnosis of gastric HCMV infection.

Conclusion.—These 11 cases of HCMV infection of different portions of the gastrointestinal tract appeared in patients with no obvious cause of immunosuppression. Atypical HCMV inclusions, not reported previously in immunocompetent hosts, were noted in 5 cases. Particularly in elderly patients, HCMV infection in the gastrointestinal tract may suggest immunologic defects caused by an undetected malignant tumor.

▶ There have been several individual case reports but very few series of HCMV infection in nonimmunocompromised patients. The viral inclusions are predominantly seen in the stromal and endothelial cells, with epithelial and smooth muscle cells affected less frequently. Those studies described the histologic features, but detailed follow-up was not available. The current study by Maiorana et al has the longest and most informative follow-up to date. They found that about 36% of immunocompetent individuals who have HCMV infection in the alimentary tract were eventually found to have a malignant tumor. Thus, HCMV infection in otherwise healthy elderly men might serve as a biologic marker for malignancy. Therefore, the search for a tumor may be warranted. Since the pathology literature is sparse in this subject, the message for the pathologists is to become aware that we can encounter this scenario in our practices. However, in a separate study Wreghitt et al[1] analyzed 124 patients who had serologic evidence of HCMV infection in that they had high levels of anti-HCMV immunoglobulin M. The initial population consisted of 7630 patients. Thus, the incidence was low at 1.63%. Their patients had no documented tissue diagnosis of HCMV. Different from Maiorana et al's group of patients, 90% of Wreghitt et al's patients were aged 20 to 59 years. In addition, no malignancy was found in up to 12 months of follow-up.

P. A. Bejarano, MD

Reference

1. Wreghitt TG, Teare EL, Sole O, et al: Cytomegalovirus infection in immunocompetent patients. *Clin Infect Dis* 37:1603-1606, 2003.

A Schema for Histologic Grading of Small Intestine Allograft Acute Rejection

Wu T, Abu-Elmagd K, Bond G, et al (Univ of Pittsburgh, Pa)
Transplantation 75:1241-1248, 2003   3–6

Background.—Small bowel transplantation is increasingly performed for the treatment of irreversible intestinal failure or short-bowel syndrome. Acute cellular rejection is the major cause of intestinal graft failure after transplantation. Acute cellular rejection can rapidly increase in severity if not treated early, causing graft failure and death. An accurate diagnosis and the treatment of acute rejection are, therefore, critical for the care of patients who have undergone small intestine transplantation. Histologic evaluation of small bowel allograft biopsy specimens is important for the diagnosis of acute rejection, but a standard histologic schema for grading the severity of intestinal acute rejection is not available at present. A histologic grading system was developed for the diagnosis of small bowel allograft acute rejection.

Methods.—A total of 3268 small bowel allograft biopsy specimens were obtained from adult patients who underwent small bowel transplantation at one center from 1990 to 1999. A histologic grading system was proposed and validated by retrospective correlation with clinical outcomes.

Results.—There were 180 acute rejection episodes diagnosed among the 3268 biopsy specimens, including 4 episodes of severe rejection. All 4 of these histologically diagnosed episodes of severe acute rejection resulted in graft failure before resolution, despite aggressive immunosuppressive ther-

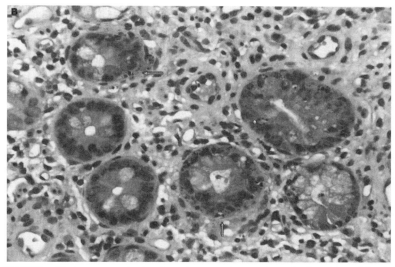

FIGURE 3.—Moderate acute rejection. Crypt damage and apoptosis are distributed more diffusely than in mild acute rejection. The number of apoptotic bodies is greater than in mild acute rejection, with focal confluent apoptosis (*arrows*). The mucosa is usually intact, without ulceration; hematoxylin-eosin; original magnification, ×200. (Courtesy of Wu T, Abu-Elmagd K, Bond G, et al: A schema for histologic grading of small intestine allograft acute rejection. *Transplantation* 75(8):1241-1248, 2003.)

apy. Of the 14 moderate acute rejection episodes, 4 were associated with unfavorable clinical outcomes (Fig 3). In contrast, the 74 mild and 88 indeterminate acute rejection episodes were not associated with unfavorable clinical outcomes. Statistical analyses demonstrated that grades indicative of more severe acute rejection episodes were associated with a greater probability of unfavorable outcomes. Good overall agreement was present among different pathologists involved in this study in diagnosing acute rejection with the use of the proposed schema, which was indicative of the practicality of this system.

Conclusions.—A reliable, predictive schema for the assessment of the severity of human small bowel acute rejection is provided.

▶ In some large academic centers, intestinal transplantation is being performed on a routine basis. The patients undergoing this procedure have irreversible intestinal failure or short-bowel syndrome as a consequence of number of conditions. These include abdominal trauma, Crohn's disease, vascular thrombosis, adhesions, volvulus, radiation enteritis, familial polyposis, necrotizing enterocolitis, and mesenteric fibromatosis, among others. In addition to intestine transplantation, stomach transplantation is also being performed. The histologic hallmark of intestinal rejection is the presence of apoptosis in the crypts. It is accompanied by architectural distortion and crypt epithelial injury in the form of cytoplasmic basophilia, nuclear enlargement, hyperchromasia, decreased cell height, mucin depletion, and loss of Paneth's cells. Mixed infiltrates with activated lymphocytic infiltrates in the lamina propria are also seen. Clinical symptoms include a fever, nausea, vomiting, increased stomal output, abdominal pain, and distension. When rejection is severe, patients may present with a picture of sepsis. It has been postulated that rejection can be diagnosed when there are 6 or more apoptotic bodies per 10 crypt cross-sections. Thus, the larger the piece obtained, the greater the information it may yield. A consensus is being obtained among the transplant centers on the nomenclature of the degrees of rejection. Such consensus was studied at the VIII International Small Bowel Transplant Symposium held in Miami at the end of 2003, and the results are in the process of being published.

P. A. Bejarano, MD

CDX2, a Highly Sensitive and Specific Marker of Adenocarcinomas of Intestinal Origin: An Immunohistochemical Survey of 476 Primary and Metastatic Carcinomas
Werling RW, Yaziji H, Bacchi CE, et al (PhenoPath Labs and IRIS, Seattle, Wash; UNESP-Botucatu, Brazil)
Am J Surg Pathol 27:303-310, 2003   3–7

Background.—CDX2 is a recently cloned caudal-type homeobox gene that encodes a transcription factor that plays an important role in the proliferation and differentiation of intestinal epithelial cells. This protein is normally present throughout embryonic and postnatal life within nuclei of epithelial cells of the intestine from the proximal duodenum to the distal rectum. Expression of the CDX2 protein in primary and metastatic colorectal carcinomas has been previously documented, but neither the sensitivity nor the specificity of CDX2 expression, as determined by immunohistochemical analysis, has been determined. Whether immunohistochemically detected CDX2 expression could be a sensitive and specific marker of adenocarcinomas of intestinal origin in both the primary and metastatic setting was determined.

Methods.—An immunohistochemical survey of 476 tumors was performed with a monoclonal antibody, CDX2-88, and included 89 tumors from the colon and duodenum and 95 tumors from other gastrointestinal sites.

Results.—CDX2 was expressed uniformly (in 76%-100% of tumor cells) in all but 1 of the colorectal and duodenal tumors evaluated. However, high-level overexpression of CDX2 was also found in mucinous ovarian carcinomas and in adenocarcinomas primary to the urinary bladder, of which 64% and 100%, respectively, were positive. Gastric, gastroesophageal, and pancreatic adenocarcinomas and cholangiocarcinomas all showed similar heterogeneous patterns of CDX2 expression. Most tumors in each group showed CDX2 expression by a minority of cells; however, a significant minority of cases in each group were completely negative and a smaller minority were uniformly positive. No expression of CDX2 was seen in hepatocellular carcinomas, and only very rare examples of carcinomas of the genitourinary and gynecologic tracts, breast, lung, and head and neck showed significant levels of CDX2 expression.

Conclusions.—Uniform expression of CDX2 was found to be an exquisitely sensitive and highly but incompletely specific marker of intestinal adenocarcinomas. CDX2 was shown to provide superior sensitivity and comparable specificity to villin, a previously described marker of gastrointestinal adenocarcinomas. However, CDX2 expression can also be seen in select nongastrointestinal adenocarcinomas, such as mucinous ovarian carcinomas and adenocarcinomas of the urinary bladder.

▶ There are few intestinal immunohistochemical markers that can be used on a regular basis in the daily practice of a surgical pathologist. Among them, villin and CK20 are the better studied. However, CDX2 is a more robust marker, in particular for colorectal adenocarcinomas, for which it shows great sensitivity and specificity when the differential morphological diagnosis includes extraintestinal adenocarcinomas. Notable exceptions include mucinous ovarian adenocarcinomas and bladder adenocarcinomas. I would also not count on it to distinguish pancreatic, esophageal, or gastric tumors from intestinal adenocarcinomas. I find CDX2 helpful when I am dealing with tumors that I expect to be negative for it. These tumors include nonmucinous carcinomas of the ovary, carcinomas from the lung, breast, salivary gland, urothelium, kidney, and liver cell, and mesothelioma. However, it is wise not to rely on a single antibody to make a definitive diagnosis. Transcription factors such as CDX2 have several advantages over cytoplasmic or membranous markers because they tend to have an "all or none" signal, as the authors stated, which means that a majority of cells will be stained if a tumor is, indeed, positive. As with other transcription factors, including thyroid transcription factor-1 for the lung and myoD1 and myogenin for skeletal muscle, the nuclear immunoreactivity of CDX2 makes it easier to interpret than cytoplasmic markers. Also, transcription factors mark tumors independently of the degree of differentiation. I think this an important antibody to have in the immunohistochemical armamentarium of a diagnostic laboratory.

P. A. Bejarano, MD

Significance of Intraepithelial Lymphocytosis in Small Bowel Biopsy Samples With Normal Mucosal Architecture
Kakar S, Nehra V, Murray JA, et al (Mayo Clinic, Rochester, Minn)
Am J Gastroenterol 98:2027-2033, 2003   3–8

Background.—The finding of intraepithelial lymphocytosis is not specifically diagnostic of gluten sensitivity (GS). The specificity of an increase in intraepithelial lymphocytes (IELs) for diagnosing GS and the significance of increased IELs in the absence of GS were determined.

Methods.—Small-bowel biopsy specimens from 43 patients with increased IELs, no previous diagnosis of GS, and no other pathology were analyzed. Forty-six patients with normal duodenal biopsy results composed a control group. The clinical records of the 2 groups were also reviewed. In 13 patients, immunohistochemical characterization of IELs was performed.

Findings.—Based on positive immunoglobulin A antiendomysial antibodies and a favorable response to gluten-free diet, GS was diagnosed in 9.3% of the patients. One patient had partially treated tropical sprue. Another 6 patients had disorders of immune regulation, including Hashimoto's thyroiditis, Graves' disease, rheumatoid arthritis, psoriasis, and multiple sclerosis. Six patients were receiving nonsteroidal anti-inflammatory drugs (NSAIDs). However, none of the control subjects had GS, tropical sprue, or immunoregulatory disorders, and only 1 was receiving NSAIDs.

Increased IELs were also documented in patients with Crohn's disease, lymphocytic/collagenous colitis, and bacterial overgrowth, although this correlation was not statistically significant. Histologic features—such as the number and distribution of IELs and crypt mitoses—and immunophenotypic analysis of IELs did not reliably differentiate GS-related from non–GS-related causes of increased IELs.

Conclusion.—The finding of IELs in an otherwise normal small-bowel biopsy sample is somewhat nonspecific. However, it may be the initial presentation of GS in almost 10% of patients. Thus, clinicians should further investigate all patients with a finding of IELs for GS. Increased IELs may also correlate with autoimmune disorders and NSAIDs.

▶ Biopsy tissues of the duodenum or the jejunum usually show small lymphocytes in the epithelium. The normal range is 6 to 40 lymphocytes per 100 epithelial cells. Larger numbers of IELs can be seen in GS, immunologic diseases (Hashimoto's thyroiditis, Graves'disease, rheumatoid arthritis, psoriasis, multiple sclerosis, etc), dermatitis herpetiformis, intake of NSAIDs, inflammatory bowel disease, and even in first-degree relatives of persons with GS.

In this study, the patients had epithelial lymphocytosis with normal villous architecture, thus showing that these patients may have symptomatic disease. Among them, 4 were found to have GS as they responded to gluten-free diet or had immunoglobulin A endomysial antibodies in serum. The authors' counted lymphocytes in 300 epithelial cells in at least 3 different villi in each case. The cut-off was 40 lymphocytes per 100 epithelial cells.

Increased epithelial lymphocytosis occurs in GS and other enteropathies with villous atrophy, such as food allergy and giardiasis. Immunohistochemically, the lymphocytes in GS are $\gamma\delta$ T cells. However, the stain for this type of lymphocyte is not readily available for formalin-fixed, paraffin-embedded tissues. In summary, increased lymphocytosis with normal architecture is not a specific finding, but its presence should prompt the clinical investigation for some of the disorders mentioned, although with only a few patients being identified as having GS.

P. A. Bejarano, MD

Lymphocytic Colitis: A Retrospective Clinical Study of 199 Swedish Patients
Olesen M, Eriksson S, Bohr J, et al (Örebro Univ, Sweden)
Gut 53:536-541, 2004   3–9

Background.—Diagnosing lymphocytic colitis (LC) depends on microscopic analysis of colonic mucosal biopsy specimens in which characteristic abnormalities are observed in a macroscopically normal or near-normal colonic mucosa. The clinical features of LC and treatment outcomes in 1 large cohort were reported.

Methods.—One hundred ninety-nine patients seen in 24 Swedish gastroenterology clinics were included. Biopsy material was reexamined using strict histopathologic criteria. Medical records were also reviewed.

Findings.—The ratio of female to male patients was 2.4 to 1. Patient age at diagnosis ranged from 48 to 70 years, with a median of 59 years. The most common symptoms were diarrhea, in 96%; abdominal pain, in 47%; and weight loss, in 41%. Thirty percent of patients had a chronic-intermittent disease course. In 7%, the course was chronic continuous. Sixty-three percent of patients had a single attack. Disease duration in these cases was 1 to 11 months. Forty percent of patients had associated diseases, such as thyroid disorders, celiac disease, and diabetes mellitus. Thirty-four first- or second-degree relatives of 24 patients had a family history of ulcerative colitis, Crohn's disease, collagenous colitis, or celiac disease. In 10% of patients, drug-induced disease was suspected. Corticosteroids, including budesonide, resulted in improvement in more than 80% of patients treated.

Conclusion.—This retrospective study of patients with LC revealed a new finding of family history of other bowel disorders. Sudden onset and single attacks of limited duration suggest an infectious cause in some cases. Drug use may induce LC.

▶ LC and collagenous colitis are the 2 entities that form the group of microscopic colitis. The diagnosis is primarily histologic because the endoscopic appearance can be normal or near normal. This is the largest clinico-pathologic study to date on LC and the authors had these parameters for inclusion: More than 20 intraepithelial lymphocytes per 100 surface epithelial cells, flattening of mucosa, mucin depletion, inflammation of lamina propria with predominately mononuclear cells, and a subepithelial collagen layer less than 10 µm thick. Patients with infection were excluded.

This article is a good summary of the current information on LC, whose etiology still is unknown. The theory of an infectious cause is supported by a sudden onset in 25% of patients, a clinical course with a single extended attack of diarrhea in 63% of cases, and response to metronidazole in some patients. In 10% of cases, some drugs have been also implicated, in particular, ticlopidine, a component used in the management of thrombotic stroke. The possibility of a genetic factor is unknown, but it is suggested since the authors' found that about 12% of the patients had relatives with inflammatory bowel disease, collagenous colitis, or celiac disease. LC affects women more frequently than men.

P. A. Bejarano, MD

Cdx2 as a Marker of Epithelial Intestinal Differentiation in the Esophagus
Phillips RW, Frierson HF Jr, Moskaluk CA (Univ of Virginia, Charlottesville)
Am J Surg 27:1442-1447, 2003   3–10

Background.—The presence of goblet cells is required to establish the histologic diagnosis of Barrett's esophagus, but this finding may not be the earliest indicator of intestinal metaplasia. The human *Cdx2* gene is a member of the caudal type of homeobox gene family, whose members are homologs of the caudal gene of *Drosophila melanogaster*. The *Cdx2* gene is expressed throughout the large and small intestine, with its proximal limit at the gastroduodenal junction. Cdx2 has recently been shown to be present in metaplasic intestinal-type epithelium within the stomach. It was hypothesized that expression of the *Cdx2* gene occurs in the development of intestinal metaplasia of the esophagus and that its encoded protein might be a marker for the histopathologic diagnosis of Barrett's esophagus.

Methods.—Immunohistochemistry was used to detect Cdx2, a transcriptional regulator important in the early differentiation and maintenance of intestinal epithelium, in 134 esophageal biopsy or resection specimens, including 62 specimens with junctional-type epithelium, 34 with Barrett's epithelium without dysplasia, and 38 with Barrett's epithelium and dysplasia or carcinoma. In addition, periodic acid–Schiff alcian-blue staining (pH 2.5) was performed on adjacent sections.

Results.—There was diminution or focal loss of detectable protein in some dysplasias (primarily high-grade) and adenocarcinomas. Cdx2 was detected in 20 of 62 cases (30%) of junctional-type epithelium. Acid mucin was present in goblet cells and nongoblet columnar cells in 48 of 62 cases (77%) with junctional-type epithelium only, including 17 of 20 (85%) that were Cdx2 positive and 31 of 42 (74%) that were Cdx2 negative.

Conclusions.—Cdx2 protein appears to be a sensitive marker of intestinal metaplasia in the upper gastrointestinal tract and may be useful for the detection of histologically equivocal cases of Barrett's esophagus.

▶ The American College of Gastroenterology defines Barrett's esophagus as "a change in the esophageal epithelium of any length that can be recognized at endoscopy and is confirmed to have intestinal metaplasia at biopsy." The latter specialized-type glandular epithelium presents an increased risk for the development of adenocarcinoma. This epithelium appears as goblet cells that contain acid-mucin, detectable with an alcian-blue stain. Any pathologist dealing with lower esophagus biopsy tissues has likely encountered cases of equivocal goblet cells and alcian-blue staining results. The use of Cdx2 as a marker for intestinal metaplasia is based on the fact that it is a transcription factor in the development of intestine during embryogenesis. Its presence has been studied in the stomach in cases of intestinal metaplasia as well. In the esophagus, Cdx2 immunostaining would indicate the presence of Barrett's esophagus. One advantage of this stain over alcian-blue is that its nuclear immunostaining facilitates interpretation, and since it is a transcription factor, it can be interpreted as positive or negative because it lacks the subjective variability in intensity that cytoplasmic histochemical stains show. The authors found that 30% of cases of junctional-type esophageal epithelium showed Cdx2 immunoreactivity. Apparently, this would be evidence for the lack of specificity. However, they interpreted this finding as evidence that Cdx2 staining is more sensitive for the diagnosis of Barrett's esophagus than routine hematoxylin/eosin, and alcian-blue evaluation. They argue that in these cases, the molecular process of intestinal differentiation already took place, even when routine histology does not show it yet. While this is possible, a definitive proof for this assumption would require follow-up on these patients to see which ones actually develop morphologic evidence of intestinal metaplasia. The lack of expression of Cdx2 in some high-grade dysplasia and adenocarcinoma cases is explained by downregulation with decreased cellular differentiation, as it has been observed in colorectal and gastric adenocarcinomas.

P. A. Bejarano, MD

Role of Lymphocytic Immunophenotyping in the Diagnosis of Gluten-Sensitive Enteropathy With Preserved Villous Architecture

Mino M, Lauwers GY (Harvard Med School, Boston)
Am J Surg Pathol 27:1237-1242, 2003   3–11

Background.—Gluten-sensitive enteropathy (GSE) is reported to be frequently underdiagnosed, with 20% to 50% of patients, mainly adults, failing to present with frank malabsorptive symptoms. Clinically significant GSE can be associated with architecturally normal small bowel villi and evenly distributed increased intraepithelial T lymphocytes (IELs). The distribution pattern of IELs has been shown to be a sensitive feature of GSE but to be of relatively low specificity, which has limited its usefulness as a diagnostic marker. In these patients, a delay in diagnosis and early initiation of treatment may prolong their symptoms and put them at risk for the development of complications, including autoimmune disorders. The role of histology in the detection of GSE with preserved villi and increased IELs was further refined by evaluating the immunophenotype of IELs with antibodies readily available to practicing pathologists.

Methods.—Twenty-eight cases of architecturally normal duodenal biopsies with increased IELs were retrieved from the archival files of one hospital. All the biopsy specimens demonstrated well-oriented, elongated, thin villi with the number of IELs greater than 20 per 100 surface enterocytes. The control group consisted of 11 age- and sex-matched patients with duodenal biopsy specimens obtained during upper endoscopy for esophageal and gastric symptoms, and that demonstrated normal villi and no increased IELs. Three well-oriented villi were randomly chosen for each antibody, and the numbers of immunoreactive IELs per 20 enterocytes were counted separately in the tip and base of each villus, then added to obtain the complete villi score.

Results.—Of the GSE patients, 87.5% showed a tip-to-base ratio of greater than 1.7, compared with only 12.5% of non-GSE patients and none in the controls. This pattern persisted in 50% of treated GSE patients, although the CD3+ tip-IEL scores were significantly smaller. The CD8 immunostaining would appear to be of little value.

Conclusions.—IEL immunophenotyping has a potential role in the detection of GSE with preserved villi and increased IELs. The top-heavy distribution pattern of CD3+ IELs is a sensitive diagnostic feature of GSE.

▶ Historically, the histopathologic diagnosis of GSE has been based on the presence of abnormalities in small intestine biopsy specimens. These alterations include blunting or absence of villi, elongated hyperplastic crypts, cuboidal enterocytes, heavy lymphocytic infiltrates of the lamina propria, and significant numbers of intraepithelial lymphocytes. In general, these histologic features need to be correlated with antibodies in serum, of which the most sensitive and specific for GSE are IgA antiendomysium and antitissue transglutaminase antibodies. However, there are patients whose biopsy specimens may not show architectural abnormalities or who may have absent antibodies in serum, but still suffer from GSE. In these patients, prompt diagnosis and early initiation of treatment may be delayed, prolonging the symptoms and putting them at risk for developing complications such as malignancies, osteoporosis, and autoimmune disorders. The authors counted IELs per 20 enterocytes that stained for CD3 in 3 well-oriented villi. They counted lymphocytes separately in the tip (distal half segment) and base (proximal half segment) in each villus. The ratio of each separate count to the total of villi T-lymphocytes in the villi served as the score for further calculations. A higher ratio at the tip of villi, that is, a top-heavy pattern, correlated with the diagnosis of GSE made clinically by serologic markers and improvement of symptoms while on a gluten-free diet. This is an interesting study whose findings could be applied to either histologically borderline cases of GSE or in those in which there is clinical evidence of the disease, but the architecture of the villi is not affected yet.

P. A. Bejarano, MD

4 Hepatobiliary System and Pancreas

Sampling Variability of Liver Fibrosis in Chronic Hepatitis C
Bedossa P, Dargère D, Paradis V (Hôpital Bicêtre, France; Centre Natl de la Recherche Scientifique, Paris; Hôpital Beaujon, Clichy, France)
Hepatology 38:1449-1457, 2003   4–1

Introduction.—Fibrosis is a frequently used end point in clinical trials of chronic hepatitis C. Liver biopsy continues to be the gold standard for fibrosis evaluation in hepatitis C. Yet, this procedure has several limitations, including morbidity and mortality, observer variability, and sampling variation. To optimize results, a biopsy specimen of sufficient length and an adequate number of portal tracts is usually recommended. The heterogeneity of liver fibrosis and its influence on the accuracy of evaluation of fibrosis with liver biopsy was examined by using surgical samples of livers from patients with chronic hepatitis C.

Methods.—Both image analysis and METAVIR score (reference value) were used to measure fibrosis on the whole biopsy section. With the digitized image of the whole section, virtual biopsy specimens of increasing length were composed. Fibrosis was evaluated independently on each biopsy specimen. Findings were compared with the reference value according to the length of the biopsy specimen. Imaging analysis revealed that the coefficient of variation of fibrosis measurement with 15-mm long biopsy specimens was 55%; for specimens of 25-mm length, it was 45%. With the METAVIR scoring system, 65% of biopsies 15 mm in length were categorized correctly according to the reference value. This rose to 75% for a 25-mm specimen, without any marked benefit for longer biopsy specimens.

Conclusion.—Sampling variability of fibrosis is an important limitation in the evaluation of fibrosis with liver biopsy. A length of a minimum of 25 mm is necessary to assess fibrosis accurately with a semiquantitative score. Sampling variability becomes a major limitation when more accurate methods are used, such as automated image analysis.

▶ Histologic examination of liver biopsy tissues is the gold standard to assess fibrosis in chronic hepatitis. The amount of fibrosis determines the stage of the disease, and in general, there is good reproducibility among pathologists when staging liver biopsies. However, variability in the sample remains a limiting factor in staging accurately these livers. This study uses a digital approach to reconstitute virtual biopsy specimens of different sizes artificially created from a block of tissue obtained from 17 hepatectomy specimens. The scoring system used was the French METAVIR system, which scores fibrosis in 5 categories: 0, no fibrosis; 1, portal fibrosis; 2, portal fibrosis with a few septa; 3, septal fibrosis; and 4, cirrhosis. Fortunately, this scoring system is similar to other systems of more popular use in the United States. Therefore, the data can be extrapolated to general practice. Most studies have suggested that 15-mm long biopsy tissues would be appropriate. Bedossa et al prefer 25 mm, thus lending support to us, the pathologists, who like and think that the larger the better. The authors stated that automated image analysis is a more accurate method to assess fibrosis and to overcome sampling variability. However, it requires special equipment and may not be suitable for daily practice. Therefore, staging by light microscope with a trichrome stain will remain the way to assess fibrosis. Image analysis perhaps will be limited to research projects.

P. A. Bejarano, MD

Reversibility of Hepatitis C Virus-Related Cirrhosis
Pol S, Carnot F, Nalpas B, et al (Hôpital Necker, Paris; Hôpital Georges Pompidou, Paris; Hôpital Saint-Antoine, Paris; et al)
Hum Pathol 35:107-112, 2004   4–2

Background.—Cirrhosis is the end stage of chronic hepatitis of any cause, whether alcoholic, viral, autoimmune, drug related, or metabolic. Cirrhosis is a diffuse process that is characterized by fibrosis and a conversion of normal architecture into structurally abnormal nodules. Cirrhosis is usually thought to be an irreversible lesion; however, complete disappearance of cirrhosis has recently been reported in patients with autoimmune cirrhosis that was efficiently inactivated by immunosuppressive treatments. The purpose of this retrospective study was to determine the potential reversibility of hepatitis C virus (HCV) cirrhosis with the combined antifibrotic effects of interferon-α and the increasing frequency of sustained virologic response.

Methods.—The study group was composed of 64 HCV-cirrhotic immunocompetent patients who underwent antiviral therapies (interferon-α with or without ribavirin) and pretreatment and posttreatment biopsies (group 1). Resolution of cirrhosis was defined as a decrease in the fibrosis score (F) from 4 to 2 or less by the Metavir score after blinded analysis by 2 independent pathologists. A second group of 4 HCV-infected dialysis patients was also studied. Patients in group 2 had received antiviral treatment, and 3 of these patients underwent combined renal and liver transplantation, which allowed analysis of the whole liver.

Results.—In the first group, the final biopsy in 5 (7.8%) of 64 cirrhotic patients showed only F2 to portal and periportal fibrosis with rare fibrous septa without nodule formation. Four of these 5 patients were patients who achieved complete sustained response (negative polymerase chain reaction results and normal alanine aminotransferase levels); the remaining patient was a relapsing patient. In the second group, reversibility of cirrhosis was observed in 3 of the 4 patients and was clearly demonstrated in 2 patients after analysis of the whole-liver examination at the hepatectomy that preceded the transplant procedure.

Conclusions.—Regression of cirrhosis may be obtained with long-lasting suppression of the necroinflammatory activity of liver disease or the antifibrogenetic effects of interferon-α administration.

▶ The initially reported patients whose cirrhosis disappeared had an etiology of autoimmune disease. This study from France shows that cirrhosis from HCV can reverse in about 8% of patients. This finding is accompanied by a sustained virologic response that is reflected also in the suppression of the necroinflammatory damage to the liver as seen in tissue sections. The improvement is attributed in part to the antifibrogenetic activity of interferon-α, which appears to limit the activation of stellate cells. Thus, these cells do not transform into myofibroblasts to produce collagen. It is also possible that interferon increases the production of collagenase, which lyses fibrous tissue. Normally, a patient diagnosed as having cirrhosis clinical and histologically does not undergo future biopsies for follow-up unless a malignancy is suspected. However, the increasing concept of reversible cirrhosis in patients with hepatitis C may lead to the performance of liver biopsies in these patients previously diagnosed with cirrhosis and receiving interferon. The purpose of these follow-up biopsies would not only evaluate the degree of inflammatory activity in a cirrhotic liver, but also assess any improvement in the amount of fibrosis. In this study, 3 of 5 patients had HCV genotype 3 and 2 had genotype 1. The cumulated duration of the treatment was long (60 ± 19 weeks). In this European study the French Metavir scoring system was utilized, which has a scale from 0 to 4 for fibrosis. This is similar to the Batts-Ludwig system, which tends to be used in the daily pathology practice in the United States.

P. A. Bejarano, MD

Pathologic Features Associated With Fibrosis in Nonalcoholic Fatty Liver Disease

Gramlich T, Kleiner DE, McCullough AJ, et al (Cleveland Clinic Found, Ohio; NIH, Bethesda, Md; Metro-Health Med Ctr, Cleveland, Ohio; et al)
Hum Pathol 35:196-199, 2004   4–3

Background.—Nonalcoholic fatty liver disease (NAFLD) is the designation used for a spectrum of clinicopathologic conditions that ranges from steatosis to nonalcoholic steatohepatitis (NASH). Across this spectrum of disease there is a varying risk for progression to cirrhosis. NAFLD is increasingly recognized as a common form of liver disease in the United States. Although NASH can progress to cirrhosis, it would appear that steatosis alone is nonprogressive, and only 15% to 20% of patients with NASH will progress to cirrhosis in 1 or 2 decades. The clinical and pathologic features of patients with NAFLD and the association of these features with histologic fibrosis were studied.

Methods.—An NAFLD database was used to identify patients with an established diagnosis of nonalcoholic fatty liver. This database was based on liver biopsy specimens and contained extensive clinical, demographic, and laboratory data. Liver biopsy specimens were read blindly by 1 hepatopathologist with a 19-item pathologic protocol and by another hepatopathologist with a second pathologic protocol. Clinical and pathologic data were matched to the presence of different types of histologic fibrosis. Univariate and multivariate analyses were used to determine all the variables independently associated with histologic fibrosis.

Results.—Of the 132 NAFLD patients identified, 21.2% had advanced fibrosis. Sinusoidal fibrosis was present in 20.3% of patients, whereas periventricular fibrosis was seen in 17.2% of patients. Ballooning degeneration and Mallory bodies were independently associated with both sinusoidal fibrosis and perivenular fibrosis. In addition, aspartate aminotransferase/alanine aminotransferase ratio and ballooning degeneration were also independently associated with periportal-portal fibrosis.

Conclusions.—The presence of hepatocyte injury in NAFLD is associated with fibrosis. These pathologic features could be useful for establishing the pathologic criteria for the diagnosis of the progressive form of NAFLD or NASH.

▶ The authors analyzed liver biopsies with steatosis by looking at 32 histologic variables separated in 2 protocols. The purpose of the study was to determine what features are more strongly associated with NASH and therefore with fibrosis. The distinction between NASH and simple steatosis has prognostic importance because in the former 15% to 20% of patients will develop fibrosis, whereas in the latter 2% to 5% do. In fact it is now believed that some patients labeled to have cryptogenic cirrhosis in reality had NASH as the underlying liver disease. This study confirms that the pattern of fibrosis seen in NASH is predominately sinusoidal or perivenular. In addition to steatosis, the 2 main features in multivariate analysis that are present in NASH are ballooning degeneration and Mallory bodies. These 2 findings indicate that there was liver cell injury. The former is also known, as hydropic degeneration and the liver cell appears swollen. Mallory bodies represent damage of the cytoskeleton and they are seen as irregular, pink, ropy, cytoplasmic inclusions. When we are examining a liver biopsy with steatosis in which a diagnosis of NASH needs to be documented or ruled out, we have to determine the presence or absence of ballooned cells, Mallory bodies, and pericellular (sinusoidal) fibrosis.

P. A. Bejarano, MD

Detection of Hepatitis C Virus RNA in Formalin-Fixed, Paraffin-Embedded Thin-Needle Liver Biopsy Specimens

Vogt S, Schneider-Stock R, Klauck S, et al (Otto-von-Guericke Univ, Magdeburg, Germany)

Am J Clin Pathol 120:536-543, 2003   4–4

Background.—Typically, acute or chronic hepatitis C virus (HCV) infection is detected by elevated levels of alanine aminotransferase and aspartate aminotransferase and the presence of HCV RNA in serum. In some patients with HCV, however, such as liver transplant recipients, serologic testing results may be ambiguous or negative because of immunosuppression. Whether HCV RNA could be detected in formalin-fixed, paraffin-embedded (FFPE) thin-needle liver biopsy (TNB) specimens from liver transplantation patients was examined.

Methods.—A total of 23 FFPE liver specimens (13 obtained by TNB, 10 obtained by large-needle biopsy [LNB]) and 15 snap-frozen, unprocessed liver specimens (8 obtained by TNB, 7 obtained by LNB) were taken from 20 patients with chronic HCV infection (14 men and 6 women 27-66 years of age). LNB needles have an internal diameter 1.0 mm or greater, while TNB needles have an internal diameter of less than 1.0 mm.

According to the Ishak score, most patients (16) had grade 0-5 chronic hepatitis, but 4 patients had grade 6 disease (cirrhosis). HCV RNA expression in these samples was analyzed by nested reverse transcription–polymerase chain reaction. All patients also underwent serologic testing to detect HCV RNA.

Results.—Serum samples were positive for HCV RNA in all cases, and all but 1 patient had HCV genotype 1b (the exception had genotype 3a). HCV RNA was found in 11 of 13 FFPE TNB specimens (85%) and in 7 of 10 FFPE LNB specimens (70%). These findings in archival specimens were similar to those in unfixed tissues, in which HCV RNA was found in 7 of 8 TNB specimens (88%) and 6 of 7 LNB specimens (86%). HCV RNA could be detected in fragmented biopsy specimens and in specimens showing advanced fibrosis or cirrhosis.

Conclusion.—Neither fragmentation of the core cylinder, the presence of advanced fibrosis or cirrhosis, nor processing and storage of the specimen affected the detection of HCV RNA in these TNB and LNB samples. Reverse transcription–polymerase chain reaction provided sufficient material for the detection of HCV RNA in these samples. Thus, TNB can be used to detect HCV RNA in liver transplant patients and reduces the risk of complications associated with larger-bore needles.

▶ The applicability of the findings in this study would be more appreciated in the transplant population. Patients who undergo liver transplantation for HCV are immunosuppressed and thus may yield nondetectable antibodies in serum. Therefore, testing liver biopsy tissues for HCV can help in the distinction between rejection and recurrent viral infection. Unfortunately, this study did not focus on this matter of analyzing difficult cases after liver transplantation.

Nonetheless, the point is that HCV RNA can be found in FFPE tissue in TNB and LNB specimens in similar percentages to unfixed tissues. In fact, the results are comparable to other studies in which RNA was found in 60% to 84% of FFPE specimens.

Paradoxically, TNB specimens demonstrated higher increased detection of HCV RNA than LNB specimens, but the difference was not significant and it was attributed to coincidence. Negative results in the formalin-fixed tissue is explained by cross-linking RNA with proteins leading to degradation of RNA, which is influenced by prolonged time fixation. Failure to detect RNA in the unfixed samples can be due to the fact that they are not snap-frozen immediately following the biopsy procedure, thus leading to degradation of the tissue by proteases present in the liver parenchyma.

It is also possible that the samples submitted for RNA analysis did not contain liver parenchyma but connective tissue only. Another factor that influences detection of HCV RNA is that the viral load in the liver may vary from area to area, resulting in false-negative results. Lastly, the primers utilized may not detect all 6 HCV genotypes known to date.

P. A. Bejarano, MD

Autoimmune Hepatitis With Centrilobular Necrosis
Misdraji J, Thiim M, Graeme-Cook FM (Harvard Med School, Boston)
Am J Surg Pathol 28:471-478, 2004   4–5

Background.—The typical histologic findings in autoimmune hepatitis (AIH) include interface hepatitis with portal and periportal plasma cells, hepatocyte rosettes, bridging necrosis, acinar collapse, and lobular inflammation. Centrilobular necrosis (CN) is rare in AIH, and pathologists examining liver biopsy specimens showing zone 3 hepatitis might not consider AIH in the differential diagnosis. But recognizing AIH as a cause of zone 3 hepatitis is important, as the condition typically responds to steroid therapy. To aid in the recognition of this entity, the clinicopathologic features of 6 patients with AIH with a predominantly zone 3 hepatitis were described.

Methods.—The subjects were 3 men and 3 women 32 to 66 years of age (average age, 48 years) with AIH with CN as the predominant histologic feature. Their medical records and biopsy specimens (total of 9) were reviewed.

Results.—All 6 patients had elevated levels of alanine transaminase and positive antinuclear antibody or anti–smooth muscle antibody test results, but they had negative findings for viral hepatitis B and C on serologic testing. Four patients had a history of autoimmune disorders. One had a history of ethanol use, 1 had previously been treated with interferon-β, and 1 was taking atorvastatin. Drug hypersensitivity hepatitis was ruled out in all 6 cases.

All patients responded to standard immunosuppressive therapy. Biopsy specimens revealed confluent zone 3 necrosis in 4 cases and spotty CN in 2. Plasma cells in both zone 3 and portal tracts were seen in 4 cases, but were absent in 2 cases. AIH was not considered in the initial diagnosis in 2 of these cases and was not identified until subsequent biopsy specimens showed characteristics more commonly associated with AIH.

Conclusion.—As with classical AIH, most of these patients with AIH with CN had serologic and clinical evidence of autoimmune disease. Unlike other causes of zone 3 hepatitis, however, AIH with CN responds to steroids. Pathologists should thus consider this entity when examining liver biopsy specimens with predominantly zone 3 hepatitis.

▶ Although CN is an unusual pattern in AIH, its recognition on liver biopsy tissues is important in order to initiate adequate therapy promptly. This pattern of confluent loss of hepatocytes in zone 3 raises the possibility of a vascular problem of either ischemic or venous outflow nature. However, in these latter events the amount of chronic inflammatory infiltrates in central areas would be essentially minimal to absent.

The presence of chronic inflammation should alert the pathologist that the case may represent hepatitis—in particular, AIH—thus requiring correlation with autoimmune markers in serum. The presence of numerous plasma cells is helpful in suggesting an autoimmune process, but their absence does not argue against the diagnosis of AIH, as the infiltrates can be solely lymphocytic. Centrilobular inflammation with some necrosis is also occasionally observed in the transplant population as a pattern of rejection. In these situations, the injury has greater affinity for central veins than bile ducts and veins in the portal tracts, opposite to the classic histology of acute cellular rejection.

P. A. Bejarano, MD

Liver Transplantation for Primary Sclerosing Cholangitis: A Long-Term Clinicopathologic Study
Khettry U, Keaveny A, Goldar-Najafi A, et al (Lahey Clinic Med Ctr, Burlington, Mass; Tufts Univ, Boston; Beth Israel Deaconess Med Ctr, Boston; et al)
Hum Pathol 34:1127-1136, 2003   4–6

Background.—Patients' course and outcomes after liver transplantation (LT) for primary sclerosing cholangitis (PSC) have not been established. Types of liver transplant dysfunction were delineated, and clinical and pathologic features of diagnostic and prognostic importance were determined.

Methods and Findings.—Fifty-one patients with PSC followed up for 2 to 14 years were included in the retrospective study. Sixteen patients with native liver hilar xanthogranulomatous cholangiopathy (XGC) had a median graft survival of 573 days and a median patient survival of 835 days. In the 35 patients without XGC, these medians were 2489 and 2794 days, respectively. Nine early deaths resulted from perioperative complications. Of the remaining 42 patients, 6 had recurrent PSC with typical histologic and cholangiographic results; 12 had autoimmune liver disease not otherwise specified with histology of autoimmune hepatitis/overlap syndrome; 3 had chronic rejection; 4 had ischemic cholangiopathy; and 17 had no recurrence.

Outcomes after LT were not influenced by the presence of inflammatory bowel disease, total ischemia time of 11 hours or more, recipient-donor ABO and HLA class I and II matches, or type of immunosuppression. A recipient-donor sex mismatch was more common in patients with recurrent PSC than in those free from recurrence. Post-LT malignancies were significantly more common in patients without recurrences, compared with all others combined, and caused 4 deaths. In the other groups, 11 of the 13 deaths were caused by sepsis complicating graft dysfunction.

Conclusion.—Allograft autoimmune liver disease occurred in 43% of long-term post-LT patients with PSC. Features of PSC were observed in 33%. Native liver XGC had a negative effect on post-LT graft and patient survival. The increased incidence of malignancies in patients without recurrence may indicate overimmunosuppression.

▶ This study shows that the graft and patient survival are decreased when the native liver of these patients shows XGC. Liver hilar XGC is a marked inflammatory reaction with abundant macrophages and foamy histiocytes associated with destruction, dilation, and distortion of bile ducts with bile leakage. It is postulated that the inflamed hilar field predisposes intraoperative and/or early posttransplant vascular and biliary anastomotic complications. There are not many articles on the significance of XGC in the transplant population. Therefore, additional studies on this area are needed.

It is interesting that the authors found posttransplant biopsies showing features of hepatitis in some of the PSC patients. It is possible that they developed a picture of autoimmune hepatitis after the transplant. This is similar to the so-called overlap syndrome in which some patients with primary biliary cirrhosis develop autoimmune hepatitis as well. Thus, autoimmunity enters in the differential diagnosis of acute cellular rejection in a PSC transplant patient. Since recurrent PSC is characterized by the absence of interlobular in a similar fashion to chronic rejection, the distinction between the 2 processes requires evaluation of sequential liver biopsies over a period of time with correlation with cholangiographic studies. The characteristic features of narrowing and dilatation in the latter imaging studies would orient toward a recurrence of PSC.

P. A. Bejarano, MD

Cytoplasmic Immunoreactivity for Thyroid Transcription Factor-1 in Hepatocellular Carcinoma: A Comparative Immunohistochemical Analysis of Four Commercial Antibodies Using a Tissue Array Technique
Pan C-C, Chen PC-H, Tsay S-H, et al (Natl Yang-Ming Univ, Taipei, Taiwan)
Am J Clin Pathol 121:343-349, 2004   4–7

Background.—Thyroid transcription factor (TTF)-1 is one of the NKx2 family of homeodomain transcription factors and is expressed selectively in the thyroid, lung, and CNS. TTF-1 has been widely used by pathologists as an immunohistochemical marker to distinguish pulmonary and thyroidal tumors from tumors of other origins. The immunoreactivity of tumors originating from lung or thyroid tissue typically is nuclear. Cytoplasmic staining, which occasionally occurs with or without nuclear staining, has been reported. The major tissues revealing this cytoplasmic immunoreactivity are the liver and hepatocellular carcinoma (HCC). However, the significance of this immunoreactivity and its diagnostic usefulness for HCC are uncertain. The consistency of cytoplasmic immunoreactivity in HCC was evaluated.

Methods.—Immunohistochemical stains for 4 commercial anti-TTF-1 antibodies (DAKO, Zymed, Novocastra, and Santa Cruz Biotechnology) were performed on 77 HCCs and 334 nonhepatic epithelial tumors. The HCC tumors were submitted for hepatocyte antigen immunohistochemical stain. Heat-induced epitope retrieval (HIER) methods were used.

Results.—With the DAKO Target Retrieval Solution, the positive rates of cytoplasmic TTF-1 in HCC for DAKO, Zymed, Santa Cruz, and Novocastra antibodies were 58%, 14%, 6%, and 0%, respectively. With ethylenediamine tetraacetic acid (EDTA) buffer the positive rates increased to 70%, 40%, 69%, and 0%, respectively. Immunoreactivity for the DAKO anti-TTF-1 antibody generally correlated with that for hepatocyte antigen. Among nonhepatic tumors, 2 of 6 ovarian mucinous carcinomas and 2 of 11 pancreatic adenocarcinomas showed cytoplasmic reactivity for the DAKO antibody; 28 cases showed nonspecific cytoplasmic staining for the Santa Cruz antibody with EDTA HIER. Zymed and Novocastra antibodies did not show cytoplasmic staining in nonhepatic tumors.

Conclusions.—These findings are not supportive of thyroid transcription factor-1 as a reliable marker for HCC. The Novocastra antibody with EDTA heat-induced epitope retrieval methods was found to be superior because of its consistent nuclear positivity and the absence of erratic cytoplasmic staining.

▶ This article is important because the widespread use of TTF-1 antibodies in diagnostic surgical disease has revealed that occasional cytoplasmic immunoreactivity can be observed. This phenomenon is more common in liver cells and their tumors. The only reliable and unequivocal pattern of immunoreactivity had been nuclear until an article published in 2002 brought up the finding of cytoplasmic pattern and attempted to dispute this view.[1] Its authors wrongly concluded that cytoplamic TTF-1 staining was highly specific for HCCs. Later, we found that cytoplasmic staining for TTF-1 was not specific as some lung, colon, breast and larynx carcinomas, and a meningioma showed cytoplasmic immunostaining.[2] Moreover, Hecht et al[3] found cytoplasmic immunoreactivity in 13% of their lung adenocarcinomas. We agreed with the latter authors that this pattern should be considered negative. Others have seen perinuclear or cytoplasmic staining in intestinal epithelium, pancreatic ductal and acinar cells, carcinoids, and squamous cell carcinomas of the lung, head and neck, and cervix. In addition, the cytoplasm of benign hepatocytes, rare plasma cells, and histiocytes also stain. We believed that cytoplasmic staining should not be considered diagnostic, and that only nuclear staining is indicative of either lung or thyroid origin among non–small-cell carcinomas.

This study from China supports the view that cytoplasmic TTF-1 should not be used in the diagnosis of HCC, and for that matter, of any tumor. The authors were meticulous in the methods used at comparing 4 types of TTF-1 antibodies. All of them are reliable for the diagnosis of lung adenocarcinomas, and although the antibody manufactured by DAKO showed the highest rate of erratic nonspecific cytoplasmic staining, its nuclear staining is still as sensitive and specific as the other 3 antibodies used in this study. The different species and sizes of the immunogens of the antibodies might account for the inconsistencies among the 4 antibodies. One way to determine the true presence or absence of TTF-1 antigen in liver cells would be performing Western blotting, immunoprecipitation, or in situ hybridization in future studies.

P. A. Bejarano, MD

References

1. Wieczorek TJ, Pinkus JL, Glickman JN, et al: Comparison of thyroid transcription factor-1 and hepatocyte antigen immunohistochemical metastatic adenocarcinomas, renal cell carcinoma, and adrenal cortical carcinoma. *Am J Clin Pathol* 18:911-921, 2002.
2. Bejarano PA, Mousavi F: Incidence and significance of cytoplasmic thyroid transcription factor-1 immunoreactivity. *Arch Pathol Lab Med* 127:193-195, 2003.
3. Hecht JL, Pinkus JL, Weinstein LJ, et al: The value of thyroid transcription factor-1 in cytologic preparations as a marker for metastatic adenocarcinomas of lung origin. *Am J Clin Pathol* 116:483-488, 2001.

Clinicopathological Correlates of Pancreatic Intraepithelial Neoplasia: A Comparative Analysis of 82 Cases With and 152 Cases Without Pancreatic Ductal Adenocarcinoma
Andea A, Sarkar F, Adsay VN (Harper Hosp, Detroit; Wayne State Univ, Detroit)
Mod Pathol 16:993-1006, 2003   4–8

Background.—Pancreatic ductal carcinoma is 1 of the most aggressive cancers and ranks fifth as the cause of cancer-related deaths in the United States. One of the approaches to improving the dismal survival rates in this disease would be the development of a reliable screening test capable of detecting precursor lesions. Pancreatic intraepithelial neoplasia is often associated with pancreatic ductal adenocarcinoma and is presumed to be its precursor. However, it has been difficult to determine the frequency of these lesions because, until recently, there was no consensus regarding the terminology and criteria for grading of these lesions. The frequency and clinical correlates of pancreatic intraepithelial neoplasia in pancreata involved by ductal adenocarcinoma and in benign pancreata using recently proposed criteria were compared.

Methods.—Pancreatectomy specimens from 82 patients with ductal adenocarcinoma and from 152 patients who underwent pancreatectomy for reasons other than primary malignancy were evaluated for the presence, grade, and number of foci of pancreatic intraepithelial neoplasia. Cases were graded by the highest grade of intraepithelial neoplasia focus identified.

Results.—The overall frequency of pancreatic intraepithelial neoplasia lesions in ductal adenocarcinoma patients, including grade 1A, was 82%, which was significantly higher than the frequency in patients with benign reasons for pancreatectomy. There was a progressive increase from normal pancreata to pancreatitis to ductal adenocarcinoma in the frequency of overall pancreatic intraepithelial neoplasia lesions (16%, 60%, and 82%, respectively) and grade 3 pancreatic intraepithelial neoplasia (0%, 4%, and 40%, respectively). The frequency of higher-grade pancreatic intraepithelial neoplasia lesions in pancreata resected for ductal adenocarcinoma was 59%, which was significantly higher than those without primary carcinoma (17%).

Conclusions.—The progressive increase in the frequency of pancreatic intraepithelial neoplasia from incidental pancreatectomies to pancreatitis and to ductal adenocarcinoma is thought to provide indirect support for the precancerous role attributed to pancreatic intraepithelial neoplasia lesions. It is suggested by the relatively high absolute occurrence of pancreatic intraepithelial neoplasia grade 1A in benign conditions that this group is representative of a combination of neoplastic and non-neoplastic lesions.

▶ The 5-year survival in patients with pancreatic carcinoma is about 4%. Theoretically, early detection or better identification of precursor lesions would improve the ominous prognosis of this disease. Unfortunately, the inaccessibility of the pancreas by routine biopsy and the lack of understanding of precursor lesions on the pathogenesis of carcinoma present a challenge for the detection of early lesions. In 2001 a consensus was reached that coined the term pancreatic intraepithelial neoplasia (Pan IN), which was then classified in 4 degrees.[1] In grade 1A, there is flat epithelium with tall columnar cells and abundant supranuclear mucin, and the nuclei are basally located and bland. In grade 1B, the cytology is the same as in grade 1A, but papillary, micropapillary, or basally pseudostratified architecture is present. In grade 2, the epithelium is often papillary, but rarely can be flat; it shows loss of cellular polarity nuclear stratification, crowding, enlarged nuclei, and hyperchromasia. Mitosis can be seen and not abnormal. In grade 3, the changes are equivalent to carcinoma in situ with papillary, micropapillary, or cribriform architecture. It shows budding off of small clusters of cells into the lumen and luminal necrosis. The atypia is significant and the mitosis is abnormal. The higher incidence of dysplasia in the ducts of the head of the pancreas compared with in the tail may explain the higher frequency of adenocarcinoma in the head than in the tail. This article sets guidelines for future studies and explores the progression of epithelial changes that may occur in the sequence from normal pancreas to pancreatitis to adenocarcinoma.

P. A. Bejarano, MD

Reference

1. Hruban RH, Adsay NV, Albores-Saavedra J, et al: Pancreatic intraepithelial neoplasia: A new nomenclature and classification system for pancreatic duct lesions. *Am J Surg Pathol* 25:579-586, 2001.

Cellular Proliferative Fraction Measured With Topoisomerase IIα Predicts Malignancy in Endocrine Pancreatic Tumors

Diaz-Rubio JL, Duarte-Rojo A, Saqui-Salces M, et al (Instituto Nacional de Ciencias Medicas y Nutricion "Salvador Zubrian," Mexico City)
Arch Pathol Lab Med 128:426-429, 2004   4–9

Background.—Endocrine pancreatic tumors (EPTs) account for 1% to 2% of all pancreatic tumors. They usually manifest in adults, and the clinical picture associated with EPTs can vary widely. The growth pattern and benign course of EPTs are slow, but malignancy occurs in 5% to 10% of insulinomas and in up to 60% of gastrinomas. In nonfunctional tumors, the frequency of malignancy can be as high as 90%. Several predictive markers for malignancy and/or survival have been investigated, but the results have been inconsistent. Angiogenesis and vascular endothelial growth factor (VEGF) have been recognized as necessary for tumor growth and invasion, and sex-hormone receptors have been identified in pancreatic islet cells and tumors; a prognostic role for the progesterone receptor in EPTs has been investigated, with uncertain results. The role of proliferative, apototic, angiogenic, and hormonal markers as predictors of malignancy in EPTs was determined.

Methods.—Paraffin-embedded EPT samples from 21 consecutive patients were studied for prognostic markers. The main outcome measures were the proliferative fraction (topoisomerase IIα), microvascular density (CD34), VEGF expression, and estrogen receptor-β (ERβ) expression, which were assessed with immunohistochemistry. Apoptosis was also evaluated with terminal deoxynucleotidyl transferase nick-end labeling.

Results.—There were 13 benign and 8 malignant tumors. Topoisomerase IIα was significantly increased in malignant tumors, but there were no differences between benign and malignant tumors in apoptosis, microvascular density, or VEGF expression in association with malignancy. No correlation was evident between microvascular density and VEGF expression, and ERβ was not detected. The test was found to have 88% sensitivity and 100% specificity for the prediction of malignancy.

Conclusions.—Measurement of cell proliferation with topoisomerase IIα is a simple prognostic marker for malignancy in endocrine pancreatic tumors. Other potential markers, including angiogenesis, apoptosis, and the presence of ERβ, were not associated with malignant behavior.

▶ DNA topoisomerases maintain cells in a normal state controlling DNA conformation, replication, recombination, and other transcriptional events. Proliferating cells are rich in topoisomerase IIα, and thus it serves as a marker of cell proliferation. It is associated with aggressive behavior in thyroid and lung small-cell carcinomas. The biologic behavior of endocrine pancreatic tumors is essentially impossible to predict on histomorphologic grounds alone, as criteria for malignancy include invasion of adjacent organs and metastasis. In this study from Mexico, a high-labeling index for topoisomerase IIα by immunohistochemistry was associated with malignant behavior in pancreatic endocrine tumors. This is interesting because the results apply not only to nonfunctional tumors that are already known to behave in a malignant fashion in about 90% of cases, but also to functioning tumors. The latter are more frequently encountered and display more erratic behavior. Thus, the data in this article apply mainly to functioning tumors. The information obtained by staining endocrine tumors of the pancreas may help clinicians to perform a more diligent search for metastasis or to decide on the administration of adjuvant chemotherapy. Eventually, drugs targeting topoisomerase II may be developed. Additional studies are needed to better define a cutoff index because in this single study there is overlap with some tumors showing low index that behaved aggressively.

P. A. Bejarano, MD

Diffuse Lymphoplasmacytic Chronic Cholecystitis Is Highly Specific for Extrahepatic Biliary Tract Disease but Does Not Distinguish Between Primary and Secondary Sclerosing Cholangiopathy
Abraham SC, Cruz-Correa M, Argani P, et al (Mayo Clinic, Rochester, Minn; Johns Hopkins Univ, Baltimore, Md; Univ of Pennsylvania, Philadelphia)
Am J Surg Pathol 27:1313-1320, 2003   4–10

Background.—A distinctive histologic triad of findings relatively specific for primary sclerosing cholangitis (PSC) is reportedly common in the gallbladders of patients with PSC. This triad—consisting of diffuse, mucosal-based, dense lymphoplasmacytic infiltrates—is called "diffuse lymphoplasmacytic acalculous cholecystitis." The authors of this article recently observed cases of diffuse lymphoplasmacytic chronic cholecystitis in a group of patients with biliary tract disease associated with lymphoplasmacytic sclerosing pancreatitis as well as in patients undergoing Whipple resection for pancreatic head malignancy.

Methods.—The authors examined 20 gallbladders from patients with obstructive jaundice caused by malignancies of the pancreatic head, duodenum, or ampulla; 5 from patients with choledocholithiasis; 20 from patients with PSC; and 20 from patients with cholelithiasis. The histologic features assessed were degree of mucosal and deep inflammation, lymphoid nodules, epithelial metaplasia, muscular hypertrophy, Rokitansky-Aschoff, sinuses, fibrosis, and cholesterolosis.

Findings.—Gallbladders in malignancy-related obstructive jaundice and gallbladders with PSC were almost identical in scores for mucosal inflammation, lymphoid nodules and frequency of diffuse lymphoplasmacytic chronic cholecystitis. However, gallbladders from patients with PSC were significantly more likely to have focal or extensive epithelial metaplasia. Gallbladders from patients with cholelithiasis were characterized by a lack of significant mucosal inflammation in most cases and frequent Rokitansky-Aschoff sinuses, fibrosis, and muscular hypertrophy. The histologic features of gallbladders from the choledocholithiasis group overlapped with those of PSC/malignancy-related obstructive jaundice and cholelithiasis.

Conclusion.—Diffuse lymphoplasmacytic chronic cholecystitis may be highly specific for extrahepatic biliary tract disease. However, it does not appear to differentiate between primary and secondary cholangiopathies.

▶ According to the criteria used by the authors of this study and proposed by others, diffuse lymphoplasmacyctic chronic cholecystitis is characterized by intense mucosal or deep lymphoid aggregates and epithelial metaplasia. Metaplasia can be intestinal, pyloric, or gastric types. Sometimes, a transmural inflammation involving the muscularis propria can be seen. Previous studies have revealed that diffuse lymphoplasmacytic cholecystitis in the absence of lithiasis was about 45% sensitive and 100% specific for PSC. However, and in contrast to the current study, other published series lacked controls from patients with other extrahepatic biliary tract diseases not related to PSC.

This study is different in that it included 65 gallbladders from patients with PSC, uncomplicated chronic cholecystitis, choledocolithiasis, and obstructive jaundice secondary to ampullary or pancreatic carcinoma. It is shown that diffuse chronic lymphoplasmacytic cholecystitis affects many gallbladders with extrahepatic biliary tract disease, regardless of its etiology. In fact, the authors of this article showed in a previous publication[1] that inflammatory infiltrates and lymphoid nodules are present in the gallbladders of patients suffering from lymphoplasmacytic sclerosing pancreatitis. However, this pattern of cholecystitis is much less frequent in patients with cholelithiasis or hepatitic processes. The message is that if diffuse lymphoplasmacytic chronic cholecystitis is encountered, the possibility of extrahepatic biliary tract disease, primary or secondary, can exist.

P. A. Bejarano, MD

Reference

1. Abraham SC, Cruz-Correa M, Argani P, et al: Lymphoplasmacytic chronic cholecystitis and biliary tract disease in patients with lymphoplasmacytic sclerosing pancreatitis. *Am J Surg Pathol* 27:441-451, 2002.

Eosinophilic Pancreatitis and Increased Eosinophils in the Pancreas
Abraham SC, Leach S, Yeo CJ, et al (Mayo Clinic, Rochester, Minn; Johns Hopkins Univ, Baltimore, Md; Armed Forces Inst of Pathology, Washington, DC; et al)
Am J Surg Pathol 27:334-342, 2003   4–11

Background.—Prominent eosinophilic infiltrates in the pancreas are unusual. The clinicopathologic features of 3 patients with eosinophilic pancreatitis were described, along with a retrospective 18-year institutional review of disease processes associated with pancreatic eosinophilia.

Methods and Findings.—In the 18-year period studied, less than 1% of all pancreatic specimens at Johns Hopkins Hospital had been noted to demonstrate increased numbers of eosinophils. Eosinophilic pancreatitis itself rarely caused pancreatic eosinophilia. Only 3 such cases were seen at Johns Hopkins. Other disease processes were more commonly associated with prominent eosinophilic infiltrates and included pancreatic allograft rejection (14 patients), lymphoplasmacytic sclerosing pancreatitis (LPSP) (5 patients), inflammatory myofibroblastic tumor (4 patients), and systemic mastocytosis (1 patient).

Two distinct histologic patterns observed in the patients with eosinophilic pancreatitis were as follows: (1) a diffuse periductal, acinar, and septal eosinophilic infiltrate with eosinophilic phlebitis and arteritis and (2) localized intense eosinophilic infiltrates associated with pseudocyst formation. Peripheral eosinophilia was noted in all 3 patients with eosinophilic pancreatitis. All 3 also had multiorgan involvement. A patient with LPSP also had substantial peripheral eosinophilia. Five of the 24 patients with LPSP had prominent eosinophilic infiltrates in the gallbladder, biliary tree, or duodenum. Not all patients with LPSP and prominent eosinophils in other organs had increased eosinophils in the pancreas.

Conclusion.—Pancreatic eosinophilia is uncommon. It may be associated with many diseases. Although true eosinophilic pancreatitis is an interesting clinicopathologic entity, it is one of the rarest etiologies of pancreatic eosinophilia.

▶ Prominent eosinophilia in the pancreas is a rare observation with an estimated frequency of less than 1% of examined pancreatata. The causes of eosinophilic pancreatitis include parasitic infection, medication hypersensitivity, toxin injection, association with malignancies, milk allergy, and peri-insular eosinophilic infiltration associated with islet cell hypertrophy in infants of diabetic mothers. However, other processes may produce increased numbers of eosinophils to lesser extent. They include pancreatic allograft rejection, inflammatory myofibroblasts tumor, LPSP, alcoholic and nonalcoholic pancreatitis with pseudocyst formation, and Langerhans' histiocytosis.

By itself, eosinophilic pancreatitis is even more infrequent with fewer than 12 cases reported, as the authors' review of the literature revealed. In this entity, the inflammatory infiltrate is composed purely or nearly purely of eosinophils. This article describes 3 additional patients whose symptoms and preoperative clinical impression indicated that they had pancreatic tumors. The gross appearance of eosinophilic pancreatitis may mimic a malignancy. However, it is ruled out microscopically. This is also similar to pure eosinophilia in other organs, in particular eosinophilic esophagitis that clinically resembles a malignant tumor.

P. A. Bejarano, MD

5 Dermatopathology

Classifying Melanocytic Tumors Based on DNA Copy Number Changes

Bastian SC, Olshen AB, LeBoit PE, et al (Univ of California, San Francisco)
Am J Pathol 163:1765-1770, 2003   5–1

Background.—Melanocytes may give rise to many different benign and malignant neoplasms that differ in their clinical and histopathologic appearance but more importantly in their biologic behavior. The benign melanocytic tumors are referred to as melanocytic nevi, and the malignant tumors are termed melanoma. Histopathology is the present gold standard for the diagnostic classification of melanocytic neoplasms. However, there can be significant overlap in the histopathologic presentation of melanoma and benign melanocytic nevi, and misdiagnoses are common. Whether genetic criteria can aid in the diagnosis of benign melanocytic nevi from melanoma was determined.

Methods.—DNA copy number changes were determined in 186 melanocytic tumors (132 melanomas and 54 benign nevi) by using comparative genomic hybridization.

Results.—There were significant differences between melanoma and nevi. A total of 127 (96.2%) of the melanomas had some form of chromosomal aberration, but only 7 (13%) of the benign nevi cases manifested aberrations. All 7 cases with aberrations were Spitz nevi, and in 6 of these cases the aberration was an isolated gain involving the entire short arm of chromosome 11. This aberration was not observed in any of the 132 melanomas. The 132 melanomas were also analyzed for genetic differences depending on anatomic site, Clark's histogenetic type, and sun-exposure pattern. It was found that melanomas on acral sites have significantly more aberrations involving chromosomes 5p, 11q, 12q, and 15 as well as focused gene amplifications. Melanomas that were classified as lentigo maligna melanomas or as occurring on severely sun-damaged skin showed significantly more frequent losses of chromosomes 17p and 13q.

Conclusions.—A pattern of chromosomal aberration in melanoma, distinct from melanocytic nevi, was identified in this study. This pattern should be evaluated further as a diagnostic test for melanocytic lesions that are now ambiguous. This study also found significant differences in the genetic composition of melanomas that depend on anatomic location and sun-exposure pattern, findings that indicate possible variation in potential therapeutic targets among melanoma types.

► There seems to be a growing body of literature that centers around Drs Bastian and Pinkel on the molecular characteristics of melanocytic tumors. They seem to understand that our diagnostic criteria for distinguishing melanomas from nevi are imperfect; rather than trying to write sets of criteria that would fit their personal beliefs, they are trying to develop an objective assessment. They discuss whether the current clinicopathologic differences are due to the biologic differences or depend on the skin architecture or even different anatomic sites.

The authors analyzed 132 malignant melanomas and 54 benign melanocytic neoplasms; DNA was retrieved from paraffin-embedded tissue and comparative genomic hybridization (CGH) was performed. Interpretation of CGH was performed blindly to histopathologic diagnosis. Melanomas and nevi revealed highly significant aberration differences; what is interesting is the fact that 5 melanomas (2 of which metastasized) showed no aberrations by CGH. Further comparison was carried out between melanomas on acral skin versus nonacral skin; differences (statistically significant) were found there also. Further, nonacral melanomas were divided between superficial spreading and lentigo maligna types; differences were found but were not statistically significant.

In conclusion, the vast majority of melanomas examined had at least 1 aberration (>92%), but benign nevi had none. The subset of Spitz nevi showed no aberration; this aberration was not seen in any of the melanomas.

These findings show promise for diagnosis of so-called borderline neoplasms, especially those of the "Spitzoid" variety; however, it would be of interest to correlate those with follow-up and sentinel node status.

D. M. Jukic, MD, PhD

Mechanisms of Cell-Cycle Arrest in Spitz Nevi With Constitutive Activation of the MAP-Kinase Pathway
Maldonado JL, Timmerman L, Fridlyand J, et al (Univ of California, San Francisco)
Am J Pathol 164:1783-1787, 2004   5–2

Background.—Melanocytic nevi typically develop on sun-exposed skin during childhood and adolescence but may be present at birth. After an initial period of gradual expansion of the nevus, it stabilizes in size and may undergo changes of involution later in life. Melanocytes must undergo a number of cell divisions to form a clinically noticeable lesion. However, distinct from the setting of melanoma, the proliferation of melanocytes in nevi eventually ceases. Recent studies have shown that activating mutations of genes within the RAS-RAF-MEK-ERK-MAP-kinase pathway occur in nevi as well as in melanoma. Mutations of *NRAS* have been described in congenital nevi, and mutations of *HRAS* have been reported in Spitz nevi. A previous study found copy number increases of chromosome 11p that were frequently paralleled by mutations in the HRAS oncogene mapping to this region. The mechanisms that inhibit proliferation in the presence of HRAS activation were explored.

Methods.—MAP-kinase activation was analyzed by immunohistochemistry for phospho-ERK, cyclin D1, and microphthalmia transcription factor expression in 17 Spitz nevi and 18 Spitz nevi without 11p copy number increase.

Results.—Relatively high levels of phospho-ERK and cyclin D1 were found, which is suggestive of MAP-kinase pathway activation in both groups of Spitz nevi. However, Spitz nevi with 11p copy number increases were found to have significantly higher levels of cyclin D1 expression and lower levels of microphthalmia transcription factor, a finding that is suggestive of stronger MAP-kinase pathway activation in this group. In contrast to this apparent activation, the proliferation rate as assessed by Mib1 expression was low in both groups. An analysis of cell-cycle inhibitory proteins, including p16, p21, and p27 showed that the majority of Spitz nevus cells expressed high levels of p16, with cells of the cases that had increased copy number of 11p expressing significantly higher levels compared with those of Spitz nevi with normal copy number of 11p.

Conclusions.—It appears that in benign nevi with constitutive activation of the MAP-kinase pathway, the function of p16 is that of an essential mediator of oncogene-induced senescence, preventing progression to melanoma.

▶ This is a recent journal article that is a logical extension of the one previously reviewed (Abstract 5–1). However, here the authors focus of intricacies seen in Spitz nevi; they are also dealing with the RAS-RAF-MEK-ERK-MAP-kinase pathway, as several studies have described mutations of constituents of this pathway in melanomas and nevi.[1]

The authors describe an increase in the number of copies of chromosome 11p that correspond with mutations of HRAS on Spitz nevi subset. They do discuss in brief the clinicopathologic background of Spitz nevi; however, there is no mention of the so-called "Spitzoid neoplasms of uncertain biologic potential"; rather, they mention the controversial entity of metastasizing Spitz nevi.

Thirty-five Spitz nevi were investigated; 17 have shown increased number of copies of chromosome 11p and 18 had normal numbers of chromosome 11p. It would be of interest if the authors had drawn a morphologic parallel at this point: were there any histopathologic differences between these 2 groups?

The expression levels of pathway constituents were further evaluated by using immunohistochemistry; phospho-ERK was expressed in high levels in both groups of Spitz nevi, but cyclin-D1 was expressed at a higher level in a group with 11p amplification. The same was true for levels of expression of p16. Microphthalmia transcription inhibition factor revealed the opposite pattern.

In the discussion, the authors noted that the mutations of *BRAF*, frequently seen in other melanocytic nevi, is usually absent in Spitz nevi. Also, the evidence (all the data from this pattern taken together) suggests stronger activation of MAP-kinase pathway, especially with decreased levels of microphthalmia transcription inhibition factor.

This is a refreshing article that is right on the target—using molecular methods for identification of immunohistochemical substrate that will allow use of these data in everyday diagnostic dilemmas. However, it needs stronger morphologic criteria of what has been looked at (see above) and a long-term follow-up.

D. M. Jukic, MD, PhD

Reference

1. Maldonado JL, Fridlyand J, Patel H, et al: Determinants of *BRAF* mutations in primary melanomas. *J Natl Cancer Inst* 95:1878-1890, 2003.

Mutations in the Sarcoplasmic/Endoplasmic Reticulum Ca²⁺ ATPase Isoform Cause Darier's Disease

Dhitavat J, Dode L, Leslie N, et al (Univ of Oxford, England; Trousseau Hosp, Tours, France; Purpan Hosp, Toulouse, France)
J Invest Dermatol 121:486-489, 2003   5–3

Background.—Darier's disease (DD) is an autosomal dominant skin disorder that is characterized by warty papules and plaques in the seborrheic area, palmoplantar pits, and distinctive nail abnormalities. The onset of DD is usually before the third decade. Penetrance is complete in adults, although expressivity is variable. The presentation in mildly affected patients is that of scattered keratotic papules, whereas patients with more severe disease have verrucous plaques or malodorous hypertrophic flexural disease. ATPase (SERCA)2 has been identified as the defective gene in DD. A family affected with classic DD was investigated and a mutation in a region of *ATP2A2* molecule, which is specific for SERCA2b (Fig 1), was identified. The effect of this mutation on the expression of the corresponding mutant SERCA2b in COS-1 cells was also described.

Methods.—A family of French extraction affected with classic DD through 3 generations was studied. The proband was a 54-year-old man with severe extensive hyperkeratotic papules and verrucous plaques of the neck, axillae, extremities, buttocks, and perineum.

Results.—A deletion (2993delTG) in a region of exon 20 of *ATP2A2*, which is specific for SERCA2b, was identified. This heterozygous mutation is predictive of a frameshift with a premature termination codon (PTC + 32aa) in the eleventh transmembrane domain of SERCA2b and is segregated with the disease phenotype in the family members tested. Functional analysis demonstrated a drastic reduction of the expression of the mutated protein in comparison with the wild-type SERCA2b.

Conclusions.—It appears that SERCA2b is a critical component in the biology of the epidermis, and defects in SERCA2b can cause DD.

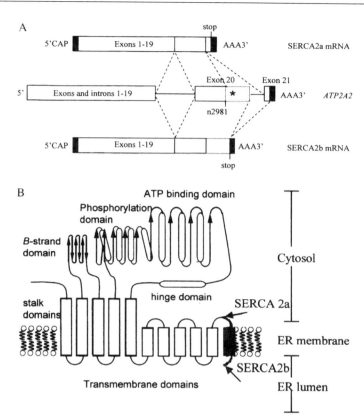

FIGURE 1.—Splicing of *ATP2A2*. **A,** Alternate splicing of *ATP2A2* transcripts at nucleotide position 2981 in exon 20 gives rise to 2 distinct isoforms, SERCA2a and SERCA2b. Mutation identified in this family (2993delTG) is indicated by an asterisk. *Black boxes* represent untranslated regions. **B,** Model of human SERCA2 polypeptide. Predicted secondary structure of SERCA2a consists of 10 transmembrane domains and tetrapeptide tail located in cytoplasm, whereas SERCA2b tail is composed of 49 amino acids extending into endoplasmic lumen. (Courtesy of Dhitavat J, Dode L, Leslie N, et al: Mutations in the sarcoplasmic/endoplasmic reticulum Ca^{2+} ATPase isoform cause Darier's disease. *J Invest Dermatol* 121:486-489, 2003. Reprinted by permission of Blackwell Publishing.)

▶ DD (keratosis follicularis) is an autosomal dominant disease that is the first and foremost differential in the cases of acantholysis of skin surfaces. The novel thing with this disease is that mutational analysis of at least 100 affected families revealed a variety of mutations in the *ATP2A2* gene.

The first articles showing this correlate appeared in 1999[1,2]; however, the value of this article is an excellent review of what has been done so far, as well as detailed explanation of alternate splicing mechanisms of this gene, as outlined in Fig 1, which also illustrates the polypeptide SERCA2 pump, which is encoded by the *ATP2A2* gene.

Furthermore, the authors have shown that a heterozygous mutation in the SERCA2b isoform is enough to cause disease; this isoform is expressed at high levels in human keratinocytes. It is also the part of the polypeptide that protrudes in the lumina of endoplasmic reticulum.

As a conclusion, next time you have a biopsy that features acantholytic dermatitis, you might want to suggest performance of mutational analysis of the *ATP2A2* gene to rule out DD.

D. M. Jukic, MD, PhD

References

1. Sakuntabhai A, Ruiz-Perez V, Carter S, et al: Mutations in *ATP2A2*, encoding a
   Ca2+ pump, cause Darier disease. *Nat Genet* 21:271-277, 1999.
2. Ruiz-Perez VL, Carter SA, Healy E, et al: *ATP2A2* mutations in Darier's disease:
   Variant cutaneous phenotypes are associated with missense mutations, but neuro-
   psychiatric features are independent of mutation class. *Hum Mol Genet* 8:1621-
   1630, 1999.

**Ki-67 and p53 Expression in Minimal Deviation Melanomas as Compared
With Other Nevomelanocytic Lesions**
Chorny JA, Barr RJ, Kyshtoobayeva A, et al (Univ of California, Orange;
Oncotech, Irvine, Calif; Reed Pathology Lab, New Orleans, La)
Mod Pathol 16:525-529, 2003   5–4

Introduction.—The classification of minimal deviation melanoma was developed to describe forms of nevomelanocytic proliferations that do not conform to generally recognized nevus or melanoma categories and are associated with a better prognosis than conventional melanomas. The distinctiveness of minimal deviation melanoma was examined by comparing Ki-67 proliferation rates and p53 expression in both lesions with those in compound nevi, Spitz nevi, and vertical growth phase superficial spreading malignant melanoma.

Methods.—Twelve cases of each of the 4 lesion types were obtained from the files of a dermatopathology laboratory. Cases of superficial spreading malignant melanomas were at least Clark's Level III and 1.1 mm or thicker. The percentage of Ki-67 and p53-immunostained cells was determined by a pathologist blinded to the diagnoses and using ×400 magnification and a cell counter. Clinical follow-up for evidence of metastatic spread was sought in cases of minimal deviation melanoma.

Results.—The mean Ki-67 (MIB-1) proliferation rates for the compound nevi, Spitz nevi, minimal deviation melanomas, and superficial spreading malignant melanomas were, respectively, 0%, 3%, 13%, and 25%. Mean p53 values for these lesions were 0%, 9%, 9%, and 26%, respectively. Differences in proliferation rates between the 2 melanoma subtypes were not statistically significant, but mean p53 values were statistically different. Both melanoma subtypes exhibited considerable case-to-case variability in the amount of Ki-67 and p53 immunostaining. Clinical follow-up, available for 7 of 12 cases of minimal deviation melanoma, showed no evidence of residual disease.

Conclusion.—Both minimal deviation melanomas and superficial spreading malignant melanomas had high rates of proliferation than the compound nevi or Spitz nevi. Immunostained cells in the latter lesions tended to be superficially located but were evenly distributed at all levels throughout the tumors in both melanoma subtypes. Minimal deviation melanoma may represent a distinct form of low-grade melanoma.

▶ The group clustered around Dr Reed is trying to evaluate the potentially useful markers in the differential diagnosis of "melanocytic tumors of undetermined malignant potential," or so-called "atypical melanocytic proliferations" (but we are not really dealing with fungi or flowers); more specifically, they address a variant of those known as minimal-deviation melanoma, or more popularly, nevoid melanoma.

Although the study deals with an adequate number of cases (12 for each category: compound nevi, Spitz nevi, nevoid melanoma, and superficial spreading [non-deviated] melanomas), all the minimal deviation/nevoid melanomas were diagnosed by one author only.

A total of 200 cells were counted in each case for positivity with p53 and Ki-67; the mean proliferation rate for minimal deviation/nevoid melanomas was statistically greater than in Spitz or banal nevi. More importantly, if present in benign nevi, Ki-67 positive cells were located superficially; but they were seen in all levels in melanomas. p53 revealed similar distribution; the staining differed, however, only between minimal deviation/nevoid melanomas and "plain" melanomas.

The conclusions of this study are somewhat blurred, as the authors go on to discuss whether minimal deviation melanomas represent what appears to be an incompletely mutated melanoma or a mixture of benign and malignant elements. They go on to say, however, that further studies are needed—and indeed they are. Also, it would be nice if we could even agree on the terminology of minimal deviation/nevoid melanomas, for a start.

D. M. Jukic, MD, PhD

Myxofibrosarcoma Presenting in the Skin: Clinicopathological Features and Differential Diagnosis With Cutaneous Myxoid Neoplasms
Mansoor A, White CR Jr (Oregon Health Sciences Univ, Portland)
Am J Dermatopathol 25:281-286, 2003   5–5

Background.—Myxofibrosarcoma is a fibroblastic neoplasm with a broad range of histologic appearance, from hypocellular low-grade myxoid to high-grade pleomorphic sarcoma. Although it is one of the most common fibroblastic sarcomas in the elderly, patients with myxofibrosarcoma typically are not seen at dermatology clinics, and thus many pathologists may have trouble differentiating it from other conditions. To help differentiate this tumor from benign inflammatory and neoplastic processes, 6 cases of myxofibrosarcoma presenting cutaneously were described.

Methods.—Paraffin-embedded sections of resected tumor from 6 patients (4 men and 2 women, aged 60-78 years) whose myxofibrosarcoma presented as a cutaneous nodule were retrieved. Specimens were stained with hematoxylin and eosin and also submitted to immunohistochemical analysis. Clinical features and follow-up information were obtained from medical records.

Results.—Four patients had a painless, slow-growing, smooth nodule suggestive of a benign lesion (such as lipomas, neurofibroma, or follicular cyst); another patient had a papulonodular lesion suspected to represent an inflammatory process. Only the sixth patient had a firm mass suspected to be malignant (ie, cutaneous leiomyosarcoma). None of the patients had other malignancies or systemic involvement at presentation. During 3 to 6 years of follow-up, 2 patients had a recurrence (1 local, 1 distant), and 1 was lost to follow-up. The 1 patient who could be followed developed a second intramuscular, high-grade, undifferentiated sarcoma with spindle cells and pleomorphic area 10 months after initial treatment but has been symptom free for 3 years after reexcision. In each case, the bulk of the tumor appeared as an ill-defined nodular lesion in the subcutaneous tissue, with the overlying epidermis being either hyperplastic or unremarkable. Three patients had high-grade tumors and 3 patients had low-grade tumors, but all tumors showed a varying proportion of hypocellular myxoid and cellular areas. Low-grade areas were hypocellular but had copious myxoid matrix, with rather uniform spindled fibroblastlike cells and stellate-shaped cells. Thin-walled blood vessels were prominent in highly myxoid areas. Many cells were hyperchromatic and had irregular nuclei. Some cells contained intracytoplasmic mucin, which made the cells resemble a pseudolipoblast. Intermediate-grade areas were also predominantly myxoid with thin capillaries, but hyperchromatism and nuclear pleomorphisms were more prominent. High-grade areas were clearly malignant, with frequent giant cells. Some of these areas contained microscopic foci consisting of spindle cells within cellular regions. Mitoses increased from 2 per high-power field in the low-grade areas to 15 mitoses per HPF in the high-grade areas. All neoplastic cells had strong, diffuse high-power field to vimentin, and some cells stained positive for smooth-muscle and muscle-specific actin. Some CD68-positive histocytes were also seen. However, there was no immunoreactivity for desmin, S-100, HBM-45, keratin cocktail, or epithelial membrane antigen.

Conclusion.—Although 5 of these 6 tumors were initially thought to represent benign dermal neoplasm or infectious processes, histologic exam showed they were dermal, predominantly myxomatous neoplasms with extension into the subcutis. The diagnosis is based on the continuous histologic spectrum from hypocellularity to pleomorphism, and thus small samples may be misleading.

▶ As a continuation of the previous review (Abstract 5–4), these authors review myxofibrosarcomas presenting in the skin and the differential diagnosis of those with benign inflammatory and benign neoplastic processes.

This study, however, suffers from a small number of cases (only 6) but does deal with a follow-up and additional clinical features. The authors further recognize the importance of the fact that each neoplasm can, in fact, be composed of components that exhibit more than 1 grade histopathologically.

More common immunohistochemical markers have been employed in this study; as expected, neoplastic cells were strongly and diffusely positive for vimentin—as expected in the neoplasm of fibroblastic origin. Some positivity was also noted for smooth muscle and muscle-specific actin. The authors note the presence of CD68-positive histiocytic cells within tumor, correctly recognizing those as nonneoplastic.

In the discussion the authors address the clinical differential: lipoma, neurofibroma, and follicular cysts (most common). Pathologic differential rests on the correct recognition of interwoven low-grade, intermediate-grade, and high-grade areas within the same neoplasm. Low-end intermediate-grade areas revealed cells with cytoplasmic mucin vacuoles resulting in a peculiar "pseudolipoblast" appearance. The authors further emphasize that any proportion of low-grade myxoid areas can, and will be, seen in a high-grade myxofibrosarcoma. This of course, is of great importance to the practicing pathologists—do not sign out definitively soft tissue sarcomas or the small biopsy (partial sampling) without noting in your report that this sample might not be representative of the entire neoplasm.

I would recommend reading this article in its entirety; the authors have done a good job of contrasting myxofibrosarcomas with an emphasis on differential diagnosis (histologically) if only a superficial shave biopsy is present. Some of the less often encountered neoplasms are also discussed, such as myxoid dermatofibrosarcoma protuberans, myxoid neurofibroma, and nerve sheath myxoma.

D. M. Jukic, MD, PhD

Cadherin Expression Pattern in Melanocytic Tumors More Likely Depends on the Melanocyte Environment Than on Tumor Cell Progression
Krengel S, Grotelüschen F, Bartsch S, et al (Med Univ Lübeck, Germany; Municipal Hosp Hildesheim, Germany)
J Cutan Pathol 31:1-7, 2004   5–6

Background.—Cadherins and their intracellular binding partners, the catenins, play an important role in intercellular adhesion between melanocytes and keratinocytes. Some evidence suggests the disappearance of E-cadherin makes melanoma cells independent of growth regulation by keratinocytes. Evidence also suggests environmental factors influence cadherin expression because UVB light induces morphologic and immunohistochemical changes in melanocytic nevi. Thus, the expression of E-, P-, and N-cadherin and α-, β-, and γ-catenin was examined in a variety of benign and malignant melanocytic neoplasms and in benign nevi after UVB exposure.

Methods.—The expression of E-, P-, and N-cadherin and α-, β-, and γ-catenin was examined by immunohistochemical analysis in formalin-fixed, paraffin-embedded specimens of benign melanocytic nevi (12 cases of compound type, 10 cases of dermal type, 6 blue nevi, and 9 Spitz nevi) and malignant melanomas (10 cases of superficial spreading melanoma [SSM] and 7 cases of nodular malignant melanoma [NMM]). Additionally, portions of 8 melanocytic nevi in healthy control subjects were irradiated with UVB light 2 or 7 days before excision. Immunoreactivity was also assessed in these specimens.

Results.—In compound, dermal, and Spitz nevi, E-cadherin expression was moderate to strong in junctional melanocytes and decreased toward the dermis. In 5 of the 6 blue nevi, E-cadherin expression ranged from weak to strong, but expression did not decrease toward the dermis. In most SSMs, E-cadherin expression in the epidermal compartment was moderate to strong, whereas E-cadherin in NMMs was only weak to moderate. Decreased E-cadherin expression in the dermis of SSMs was similar to that of the nevi, but expression in NMMs tended to persist in thicker lesions. Furthermore, NMMs tended to have a more heterogeneous pattern of E-cadherin expression, with both positive and negative areas in the same specimen. P-cadherin expression was similar to E-cadherin expression in the compound, dermal, and Spitz nevi, but blue nevi did not stain for P-cadherin. P-cadherin expression in SSMs and NMMs was moderate to strong and tended to decrease toward the deeper dermis. N-cadherin expression was found only in 1 blue nevus and 2 Spitz nevi, and only small areas of SSM and NMM expressed N-cadherin. Most benign and malignant melanocytic lesions strongly expressed α-catenin, with decreased expression at deeper levels, although expression persisted to deeper levels in blue nevi and most NMMs. Staining for β-catenin produced the most intense response, with strong staining in all the benign melanocytic lesions and most malignant ones; however, some SSMs and NMMs had negative staining for β-catenin in the epidermis and papillary dermis. All but 1 blue nevus, 2 SSMs, and 1 NMM were negative for γ-catenin. UVB irradiation of melanocytic nevi in healthy control subjects did not significantly influence cadherin or catenin expression.

Conclusion.—Most junctional melanocytic cells in both nevi and melanomas expressed E- and P-cadherin, and this expression decreases toward the dermis. However, thick NMMs remain positive for E- and P-cadherin. Still, these in vivo results cannot confirm a loss of E-cadherin as a cause of tumor progression, and further studies are needed. UVB exposure had no appreciable effect on cadherin or catenin expression.

▶ The authors have explored an old idea with a new twist: does the extracellular matrix influence growth and proliferation of neoplastic cells, and if so, in which way? They hoped to identify some sign of divergent melanocyte-matrix interaction by observing the expression patterns of cadherins (calcium-dependent cell adhesion molecules) that form a part of the adherens junction, and the molecules they bind inside the cells, catenins. The expression of cadherins E-, P-, and N- were monitored; so were the catenins α, β, and γ.

The results observed were of interest for the practicing pathologist; in the case of E-cadherin, expression was strong in the junctional component of compound melanocytic nevi and clearly decreased toward the dermis (with maturation). Strong expression was also seen in the junctional component of Spitz nevi; however, the study was hampered by the fact that only a single

Spitz nevus with dermal component was included. Superficial spreading variants of melanomas mimicked this pattern; however, the pattern of expression in nodular melanoma was varied throughout the invasive component.

The pattern of expression for P-cadherin was similar to that of E-cadherin; nevi did not stain with N-cadherin, and only focal areas of melanomas were positive with this marker. Catenin expression patterns did not change significantly with different diagnoses of melanocytic neoplasms.

It seems that the level of downregulation with E- and P-cadherin was more pronounced in benign nevi than in the comparable malignant melanocytic neoplasms. This study is interesting, as it potentially identifies a valuable tool for dermatopathologists that, for lack of a better term, could be named "abtropfung staining patterns." However, the sample size was relatively small, and what the authors call "benign nevi" was not further subdivided (congenital nevi, Clark's nevi, etc). However, the idea is fresh, and first results are promising. We should await a larger study that would further identify these patterns.

D. M. Jukic, MD, PhD

Solitary Sclerotic Fibroma of Skin: A Possible Link With Pleomorphic Fibroma With Immunophenotypic Expression for 013 (CD99) and CD34
Mahmood MN, Salama ME, Chaffins M, et al (Henry Ford Hosp, Detroit)
J Cutan Pathol 30:631-636, 2003   5–7

Background.—Sclerotic fibroma (SF) is a well-circumscribed dermal nodule consisting of hypocellular-hyalinized bundles of collagen alternating with spindle cells in a storiform pattern. Unlike multiple nodules, which are associated with Cowden's disease, solitary SFs are not associated with systemic disease. Still, both multiple and solitary SF are indistinguishable on histopathologic examination, which raises the question whether solitary SFs are a true hamartoma, or whether they represent degeneration of fibrous lesions with a high spindle cell proliferating index, such as pleomorphic fibroma (PF), dermatofibroma, or angiofibroma. Thus, the morphologic and immunohistochemical features of solitary SFs and other hyalinized or sclerotic dermal lesions were evaluated.

Methods.—Formalin-fixed, paraffin-embedded sections of resected solitary SF from 8 patients were retrieved. Specimens were stained with hematoxylin and eosin and also submitted for immunohistochemical analysis. Clinical features and follow-up data were obtained from medical records. Findings in these SF specimens were compared with those in 4 PFs, 2 angiofibromas, 2 periungual fibromas, and 1 collagenized dermatofibroma whose central sclerotic area closely resembled SF. Additionally, 2 SF specimens were examined by electron microscopy.

Results.—After the SF was excised, none of the patients had other clinical findings of Cowden's disease, nor were there any recurrences during up to 4 years of follow-up. On microscopic examination, all 8 SFs contained prominent spindle-shaped cells with fusiform nuclei and indistinct eosinophilic cytoplasm. Spindle cells alternated with wavy collagen fibers in a storiform pattern. PFs were typically more cellular than SFs and contained floret cells with hyperchromatic nuclei interspersed with hyalinized stroma. Angiofibromas and periungual fibromas contained small fibrotic foci and areas of hyalinization. Spindle cells in SF and pleomorphic cells in PF were negative for S-100, KP-1, and MIB-1 but were diffusely and strongly positive for CD34 and O13. Spindle cells in angiofibroma, periungual fibroma, and dermatofibroma did not stain for CD34 or O13. Electron microscopy showed the spindle cells in SF were embedded in collagen. There were few organelles, and no basal lamina associated with these cells. The occasional presence of slitlike rough endoplasmic reticulum and loosely arranged intermediate filaments with few dense bodies suggested differentiation from myofibroblasts, but no other features provided clues as to the lineage of SFs.

Conclusion.—Solitary SF is a fibrotic lesion that shares an immunoprofile with PF but does not appear similar to dermatofibroma and other spindle cell cutaneous lesions. It may be that both SF and PF are variants of the same pathologic process, and SF may represent an advanced, more sclerotic stage of PF.

▶ So, what is solitary SF of skin, and why would you care? It sounds just like another small papular lesion somebody invented in times of boredom. Not so, I'm afraid. Solitary SF has also been known under other names, such as hypocellular fibroma and circumscribed storiform collagenoma, and even "Cowden's fibroma"—but the most popular name is definitely that of abbreviated form, SF. Therefore, it is not exactly another fibrous papule and, in fact, as one of the eponyms suggests, the form of SF (where one encounters multiple lesions) is associated with Cowden's disease/syndrome.

As the authors implicate, Cowden's syndrome is a complex hamartomatous disorder that is associated with visceral malignancies. This syndrome may be associated with breast carcinoma (in 25%-50% of women with the syndrome) and fibroadenomas, thyroid neoplasms, and carcinoma of the endometrium (3%-10%). Other mucocutaneous findings include tricholemmomas of the face, scrotal tongue, and keratotic papules of palms and soles. An unusual hamartomatous lesion, dysplastic gangliocytoma, of the cerebellum (Lhermitte-Duclos disease) has also been recently associated with this syndrome; the mutation is harbored at the PTEN gene. SF might be a harbinger of this syndrome—indeed, a biopsied SF might be the first sign of the syndrome—and here is your chance to play a hero and save a life of a patient who would otherwise die of metastatic endometrial carcinoma, for instance, if you only alert the clinician in time.

Therefore, one needs to know intricacies of immunoprofiling and histologic diagnosis of SF. In this report, the authors expand on the immunoprofile of SF and also discuss its differential diagnosis from PF and some other dermal/epidermal lesions.

The authors have retrieved 8 cases of SF but only 4 cases of PF. This is a drawback of the study; although the study expands on the immunoprofile of SFs, the sample of PFs is less than optimal to evaluate for a definitive immunoprofile. It is also somewhat surprising that the authors have actually performed ultrastructural studies on 2 cases of SFs, which pointed toward the possible myofibroblastic differentiation, but they did not perform additional immunostains to prove or disprove it.

The article also goes on to discuss in detail possible differential diagnoses of SF and differing expression of immunostains included in the study in other tissues and neoplasms. This is written in a very detailed manner and should prove to be beneficial to a practicing pathologist. A parallel that the authors explore (is SF related to solitary fibrous tumor?) is very interesting, but needs to be (as the authors themselves point out) expanded once solitary fibrous tumors are properly (re)classified.

The fact that none of the 8 cases of SF have shown any KI67 staining is somewhat unexpected (keeping in mind other studies[1]) and would be better explained if an exact cutoff point was considering the staining negative. Although, as I already pointed out, the number of cases of PF is low, the authors note that both PFs and SFs stain with CD34 and O13 and occasionally exhibit somewhat similar histology (with an exception of bizarre cellular elements in PFs); could they be related, and are the SFs only late, involuting stages of PFs?

The authors do put in a disclaimer stating that their cases of SF were not associated with Cowden's syndrome, and that cases of SF associated with that syndrome might express differing immunophenotypes.

In summary: read this article to get familiar with the entity of SF and possibly get inspired for a more in-depth literature search and follow-up in the future.

D. M. Jukic, MD, PhD

Reference

1. McCalmont TH: Sclerotic fibroma: A fossil no longer. *J Cutan Pathol* 21:82-85, 1994.

Expression of *PAX 3* Alternatively Spliced Transcripts and Identification of Two New Isoforms in Human Tumors of Neural Crest Origin
Parker CJ, Shawcross SG, Li H, et al (Manchester Metropolitan Univ, England; Royal Liverpool Univ, England; Glasgow Univ, Scotland; et al)
Int J Cancer 108:314-320, 2004   5–8

Introduction.—The developmental gene *PAX 3* is expressed in the early embryo in developing muscle and components of the nervous system, including the brain. The expression of all the known *PAX 3* isoforms in neural crest-derived human tumor tissues has not been examined. Reverse transcriptase polymerase chain reaction (RT-PCR) was used with specific primers to identify all *PAX 3* transcript isoforms.

Findings.—A comprehensive screening for the expression of the isoforms *PAX 3a-e* was conducted by RT-PCR with specific primers in human melanoma and small cell lung cancer (SCLC) cell lines and melanoma tumor tissues, including 8 primary ocular melanomas and 12 cutaneous metastases. Two new forms of *PAX 3*, g and h, were identified, isolated, cloned, and sequenced. Sets of primers for each isoform were designed. The specificity was

TABLE 2.—PAX 3 Isoform Expression and Detection

| PAX 3 Isoform | Origin of Cell Lines | | | | | | | | | Type of Melanoma | | | | | |
| | Cutaneous Melanoma | | | Ocular Melanoma | | | SCLC | | | Cutaneous | | | Ocular | | |
	±	+	++	±	+	++	±	+	++	±	+	++	±	+	++
a	1/8	6/8	1/8	0/2	0/2	0/2	0/7	0/7	0/7	2/17	2/17	10/17	3/8	3/8	2/8
b	0/8	2/8	6/8	0/2	0/2	0/2	1/7	0/7	0/7	6/17	4/17	5/17	0/8	2/8	6/8
c	0/8	0/8	8/8	1/2	0/2	0/2	3/7	0/7	0/7	0/17	2/17	12/17	1/8	2/8	5/8
d	0/8	0/8	8/8	2/2	0/2	0/2	1/7	5/7	0/7	1/17	2/17	13/17	0/8	0/8	8/8
e	1/8	7/8	0/8	0/2	0/2	0/2	2/7	0/7	0/7	7/17	8/17	0/17	6/8	2/8	0/8
g	0/8	8/8	0/8	1/2	0/2	0/2	0/5	0/5	0/5	14/17	0/17	0/17	0/8	8/8	0/8
h	6/8	1/8	1/8	0/2	0/2	0/2	0/5	0/5	0/5	0/17	0/17	0/17	0/8	0/8	0/8

±, Faint amplicon staining; +, intermediate amplicon staining; ++, intense amplicon staining.
(Courtesy of Parker CJ, Shawcross SG, Li H, et al: Expression of PAX 3 alternatively spliced transcripts and identification of two new isoforms in human tumors of neural crest origin. Int J Cancer 108:314-320, 2004. Reprinted by permission of John Wiley-Liss, Inc., a subsidiary of John Wiley & Sons, Inc.)

verified by sequence analysis of the products. The isoforms *PAX 3a-e* were identified in all human cutaneous melanoma cell lines (8 of 8); only *PAX 3c* (1 of 2) and *PAX 3d* (2 of 2) were detected in ocular melanoma cell lines. The same *PAX 3* isoforms were identified in more than 80% of human cutaneous melanomas: *PAX 3a* and *3b* (15 of 17), *PAX 3c* (14 of 17), *PAX 3d* (16 of 17), and *PAX 3e* (15 of 17). In 7 SCLC cell lines, the results were *PAX 3a* (0 of 7), *PAX 3b* (1 of 7), *PAX 3c* (3 of 7), *PAX 3d* (6 of 7), *PAX 3e* (2 of 7); 8 of 8 cutaneous melanoma cell lines and 8 of 8 ocular melanoma tissue, along with 14 of 17 cutaneous melanoma tissues screened expressed the new isoform *PAX 3g*. All 8 cutaneous melanoma cell lines expressed *PAX 3h*; it was not identifiable in any of the tumor tissues (0 of 20). The 2 new isoforms were not expressed in either of the 2 ocular melanoma cell lines (Table 2).

Conclusion.—A comparison of the various amplicon staining on a gel indicates that *PAX 3c* and *PAX 3d* are the primary transcripts expressed, with relatively low expression of both *PAX 3e* and *PAX 3h*. The isoforms of *PAX 3*, especially *PAX 3c* and *PAX 3d*, may have an important role in the development and progression of melanoma and SCLC. *PAX 3a* and *PAX 3b* may regulate the transactivation properties of the full-length isoforms.

▶ This is an interesting molecular pathology article that would elude its significance for a practicing surgical pathologist if not read in depth. The group of authors (from the United Kingdom) investigates the significance of expression of differing isoforms of the *PAX 3* gene in neoplasms derived from neural crest origin.

As an example of these, the authors have screened cell lines derived from malignant melanomas as well as pulmonary SCLCs; in addition, tissue samples from 8 primary ocular melanomas and 12 metastatic melanomas were also investigated.

The authors discuss the background and molecular biology of the *PAX 3* gene in great detail; I feel that somebody who had no knowledge whatsoever about the topic would find this description helpful and easy to understand. As pointed out, the expression of the *PAX 3* gene has been detected in early mouse embryos, before onset of neural differentiation of brain and neural tube. It also seems to play an important role in myogenesis and is expressed along the migratory pathway of myoblasts in the limb buds; thus, it should be of no surprise that expression of *PAX 3* has been identified in childhood rhabdomyosarcomas. Additionally, the *PAX 3* gene works synergistically with insulin growth factor-2 to increase angiogenesis and inhibit apoptosis. *PAX 3* is also involved in the maturation of melanocyte, helping to create a pigment-producing cell. It seems that *PAX 3* has a direct effect on microphthalmia-associated inhibition transcription factor, which upregulates melanocyte-specific tyrosinase.

The authors have evaluated isoforms of *PAX 3a-h* and identified intense staining for *PAX 3b* in 6 of 8 cutaneous melanoma cell lines; somewhat less was seen for *PAX 3b*. SCLC cell lines have expressed predominately *PAX 3c* and *PAX 3d*. These were also strongly expressed in melanoma cell lines and tissues.

Of importance, as the authors postulate, is that as *PAX 3a* and *3b* lack transcription transactivation domain, they might in some way interact with full-length isoforms of the *PAX gene* and alter their function. One has but to wonder whether this theory would explain the negativity of certain melanoma tissues for both (or either) microphthalmia-associated inhibition transcription factor of tyrosinase by immunohistochemistry, while melanosomes stage I and II are preserved if tissue is examined by electron microscopy.

These results also implicate significant involvement of the *PAX* gene isoforms in the oncogenesis of both melanomas and SCLCs. As a caveat, one has to remember that not everything held true on cell lines implies to the tissue pathology. Therefore, I think that the article would bring even more value if the authors examined tissues of SCLCs in the same way they examined melanoma tissues.

This article is very well written; it is a result of detailed research and exhaustive literature review and will serve as a great example to anybody who wishes to pair molecular pathology research with surgical pathology research and diagnostic implications.

D. M. Jukic, MD, PhD

Epithelioid Sarcoma: New Insights Based on an Extended Immunohistochemical Analysis

Laskin WB, Miettinen M (Northwestern Univ, Chicago; Armed Forces Inst of Pathology, Washington, DC)
Arch Pathol Lab Med 127:1161-1168, 2003   5–9

Background.—In recent years, several variants of epithelioid sarcoma (ES) have been described, including the proximal type, or large cell/rhabdoid ES, the fibromalike variant, which is composed of relatively bland spindled cells arranged in a storiform and fascicular growth pattern; and the angiomatoid ES, which features cyst formation and hemorrhage within tumor nodules. ES has a distinctive epithelioid phenotype and usually exhibits immunohistochemical reactivity for epithelial markers and mesenchymal markers. These findings have led to the identification of antibodies to certain keratin subunits and other novel antigens now available to surgical pathologists. However, these have not been tested on a large number of cases. The knowledge base regarding the immunohistochemical profile of ES was expanded to aid in the differential diagnosis of ES and to elucidate its histogenesis through an expanded immunohistochemical profile.

Methods.—Immunohistochemical testing with diverse antibodies was performed on 95 archived epithelioid sarcomas, including 73 classic and 22 histologically variant subtypes retrieved from the files of the Armed Forces Institute of Pathology.

Results.—Immunohistochemical reactivity included keratin 13, gamma-catenin, keratin, calretinin, keratin 20, and p63; 9 invasive cutaneous squamous cell carcinomas showed strong p63 positivity, epithelial-specific antigen, CD117/Kit, keratin 15, mesothelin, and CD10. No reactivity was observed for keratins 2, 5, and 10.

Conclusions.—This study found that p63 and keratin 5/6 will distinguish cutaneous squamous cell carcinoma (positive) from ES (usually negative). No single immunomarker was found that could distinguish the 4 main histologic subtypes of ES, which indicated that the lesions are all related histogenically. The limited expression of specific keratin subtypes used in this study support the concept that ES is a mesenchymal neoplasm capable of partial epithelial transformation.

▶ During my residency, I remember reading review articles authored by Markku Miettinen with special joy. Those were always highly instructive, practical, and educational, with a high scientific value; as expected, this one is no less.

As most of us know, ES can pose a diagnostic headache. Not only are they sometimes hard to differentiate from carcinomas, a subset of ES mimics granuloma anulare—mimicry that can be proven to be deadly. In this article, Laskin and Miettinen aim to help distinguish ES and other neoplasms.

The authors also duly note some of the newer variants of ES, such as proximal type, fibromalike, and angiomatoid. They also outline how ES are some of the few mesenchymal neoplasms that exhibit keratin, which is also true for myoepithelial neoplasms. Further, it is clear that inclusion of p63 antibody and CK5/6 cocktail in your staining panel will reliably distinguish ES (usually negative) from squamous cell carcinoma (classically positive); CD10 should be utilized to separate it (in conjunction with factor XIIIa) from the dermatofibroma group of lesions. Only a small group of ES reacted with c-Kit (CD117); thus, the authors are of opinion that STI571 (Gleevac) would not be effective in ES therapy. The opinion of a common histogenesis of all subtypes of ES is also expressed.

Although this is an excellent article, one has to read it in conjunction with a previous article from Miettinen et al[1] that deals with an extended immunopanel of ES for the sake of completeness.

D. M. Jukic, MD, PhD

Reference

1. Miettinen M, Fanburg-Smith JC, Virolainen M, et al: Epithelioid sarcoma: An immunohistochemical analysis of 112 classical and variant cases and a discussion of the differential diagnosis. *Hum Pathol* 30:934-942, 1999.

Immunohistochemical Demonstration of EMA/Glut1-Positive Perineurial Cells and CD34-Positive Fibroblastic Cells in Peripheral Nerve Sheath Tumors

Hirose T, Tani T, Shimada T, et al (Univ of Tokushima, Japan)
Mod Pathol 16:293-298, 2003   5–10

Background.—The constituents of malignant peripheral nerve sheath tumors (MPNST) are still poorly understood. The cellular composition of various peripheral nerve tumorous lesions was clarified.

Methods.—The lesions included in this immunohistochemical study were traumatic neuroma (5 cases), schwannoma (10 cases), neurofibroma (14 cases), perineurioma (3 cases), conventional MPNST (7 cases), and MPNST with perineural differentiation (4 cases). Antigens were detected by using the catalyzed signal amplification system and the ENVISION+ system.

Results.—In normal nerves and neuromas, perineuriums were positive for Glut1 and for epithelial membrane antigen (EMA), and there were some CD34-positive fibroblastlike cells in the endoneurium (Table 1). The schwannomas were found to consist primarily of S-100 protein–positive Schwann cells, whereas a few CD34-positive fibroblastic cells were present in Antoni B areas. Neurofibromas and conventional MPNST exhibited a mixed proliferation of S-100 protein-, EMA/Glut1-, and CD34-positive cells, which indicated a heterogeneous composition of these constituents. The catalyzed signal amplification system was found to demonstrate more EMA-positive perineurial cells in neurofibromas than did the ENVISION+ method. The composition of perineurial cell tumors (benign and malignant) was found to be EMA/Glut1-positive and S-100 protein–negative tumor cells.

Conclusions.—The findings in this study provided confirmation of the characteristic cellular composition of each nerve sheath tumor immunohistochemically and demonstrated the utility of the nerve sheath cell markers. It

TABLE 1.—Immunohistochemical Profiles of Peripheral Nerve Sheath Lesions

Lesions (N)	S-100	EMA	EMA/CSA	Glut1	CD34
Neuroma (2)	+++	+	++	++	++
	(100%)	(80%)	(100%)	(100%)	(100%)
Schwannoma (10)	+++	+*	+*	+*	+
	(100%)	(70%)	(100%)	(90%)	(100%)
Neurofibroma (14)	+++	+	+	+	++
	(100%)	(43%)	(100%)	(100%)	(100%)
Perineurioma (3)	−	+	+	+	+
	(0%)	(33%)	(100%)	(67%)	(33%)
Conventional MPNST (7)	++	−	+	+	+
	(86%)	(0%)	(86%)	(33%)	(57%)
Perineurial MPNST (4)	−	+	++	+	+
	(0%)	(75%)	(100%)	(67%)	(25%)

*Immunoreactivity in capsules. *Abbreviations: N*, Case number; *CSA*, catalyzed signal amplification system; +++, many positive cells; ++, some positive cells; +, a few positive cells; −, negative; %, percentage of positive cases.

(Courtesy of Hirose T, Tani T, Shimada T, et al: Immunohistochemical demonstration of EMA/Glut1-positive perineurial cells and CD34-positive fibroblastic cells in peripheral nerve sheath tumors. *Mod Pathol* 16:293-298, 2003.)

appears that Glut1 and EMA are specific to perineurial cells, and CD34 appears to be immunoreactive to endoneurial fibroblasts.

▶ This study is worth reading for several reasons: (1) it neatly outlines differences in histoarchitecture and immunohistochemical profile of Schwann cells, perineurial cells, and endoneurial cells (fibroblasts), known under the common name of nerve sheath cells; (2) it accentuates (in the text as well as in Table 1) the immunoprofile of nerve sheath "lesions" in the authors' experience, which is useful in building an algorithm or starting your own differential staining process; (3) it introduces an additional marker (Glut1-glucose transporter protein 1) into the differential diagnosis of nerve sheath neoplasms; (4) it readdresses and clarifies (if clarification is needed) the current classification of nerve sheath neoplasms; and (5) it raises awareness for ancillary immunohistochemical methods, such as ENVISION+ and catalyzed signal amplification.

This article also features excellent-quality immunohistochemical images that, more often than not, are lacking in the publications of this type, and complement text description in an efficient way. This article thus provides an excellent reference point for pattern comparison in nerve sheath neoplasms. The results are refreshing, and the authors are reintroducing value of looking at "old" lesions (such as neurofibroma) in a new way. They acknowledge the presence of "intermediate" cell in neurofibroma, as in their experience, neurofibroma stain with S100, Glut1, and even EMA (by catalyzed signal amplification method, mainly). This prompted the authors to conclude that neurofibromas are composed of "heterogeneous cellular constituents." It would be of great interest to further this study by investigating whether dermatofibrosarcoma protuberans is composed of same type of "intermediate" cell, as previously suggested by some authors.[1,2]

D. M. Jukic, MD, PhD

References

1. Hashimoto K, Brownstein MH, Jakobiec FA: Dermatofibrosarcoma protuberans. A tumor with perineural and endoneural cell features. *Arch Dermatol* 110:874-885, 1974.
2. Fletcher CD, Theaker JM, Flanagan A, et al: Pigmented dermatofibrosarcoma protuberans (Bednar tumour): Melanocytic colonization or neuroectodermal differentiation? A clinicopathological and immunohistochemical study. *Histopathology* 13:631-643, 1988.

Lymphomatoid Papulosis: Reappraisal of Clinicopathologic Presentation and Classification Into Subtypes A, B, and C

El Shabrawi-Caelen L, Kerl H, Cerroni L (Univ of Graz, Austria)
Arch Dermatol 140:441-447, 2004   5–11

Background.—Lymphomatoid papulosis (LYP), which is characterized by spontaneously resolving papules and nodules with strikingly atypical lymphoid cells, belongs to a family of disorders with a benign clinical course but with a malignant appearance on histopathologic examination. LYP has been a mystery since it was first described in 1968. LYP was initially believed to be an inflammatory process, but it is now thought to be an indolent cutaneous lymphoma and is listed as such in the current European Organization for Research and Treatment of Cancer and the World Health Organization classifications. The clinicopathologic features of lymphomatoid papulosis were analyzed and the characteristics of histopathologic variants delineated (types A, B, and C).

Methods.—This retrospective, nonrandomized study was conducted at a university-based dermatologic referral center. The study group was composed of 85 patients with LYP. Clinical data and 1 or more biopsy specimens were available for review from all 85 patients. Immunophenotypic and molecular analyses were performed when possible.

Results.—Of the 85 patients studied, 78 had only 1 histopathologic subtype of lymphomatoid papulosis (64 with type A, 3 with type B, and 11 with type C). The remaining 7 patients had more than 1 subtype (1 with types A and B, 5 with types A and C, and 1 with all 3 types). Two patients had regional LYP, an unusual clinical presentation that was characterized by groups of lesions localized to 1 anatomic region. This was thought to be the first observation that some histopathologic patterns, such as follicular mucinosis (1 patient), syringotropic infiltrates (1 patient), epidermal vesicle formation (2 patients), and syringosquamous metaplasia (1 patient) were associated with LYP. A distribution of hair follicles, or follicular LYP, was observed in 5 biopsy specimens. A bandlike distribution of the infiltrate, rather than a wedge distribution, was observed in 5 specimens from patients with LYP type A. Of the 8 patients with associated lymphoid malignancies, 4 had Hodgkin disease and 4 had mycosis fungoides.

Conclusions.—The differentiation of LYP from mycosis fungoides and anaplastic large cell lymphoma can be difficult if not impossible because of the multiple clinicopathologic features of LYP. The boundaries between these entities are uncertain in the spectrum of CD30+ cutaneous lymphoproliferative disorders.

▶ LYP is, as our well-known group from Graz indicates, a "lymphoproliferative" disorder, currently classified in a category of indolent cutaneous lymphomas. The individual lesions wax and wane over a span of time and can be a nightmare for the patient, clinician, and (dermato)pathologist; only a small number will eventually progress to nonindolent cutaneous lymphomas, either in mycosis fungoides or anaplastic large cell lymphoma group.

This study has examined tissue from 85 patients and has stratified lesions of LYP to the accepted classification of types A, B, and C. Authors also used immunostaining with an appropriate antibody panel as well as molecular pathology methods (namely polymerase chain reaction) to investigate rearrangements of T-cell γ receptor.

This valuable study reviews histologic and immunophenotypical characteristics of each of 3 types in great detail; descriptions are accompanied by high-quality images (low-, medium-, and high-power) and immunohistochemical stain images when appropriate. The authors also outline some unusual patterns (eg, follicular mucinosis, syringotropic and syringometaplastic infiltrates, and epidermal vesiculation). Avid readers will also note the recent article by Crowson et al[1] that describes 9 additional patients with what these authors have dubbed "granulomatous eccrinotropic lymphomatoid papulosis ."

The current study also serves to reestablish the criteria needed for diagnosis of differing variants of lymphomatoid papulosis; it clearly separates "usual" variants (type A, for instance) from type C (less usual, more commonly associated with uncertain diagnosis [whether anaplastic large cell lymphoma or not]) and concurrent or resulting anaplastic large cell lymphoma of the skin. It also stresses association of these indolent lymphomas with other lymphomas, namely mycosis fungoides, anaplastic large cell lymphoma, and Hodgkin's disease (lymphoma).

Although some prognostic data are provided, I would refer the readers to another, similarly excellent article by a group from Stanford[2] for an exposé on survival and prognostic implications. As a conclusion, I recommend the current article to anyone who has ever looked at cutaneous lymphomatoid infiltrates.

D. M. Jukic, MD, PhD

References

1. Crowson AN, Baschinsky DY, Kovatich A, et al: Granulomatous eccrinotropic lymphomatoid papulosis. *Am J Clin Pathol* 119:731-739, 2003.
2. Liu HL, Hoppe RT, Kohler S, et al: CD30+ cutaneous lymphoproliferative disorders: The Stanford experience in lymphomatoid papulosis and primary cutaneous anaplastic large cell lymphoma. *J Am Acad Dermatol* 49:1049-1058, 2003.

Immunolabeling Pattern of Syndecan-1 Expression May Distinguish Pagetoid Bowen's Disease, Extramammary Paget's Disease, and Pagetoid Malignant Melanoma in situ
Bayer-Garner IB, Reed JA (Marshfield Clinic, Wis; Baylor College of Medicine, Houston)
J Cutan Pathol 31:169-173, 2004   5–12

Background.—The differential diagnosis of intraepidermal malignant cells with pagetoid spread includes pagetoid Bowen's disease (PBD), extramammary Paget's disease (EPD), melanoma in situ (MIS), and a number of entities that less commonly manifest the pattern of pagetoid spread. Morphologic clues can often aid in the differentiation of these lesions, but immunohistochemical evaluations are often necessary to obtain the correct diagnosis. Syndecan-1 is a cell-surface proteoglycan that mediates adhesion between cells and the extracellular matrix and between the cells themselves. Whether the expression of syndecan-1 could be used to distinguish PBD from EPD and pagetoid MIS was determined.

Methods.—Syndecan-1 immunoreactivity was assessed in 22 cases of PBD, 4 cases of intraepidermal EPD, and 13 cases of MIS.

Results.—Cell membrane syndecan-1 immunoreactivity was evident in PBD and cytoplasmic syndecan-1 immunoreactivity was evident in EPD; in contrast, immunoreactivity for syndecan-1 immunoreactivity was not present in MIS.

Conclusions.—It would appear from the findings in this study that the patterns of syndecan-1 expression may aid in the differentiation of PBD, EPD, and pagetoid MIS.

▶ When I initially saw this article, I approached it with great interest. In fact, the quandary above has puzzled many, and an additional immunohistochemical stain to be included in the panel above would be more than welcome. However, it is worthwhile to note that the real quandary exists between "pagetoid" (or, more correctly, "bowenoid") squamous cell carcinoma in situ (dubbed PBD by the authors) and EPD, as MIS can be more readily excluded by an extended immunopanel that would include first and foremost MELAN-A/Mart immunostain, accompanied by S100, tyrosinase, HMB45, and MITF.

The authors reviewed the expression patterns of syndecan-1 in normal tissues, focusing on the expression pattern of keratinocytes; regrettably, there is no mention of syndecan-1 expression in other glandular tissues, to include mammary gland, in this article.

The results were of value for the differential diagnosis of PBD versus EPD; malignant cells in PBD express syndecan-1 in cell-membrane bound manner, while malignant cells of EPD exhibit cytoplasmic positivity. This will likely prove valuable if an expanded investigation is carried out; however, this study suffers from the minimal number of EPD included—only 4 cases! The authors also don't attempt to make the distinction whether their cases of EPD are of presumed primary cutaneous origin (apocrine/eccrine) or have been harvested from the patients with known primary malignancies (such as transitional/urothelial bladder carcinoma or anorectal primary, to name only a few).

Further, at 2 points the authors refer to EPD as Paget's disease, creating an unnecessary confusion between extramammary variant and primary mammary variant. The study also suffers from quoting relatively old references (out of 22 included references, 15 were from before 1994); more recent literature on the subject was ignored (no reference beyond year 2000). There is no inclusion of literature on more recent melanoma-related antibodies, either.

The problems with nomenclature do not end there—it is unclear why the authors (on the first page of the article) refer to Merkel cell carcinoma and trabecular carcinoma (of skin) as separate entities, when Merkel cell carcinoma was first described by Toker[1] under the name of trabecular cell carcinoma; they also still use the term "histiocytosis X" rather than the accepted name Langerhans cell histiocytosis.

In conclusion, although syndecan-1 seems to have potential in differentiating EPD from PBD, one would have to await results from a larger study before reaching a final conclusion. Comparison studies with mammary Paget's disease as well as with EPD originating from known primary carcinomas would also be warranted.

The reader would benefit from reading more recent literature on the subject, especially from Japanese authors[2,3] and others.[4-6]

D. M. Jukic, MD, PhD

References

1. Toker C: Trabecular carcinoma of the skin. *Arch Dermatol* 105:107-110, 1972.
2. Miyakawa T, Togawa Y, Matushima H, et al: Squamous metaplasia of Paget's disease. *Clin Exp Dermatol* 29:71-73, 2004.
3. Matsumura Y, Matsumura Y, Nishigori C, et al: Y.PIG7/LITAF gene mutation and overexpression of its gene product in extramammary Paget's disease. *Int J Cancer* 111:218-223, 2004.
4. Finan MA, Barre G: Bartholin's gland carcinoma, malignant melanoma and other rare tumours of the vulva: *Best Pract Res Clin Obstet Gynaecol* 17:609-633, 2003.
5. Lau J, Kohler S: Keratin profile of intraepidermal cells in Paget's disease, extramammary Paget's disease, and pagetoid squamous cell carcinoma in situ. *J Cutan Pathol* 30:449-454, 2003.
6. Mai KT, Alhalouly T, Landry D, et al: Pagetoid variant of actinic keratosis with or without squamous cell carcinoma of sun-exposed skin: A lesion simulating extramammary Paget's disease. *Histopathology* 41:331-336, 2002.

Pathologic Review of Negative Sentinel Lymph Nodes in Melanoma Patients With Regional Recurrence: A Clinicopathologic Study of 1152 Patients Undergoing Sentinel Lymph Node Biopsy
Li L-XL, Scolyer RA, Ka VSK, et al (Royal Prince Alfred Hosp, Camperdown, NSW, Australia; Univ of Sydney, NSW, Australia)
Am J Surg Pathol 27:1197-1202, 2003   5–13

Background.—The tumor status of regional lymph nodes that drain primary melanoma sites has been advanced as the most important prognostic factor in early-stage melanomas. It has been shown that the presence of tumor cells in the nodes in which direct drainage occurs (the sentinel lymph nodes [SLNs]) are accurately predictive of the metastatic status of the regional node field. Thus, an SLN that is melanoma negative by pathologic examination implies the absence of melanoma metastasis to that regional lymph node field. However, regional lymph node field recurrence manifests in a small proportion of patients after a negative SLN biopsy. The histopathologic findings in negative SLNs from these patients were reviewed to determine whether occult melanoma cells were present in the SLNs, to characterize the pathologic features of false-negative SLNs, and to provide recommendations for the histopathologic examination of these specimens.

Methods.—From March 1992 to June 2001, 1152 patients underwent SLN biopsy for primary melanomas at an Australian melanoma unit. Of these patients 976 were diagnosed with negative SLNs by initial pathologic examination by using 2 hematoxylin and eosin-stained sections and 2 immunostained sections for S-100 protein and HMB45. Follow-up was available for 957 of these patients, of whom 26 (2.7%) had regional lymph node recurrence develop during a median follow-up period of 35.7 months. Original slides and tissue blocks were available for reexamination in 22 of these patients, and the original slides of each block were reviewed. Multiple additional sections were cut from each block and stained with hematoxylin and eosin for S-100, HMB45, and Melan A.

Results.—Deposits of occult melanoma cells were detected in 7 (31.8%) of these 22 patients. In 5 of the 7 patients, deposits of melanoma cells were present only in the recut sections. There were no significant differences in clinical and pathologic variables for patients in whom occult melanoma cells were found by reexamination of their SLNs compared with those in whom no melanoma cells were detected.

Conclusions.—It is suggested by the detection of melanoma cell deposits in only 7 of 22 patients with false-negative SLNs that mechanisms other than failure of histopathologic examination may have a role in failure of the SLN biopsy technique in some patients. In this routine pathologic examination, the failure rate for melanoma detection in SLNs was less than 1%. It is therefore difficult to justify the routine performance of more intensive histopathologic examination of SLNs from a cost-benefit perspective. It is recommended that 2 hematoxylin and eosin–stained sections and 2 immunostained sections be examined routinely in SLNs from patients with melanoma.

▶ As pointed out in the opening sentences of this article, a small proportion of patients who have negative SLNs do go on to develop regional lymph node "field recurrence." Therefore, the problem is, are those patients relapsing from the so-called "invisible" metastasis (too small to detect by microscopic methods), or because we are missing micrometastases in the SLN, either from insufficient sampling or errors?

As is pointed out, micrometastatic deposits in SLNs can be difficult to detect—even if the entire node is sectioned—up to 600 hematoxylin and eosin sections per node. Difficult, yes; but is it impossible?

The authors examined patients followed up in a Sydney melanoma unit (976 patients with initially negative SLNs, 26 of whom developed regional recurrence); however, some patients were excluded if they developed local recurrence, in-transit metastasis, or distant metastasis.

The authors do provide detailed explanations and descriptions of primary melanomas; however, the fact remains that 31.8% (7 patients) of nodes negative by initial pathologic examination were positive on reexamination (4 serial sections at 2 levels 50 μm apart, 3 of which were stained by S100, HMB45, and Melan-A); actually, 2 of 7 patients had metastatic cells in the lymph node that were missed on the initial review.

Some possible reasons for pathologic failure include presence of metastatic melanoma cells in the lymphatics that did not reach lymph node, and, as the authors point out, failure of histopathologic examination to detect metastasis, no matter how small it is. The authors further discuss that some of the deficiencies of surgery and scanning (lymphoscintigram) might contribute to relapse. The logic becomes skewed at this point: what does the node that did not even get removed have to do with lymph node that was missed by pathologic examination? The authors correctly point out that HMB45 should not be a marker of choice (as a second marker) for immunohistochemical exam of SLNs suspicious for melanoma metastasis; in fact, our own institution utilizes S100, HMB45, Melan-A, tyrosinase, and CD68.

I would not argue with the authors that examining 600 sections from each lymph node is an overkill, but are we doing enough? Should we be actually LEAVING the tissue in the block? Couldn't we be doing some more sampling, perhaps spaced more widely apart, to examine more of the node?

The authors conclude that "performance of more extensive histopathologic examination…"than "4 serial sections," 2 of which are stained with hematoxylin and eosin and 2 of which are immunostained, are "difficult to justify because of additional laboratory cost involved," and so forth.

Ladies and gentlemen, reality check: patients undergo several-thousand-dollar workups before they even have lymph nodes submitted to pathology; hundreds of dollars or so more would hardly make a difference, especially if those can save lives. And, if we keep stubbornly refusing to do this, there are people who will do it. Real-time polymerase chain reaction for detecting those intraoperatively will replace pathologic exam if we do not improve our SLN protocols.[1] Twelve percent to 80% of missed micrometastasis (as outlined in some studies) is way too much—and it is way too much if we only "scrape" the surface of each block and neatly stash the rest of tissue in the file.

If we don't react and develop precise guidelines on how to handle these issues, maybe some of our positions will be difficult to justify.

D. M. Jukic, MD, PhD

Reference

1. Ishida M, Kitamura K, Kinoshita J, et al: Detection of micrometastasis in the sentinel lymph nodes in breast cancer. *Surgery* 131(1 suppl):S211-S216, 2002.

The Prognostic Importance of Tumor Mitotic Rate Confirmed in 1317 Patients With Primary Cutaneous Melanoma and Long Follow-up
Francken AB, Shaw HM, Thompson JF, et al (Royal Prince Alfred Hosp, Sydney, NSW; Univ of Alabama, Birmingham)
Ann Surg Oncol 11:426-433, 2004   5–14

Background.—The late physician Vincent McGovern was recognized as an international authority on the pathology of melanoma. McGovern was one of the first investigators to suggest that the assessment of tumor mitotic rate (TMR) might provide useful prognostic information. Data were analyzed from a large cohort of patients in whom tumors were originally assessed by McGovern and who now have extended follow-up. The goal of this reassessment was to determine the independent prognostic value of TMR in primary localized cutaneous melanoma.

Methods.—Data were extracted from the Sydney Melanoma Unit database for 1317 patients treated by McGovern from 1957 to 1982 for whom there was complete clinical information and who primary lesion pathologic processes included tumor thickness, ulcerative status, and TMR. These assessments were performed according to recommendations of the Eighth

International Pigment Cell Conference. Factors predictive of melanoma-specific survival were analyzed with the Cox proportional hazards regression model.

Results.—According to the recently revised American Joint Committee on Cancer Staging System, which is based on tumor thickness and ulceration, stage was the factor most predictive of survival, followed in decreasing order by primary lesion site, patient age, and TMR.

Conclusions.—These findings provided confirmation that TMR is an independent predictor of survival in patients with primary cutaneous melanoma. However, the predictive value of TMR was less than it was when assessed according to the 1982 revisions of the 1957 TMR recommendations.

► This article starts with delineation of the contributions of one of the late melanoma experts to the field, Dr McGovern, therefore serving as an introductory article of the history of medicine. The authors even emulated McGovern's microscope field.

They evaluated melanomas according to the recent American Joint Committee on Cancer staging criteria; they averaged the number of mitotic figures seen in the dermal (invasive) component of melanoma (at least 10 high-power fields) and reported after being averaged as number of mitoses per 5 high-power fields.

In short, the authors confirmed the American Joint Committee on Cancer stage as the most potent survival predictor followed closely by mitotic rate. The authors do make a point of calculating the surface of each field for each microscope—otherwise, the number of mitoses might vary up to 600%.

The take-home message of this article should be that we do need to keep recording the number of mitoses in each invasive melanoma examined, but we must do it properly. Statements such as "mitotic number: slightly increased" or similar (that can often be found in reports) make no sense and offer no contribution to a patient's follow-up or therapy. For everybody—please read this article and make sure you are counting mitotic figures in the way they should be counted.

D. M. Jukic, MD, PhD

The Diagnostic Utility of p63, CK 5/6, CK 7, and CK 20 in Distinguishing Primary Cutaneous Adnexal Neoplasms From Metastatic Carcinomas
Qureshi HS, Ormsby AH, Lee MW, et al (Henry Ford Hosp, Detroit)
J Cutan Pathol 31:145-152, 2004   5–15

Background.—Adenocarcinomas from other organs can metastasize to the skin; in rare cases these cutaneous metastases can be the initial manifestation of malignancy. It can be quite difficult to differentiate cutaneous metastases of adenocarcinomas from primary cutaneous adnexal neoplasms (PCANs) with sweat gland differentiation, particularly if they are malignant. The utility of p63, CK 5/6, CK 7, and CK 20 expression in PCANs compared with metastatic carcinomas (MCs) was investigated.

TABLE 3.—Results of CK 5/6, p63, CK 7, and CK 20 Immunostains for MCs

Diagnosis	Number of Cases	Number of Positively Stained Cases and Grade			
		CK 5/6	p63	CK 7	CK 20
Pancreatic carcinoma	1	1 (1+)	0	1 (3+)	0
Ovarian carcinoma	1	0	0	0	0
Renal cell carcinoma	2	0	0	1 (3+)	1 (1+)
Urothelial carcinoma	1	1 (3+)	1 (3+)	1 (3+)	0
Lung adenocarcinoma	2	1 (1+)	0	2 (all 3+)	0
Breast ductal carcinoma	6	0	0	6 (all 3+)	0
Thyroid carcinoma	1	0	0	1 (3+)	0
Esophagus adenocarcinoma	1	1 (1+)	1 (2+)	1 (3+)	1 (3+)
Total (percent positive)	15	4 (27%)	2 (13%)	13 (87%)	2 (13%)

(Courtesy of Qureshi HS, Ormsby AH, Lee MW, et al: The diagnostic utility of p63, CK 5/6, CK 7, and CK 20 in distinguishing primary cutaneous adnexal neoplasms from metastatic carcinomas. *J Cutan Pathol* 31:145-152, 2004. Copyright Munksgaard International Publishers Ltd., Copenhagen, Denmark.)

Methods.—A review was conducted of 21 PCANs with sweat gland differentiation (6 benign and 15 malignant), 1 sebaceous carcinoma, and 15 MCs (14 adenocarcinomas, 1 urothelial carcinoma) to skin. Immunostains for p63, CK 5/6, CK 7, and CK 20 were performed. Results of the immunostains were graded as 1, less than 10%; 2, 11% to 50%; and 3, more than 50% of tumor cells stained.

Results.—The results of immunostaining were: 20 of 22 PCANs expressed p63 and CK 5/6; 4 of 15 and 2 of 15 MCs were positive for CK 5/6 and p63, respectively; and 13 of 22 PCANs and 13 of 15 MCs were positive for CK 7, respectively. All PCANs were negative for CK 20, and 2 of 15 MCs were positive (Table 3). The sensitivity and specificity for the diagnosis of PCAN were 91% and 73% for CK 5/6, 91% and 100% for p63, and 60% and 13% for CK 7, respectively.

Conclusions.—For distinguishing PCAN from MC, positivity for p63 and CK 5/6 is relatively specific and sensitive for PCAN; CK 7 and 20 are neither sensitive nor specific, and CK 7 positivity in PCAN was focal, with a specific pattern in contrast to the diffuse positivity for MC.

▶ In this study, 16 cases of PCAN were used in comparison with 15 cases of carcinomas metastatic to skin; 6 cases of benign adnexal neoplasms were included, too. The authors utilized carcinomas of various primary sites as a source of metastatic disease. However, in most of the cases of difficult differential diagnosis, one needs to differentiate metastatic ductal carcinoma (breast) from primary eccrine or apocrine carcinoma—although other cases could be diagnostically difficult, too.

The authors suggest that utilization of CK 5/6 and p63 (transcription factor used in the differential diagnosis of prostatic carcinoma from benign glands) can be effectively used to differentiate most eccrine carcinomas from metastatic disease, with exception of PCAN.

One needs to read this article in its entirety—this is a simple but to-the-point article that will prove beneficial in most of the general pathology and dermatopathology practices, despite the fact that my write-up appears relatively short.

D. M. Jukic, MD, PhD

Clear Cells of Toker in Accessory Nipples
Willman JH, Golitz LE, Fitzpatrick JE (Univ of Colorado, Denver)
J Cutan Pathol 30:256-260, 2003   5–16

Background.—Clear cells of Toker are intraepithelial cells with clear to pale staining cytoplasm and bland cytologic features in approximately 10% of normal nipples with hematoxylin and eosin staining. It has been hypothesized that the presence of Toker cells is a precursor of extramammary Paget's disease (EMPD), but there have been no studies of the distribution of Toker cells outside the nipples. Cases of accessory nipples were examined for the presence of Toker cells.

Methods.—A retrospective study was conducted of 20 cases of accessory nipples by using hematoxylin and eosin staining for CK 7, CK 20, epithelial membrane antigen, and GCDFP-15.

Results.—Of the 20 accessory nipples studies, 13 (65%) demonstrated Toker cells with CK 7 staining. Toker cells in 6 of the 13 cases were also positive for epithelial membrane antigen. Only 1 case of accessory nipple with Toker cells showed immunoreactivity for antibodies to GCDFP-15.

Conclusions.—It appears that Toker cells occur outside the normal nipple epidermis in the epidermis of accessory nipples. The distribution of Toker cells along the milk line is correlated with the distribution of most cases of EMPD along the milk line, particularly in the groin and axillae. There is a need for additional studies to define the relation between Toker cells and EMPD.

► What is a clear cell of Toker? Contrary to what it might seem, clear cell of Toker has nothing to do with Toker's carcinoma (Merkel/trabecular cell carcinoma); on the contrary, they might be precursors of EMPD.

Clear cells of Toker are found in approximately 10% of normal nipples by using plain hematoxylin and eosin staining and are distributed anywhere between basal cells of epidermis to mid-epidermis; utilization of immunohistochemical methods increases this percentage approximately 8-fold. The authors correctly point out that EMPD could have various underlying cases (rectal, cervical, transitional cell/urothelial, prostatic and apocrine carcinoma), but some of the cases are, as we like to say, "idiopathic." In fact, there are even cases of EMPD of the breast—cases without an underlying mammary carcinoma.

The authors studied 20 cases of accessory nipples for the presence of Toker cells, trying to follow the so-called nipple line. I found this study to be a very elegant and clean study trying to correlate the distribution of Toker cells to the distribution of EMPD. They utilized CK 7, CK 20, GCDFP-15, and epithelial membrane antigen; it is interesting that they did find cells otherwise indistinguishable from normal keratinocytes to stain with CK 7, likely representing Toker cells in disguise.

Of 16 cases with identifiable Toker cells (with CK 7), only 1 convincingly stained with epithelial membrane antigen; the same number (1) stained with GCDFP-15. None stained with CK 20 (some Merkel cells did). Of interest, 1 of the cases of EMPD was associated with what the authors refer to as "diffuse hyperplasia of Toker cells."

The authors did find similar distribution of Toker cells with cases of EMPD, thus supporting the notion that those 2 are related (at least, "idiopathic" cases of EMPD); in fact, as they point out, Toker cells might be related to clear cell papulosis (seen in children).

So, if one needs to know more about the disease process in EMPD, read this article—it will spark some ideas in you on how to correlate things that seem pretty obvious at first.

D. M. Jukic, MD, PhD

Differential Diagnosis of Cutaneous Infiltrates of B Lymphocytes With Follicular Growth Pattern
Leinweber B, Colli C, Chott A, et al (Univ of Graz, Austria; Univ of Trieste, Italy; Univ of Vienna)
Am J Dermatopathol 26:4-13, 2004   5–17

Background.—Primary cutaneous follicle center cell lymphoma (FCCL) and lymphocytoma cutis (LC) are the main differential diagnoses of cutaneous B-cell infiltrates with follicular pattern of growth. Additionally, some cases of marginal zone lymphoma (MZL) with reactive germinal centers (GCs) may also represent a differential diagnostic concern. Thus, the differential diagnosis of cutaneous B-cell infiltrates with follicular growth pattern is one of the most difficult problems in dermatopathology. In endemic regions such as Austria, *Borrelia burgdorferi (Bb)*-associated lymphadenosis cutis benigna is the most common type of LC. However, the detection of *Bb* DNA within such lesions is not synonymous with benign status; 2 independent studies have shown *Bb* within the infiltrates of low-grade primary cutaneous B-cell lymphoma in approximately 20% of cases. The histopathologic, immunophenotypic, and molecular diagnostic criteria between *Bb*-associated LC, FCCL, and primary MZL with reactive GCs were evaluated.

Methods.—The study included 47 patients, including 12 with LC (mean age, 38 years); 29 with FCCL (mean age, 57.5 years); and 6 with MZL (mean age, 63.8 years). Complete phenotypic data were available for all patients. The IgH gene arrangement and the t(14;18) (major and minor breakpoint regions) were analyzed by using the polymerase chain reaction technique in 41 and 18 patients, respectively.

Results.—Histologic analysis demonstrated in all cases of FCCL 1 or more atypical feature of the follicles, including the lack of or a reduced mantle zone, lack of polarization, tendency to confluence, and absence of tingible body macrophages. In most patients with *Bb*-associated LC, the GCs lacked a mantle zone, had no polarization, and demonstrated a tendency to confluence as well. However, all cases showed the presence of several tingible body macrophages. In MZL the follicles showed features typical of reactive GCs. Immunohistologic analyses showed a reduced proliferative activity of neoplastic follicles as detected by MIB-1 antibody in 23 (79.3%) of 29 patients with FCCL but in only 1 patient with LC (8.3%). Proliferation of the GCs was normal in all patients with MZL. Positivity for CD10 and/or Bcl-6 was found in small clusters outside the follicles in 19 patients with FCCL (65.5%) and in 3 patients with LC (25%) but in no patient with MZL. The intensity of CD10 staining on follicular cells was on average stronger in patients with FCCL, but overlapping features could be observed. Staining for Bcl-2 protein was consistently negative in GC cells in cases of LC and MZL and was positive on a variable proportion of the cells in 8 cases of FCCL (28.6%). There was no evidence of the t(14;18) in any of the cases tested. An analysis of the IgH gene rearrangement demonstrated a monoclonal pattern in 1 (10%) of 10 patients with CL, 15 (5.9%) of 27 patients with FCCL, and 2 (50%) of 4 patients with MZL.

Conclusions.—The diagnosis of cutaneous infiltrates of B lymphocytes with follicular growth pattern should be obtained by integration of clinical data with the lesion's histopathologic, immunohistochemical, and molecular features.

▶ So, just how do you differentiate the reactive lymphocytic cutaneous infiltrates from lymphomas of skin? As we know, the differential diagnosis includes LC, FCCL, and, as stated in this article, some cases of MZL. The authors also outline the relationship of benign and malignant cutaneous lymphoid infiltrates with *Bb*.

An appropriate and extensive panel of antibodies was used that included CD10, Bcl-6, Bcl-2, KI-67, CD 20, CD79a, and CD3; this was followed by molecular biology methods—analysis for t(14;18) by polymerase chain reaction and IgH gene rearrangement. The authors go further to describe the marked details of histologic appearance of each of the 3 main entities in the differential.

One needs to review all the tables included by authors in this article for a good review of all the features; the tables are extensive and do not allow for detailed write-up here. One additional "gold" feature of the article is inclusion of appropriate and highly informative image material.

It is thus apparent, from the work of this group and others, that old criteria (top-heavy vs bottom heavy) are not of utmost diagnostic importance, as we were taught for a long time. The authors outline a new set of morphologic criteria: reduced or absent mantle zone, monomorphism of follicles with no apparent dark and light zones, and tendency for confluence of follicles. This series also denotes an absence of tingible body macrophages within follicular structures as a more important morphologic criterion.

FCCL revealed, according to the authors, stronger CD10 staining than the lymphocytomas; follicles in FCCL revealed reduced proliferation activity with

Ki67. Other important features were presence of Bcl-6 positive clusters outside follicles, Bcl-2 within follicular cells, and monoclonality by polymerase chain reaction. Polarization of follicles (with aid from Ki67) was also found to be valuable.

As a conclusion, and to anybody who ever diagnosed an LC, please read this article so you don't have to write up a mini-series of LC progressing to cutaneous lymphomas.

D. M. Jukic, MD, PhD

Localization of a Novel Melanoma Susceptibility Locus to 1p22
Gillanders E, and The Melanoma Genetics Consortium (NIH, Bethesda, Md; et al)
Am J Hum Genet 73:301-313, 2003   5–18

Background.—Cutaneous malignant melanoma (CMM) is a significant public health problem in all populations of European origin. A positive family history of CMM is one of the best-established risk factors; it is estimated that 10% of CMM cases are inherited. Mutations in 2 genes, CDKN2A and CDK4, have been shown to increase the risk of CMM, but these mutations account for only 20% to 25% of families with multiple cases of CMM. Additional loci involved in susceptibility for CMM were localized.

Methods.—A genomewide scan was performed for linkage in 49 Australian pedigrees containing at least 3 cases of CMM in which involvement of CDKN2A and CDK4 was been excluded.

Results.—The highest 2-point parametric log odds ratio (LOD) score was obtained at D1S2726, which maps to the short arm of chromosome 1 (1p22). A parametric LOD score of 4.65 and a nonparametric LOD score of 4.19 were found at D1S2779 in 9 families selected for the study on the basis of early onset. An analysis of 33 additional multiplex families with CMM from several continents provided additional evidence for linkage in the 1p22 region; in this cohort also the linkage was strongest in families with the earliest mean age at diagnosis. A nonparametric ordered sequential analysis was used on the basis of the average age at diagnosis in each family. The highest LOD score, 6.43, was obtained at D1S2779 and occurred when the 15 families with the earliest ages at onset were included.

Conclusions.—The findings of this study have localized a novel CMM susceptibility gene to 1p22, with the strongest evidence for linkage in approximately 20% of families with the earliest age at diagnosis.

▶ By know, most of us know that CDKN2A locus accounts for melanoma susceptibility in approximately one quarter of "melanoma kindreds"; there is also some role for CDK4 and MC1R. The group performed polymerase chain reaction on the genomic DNA retrieved from the blood samples. To be included in the study, the families in question had to have at least 3 members with melanoma who had blood available for study, be CDK2NA negative and CDK4 negative, and have no haplotype sharing in the region 9p21-22 (where CDK2NA is located).

However, the highest LOD score was observed in the locus 1p22 at marker D1S2726. This locus is genetically unlinked to the previously reported candidate locus 1p36.

Most of this article will prove to be too complex and too genetically oriented for a practicing pathologist (at least it was for me), necessitating several passes for complete understanding.

The important message a reader can get from this article is that, first and foremost, this is the first complete genomewide scan for linkage of melanoma susceptibility. The region that was reported actually spans approximately 15 Mb across bands from 1p31.1 to 1p21.3. Also, this strategy was successfully used to explore other cancer families. The genes that are candidates for a role in melanoma development are 2 known to reside in the region in question—tumor growth factor-β receptor 3 and cell division cycle 7-related kinase.

It would be of interest to examine those candidates in the fixed or frozen tissue of nonfamilial melanomas.

D. M. Jukic, MD, PhD

Value of the CD8-CD3 Ratio for the Diagnosis of Mycosis Fungoides
Ortonne N, Buyukbabani N, Delfau-Larue M-H, et al (Hôpital Henri Mondor, Créteil, France; Tip Fakültesi Patoloji Anabilim Dali Capa, Istanbul, Turkey)
Mod Pathol 16:857-862, 2003   5–19

Background.—Mycosis fungoides is the most common subtype of primary cutaneous T-cell lymphoma. It has been shown that the infiltrating lymphocytes in mycosis fungoides are predominantly CD4+, with a smaller amount of CD8+ T cells, but CD4 is also expressed by histiocytes, which can abound in this context. The contribution of the CD8/CD3 ratio to the diagnosis of mycosis fungoides was determined.

Methods.—A retrospective review was conducted to compare the immunophenotypic characteristics of 30 mycosis fungoides with 28 inflammatory dermatoses. The diagnosis of mycosis fungoides was reinforced in all cases by the presence of a cutaneous dominant T-cell clonal population. CD4, which is also expressed by histiocytes, was not considered in this investigation so that the analysis could focus exclusively on the lymphocytic infiltrates. The CD8/CD3 ratio was determined separately in the epidermis and the dermis by using both quantitative and semiquantitative methods.

Results.—Concordance rates between the quantitative and semiquantitative methods were higher in epidermal than in dermal infiltrates (Table 1). The mean CD8/CD3 ratio was significantly lower for mycosis fungoides cases than in control cases, and the difference was greater in the epidermal than in the dermal component.

Conclusions.—Although a finding of a low CD8/CD3 ratio in the epidermal component of a lymphocytic infiltrate is not absolutely specific, it is supportive of the diagnosis of mycosis fungoides. It appears that the CD8/CD3

TABLE 1.—Distribution of the Cases in the 4 CD8/CD3 Ratio Categories (by Quantitative Method)

Group	CD8/CD3 Ratio (%)							
	Epidermis				Dermis			
	0-25	>25-50	>50-75	>75-100	0-25	>25-50	>50-75	75-100
Mycosis fungoides								
Typical	74	16	0	10	40	40	20	0
Suggestive	91	0	9	0	50	25	25	0
Nonspecific	100*	0	0	0	33	33	0	33
Total	81	10	3	6	51	26	20	3
Controls								
Total	24	24	19	33	21	46	29	4

Note that 91% of the patients with infiltrates suggestive of mycosis fungoides had CD8/CD3 ratios <25.
*This finding corresponds to only 1 patient and therefore cannot be interpreted.
(Courtesy of Ortonne N, Buyukbabani N, Delfau-Larue M-H, et al: Value of the CD8-CD3 ratio for the diagnosis of mycosis fungoides. *Mod Pathol* 16:857-862, 2003.)

ratio can be evaluated semiquantitatively in routine practice for the diagnosis of mycosis fungoides.

▶ Since we no longer live in the times of Brocq and Hebra, when neoplasms looked like "bumps" or tumors, it becomes more and more challenging each day to diagnose early stages of this not-so-rare lymphoid neoplasm, especially in a large academic practice.

In recent years, some of the more prominent researchers in the field have published sets of helpful morphologic criteria, but the question remains whether there is help coming from the immunohistochemical field.

The drawback of the current staining strategies is that the CD4/CD8 ratio commonly used to address this is hampered by the fact that CD4 could be expressed by histiocytes; therefore, the authors have felt that the CD3/CD8 ratio might reveal neoplastic involvement of the epidermis more accurately.

Thirty patients with mycosis fungoides were evaluated, with a control group that included 28 patients with inflammatory dermatoses (none of the disorders of so-called borderline clonality was included).

Refreshingly, the authors did not use only the semiquantitative method, but also the fully automated method by utilization of image analysis software.

Importantly, epidermal infiltrates in the mycosis fungoides 28 revealed a CD8/CD3 ratio of less than 50%; 25 had that ratio diminished to less than 25%. Indeed, if one reads the article in detail, the semiquantitative method was reliable for assessing epidermal infiltrates only.

Therefore, the authors recommend doing this set of immunohistochemical comparisons in cases of suspected mycosis fungoides with epidermotropism; however, they do agree that further studies are needed in search of better markers.

D. M. Jukic, MD, PhD

6 Lung and Mediastinum

Is High-Grade Adenomatous Hyperplasia an Early Bronchioloalveolar Adenocarcinoma?

Ullmann R, Bongiovanni M, Halbwedl I, et al (Univ of Graz, Austria; Univ of Torino, Italy; Univ of Massachusetts, Worcester; et al)

J Pathol 201:371-376, 2003   6–1

Background.—Atypical adenomatous hyperplasia (AAH) may be a precursor for bronchioloalveolar cancer (BAC) and pulmonary adenocarcinoma (AC) of mixed type. Low- and high-grade variants of AAH are distinguished by the degree of cytologic atypia, and high-grade AAH is distinguished from AC by the higher incidence of cytologic abnormalities in AC. Nonetheless, AAH has also been associated with squamous cell carcinoma, indicating that it does not always progress to AC. To help differentiate between AAH, BAC, and AC, comparative genomic hybridization was performed.

Methods.—Formalin-fixed, paraffin-embedded specimens of low-grade AAH (4 cases), high-grade AAH (13 cases), BAC (2 cases), mixed AC (9 cases), and squamous cell carcinoma (1 case) were available from 13 patients. Diagnoses were based on World Health Organization criteria. All specimens underwent comparative genomic hybridization analyses.

Results.—There were far fewer chromosomal aberrations in low-grade AAH (average, 1.2) than in high-grade AAH (9.6) or BAC (12.5). Within an individual patient, genetic alterations among the high-grade AAH, BAC, and AC specimens showed a high degree of overlap in both gains and losses. For example, in 5 of 9 high-grade AAH specimens tested, the proportion of genetic aberrations shared by high-grade AAH and AC ranged from 48% to 87%.

Conclusion.—These findings support the differentiation of AAH into low-grade and high-grade. However, the frequency of genetic aberrations and the degree of shared aberrations between high-grade AAH and BAC suggest that high-grade AAH should be considered and treated as early

BAC. Still, some cases of high-grade AAH may represent early intraepithelial spread, rather than being a true precursor of BAC or AC.

▶ AAH is noninvasive spread of atypical epithelial cells along alveolar walls. Similar to BAC, nuclear pseudo-inclusions can be present, but the cells and nuclei are smaller in AAH. AAH can be multiple and has been divided by some authors into low and high grade. In low-grade AAH, there are empty gaps between the atypical cells, but the gaps are lost in high-grade AAH, and the latter show more nuclear atypia and enlargement.

The authors in this study performed comparative genomic hybridization on laser-microdissected tissue sections. In 1999, the World Health Organization defined BAC as a tumor exhibiting a pure bronchioloalveolar growth pattern, with an increase in thickness of the alveolar septa and no evidence of stromal, vascular, or pleural invasion. I find the histologic separation between BAC and high-grade AAH very difficult in excised specimens and much more in small biopsy tissues.

This article in part explains why it is so difficult. The authors found such a high degree of overlap in the chromosomal aberrations between high grade AAH, BAC, and AC that the histologic separation between high grade AAH and BAC is not justified from the genetic point of view. Therefore, the results suggest that high-grade AAH should be considered and treated as BAC. In addition, it is postulated that multifocal high-grade AAH may represent spread of BAC within the lung. This study, however, validates the separation of low-grade AAH from BAC as the number of chromosomal aberrations is much lower in the former.

P. A. Bejarano, MD

SUGGESTED READING

Travis WD, Colby TV, Corrin B, et al: *World Health Organization international histological classification of tumours. Histological typing of lung and pleural tumours, ed 3.* Berlin, Springer-Verlag, 1999.

Immunohistochemical Analysis of Lung Carcinomas With Pure or Partial Bronchioloalveolar Differentiation
Sarantopoulos GP, Gui D, Shintaku P, et al (Univ of California, Los Angeles)
Arch Pathol Lab Med 128:406-414, 2004   6–2

Background.—Bronchioloalveolar carcinoma (BAC) was redefined by the World Health Organization (WHO) in 1999 to include only those lesions with a so-called pure lepidic (classic) growth pattern and no evidence of invasion by a tumor. The goals were to determine whether these lung cancers with a BAC component would be classified as BACs by current WHO standards, to quantitate the BAC component within these tumors, and to determine whether there are phenotypic differences between the so-called invasive and noninvasive regions of these tumors.

Methods.—A retrospective review was conducted of 45 lung cancers with a BAC component. Hematoxylin-eosin–stained slides and classification of histologic grade, tumor subtype, and percentage of pure BAC pattern were evaluated, with additional characterization by immunohistochemical staining for thyroid transcription factor 1 (TTF-1), cytokeratin 7 (CK7), cytokeratin 20 (CK20), and Ki-67 antibodies.

Results.—Only 15.6% of the tumors (7 of 45) examined could be classified as BAC by current WHO criteria. These tumors, which were classified as nonmucinous and mixed, showed similar immunohistochemical staining for CK7, CK20, and TTF-1. Mucinous tumors showed disparate staining. Significant differences in immunohistochemical staining and tumor cell proliferation were observed for the regions of tumors designated as lepidic, infiltrative, and leading edge, and for the regions of tumors with different histologic grades.

Conclusions.—Phenotypic similarities were observed between nonmucinous and mixed bronchioloalveolar carcinomas, and these 2 carcinomas show identical immunohistochemical staining patterns. In contrast, mucinous tumors show disparate immunohistochemical staining. Pulmonary neoplasms designated as adenocarcinomas with a BAC component are a heterogenous group with a range of cell types, differentiation, growth, and immunophenotypes. Regional differences in these parameters are often observed within an individual neoplasm.

▶ Pure BAC have a better prognosis than regular lung adenocarcinomas. However, one sees in the daily practice that many adenocarcinomas show areas of bronchioloalveolar pattern of growth, and they are being diagnosed as BACs, which is contrary to the guidelines defined by the WHO. For the WHO, BAC is a carcinoma with a pure lepidic growth without stromal, vascular, or pleural invasions. When any of the latter are present, the term *mixed adenocarcinomas with BAC features* is applied. According to these strict criteria, BAC that measure less than 2 cm are curable and much less likely to recur and metastasize. It is expected that a diagnosis of BAC will be made with less frequency by pathologists if the stringent criteria are followed. This article also emphasized the point that mucinous adenocarcinomas show a nonreliable immunohistochemical pattern with negative results for TTF-1 and CK7, and positivity for CK20. Therefore, this panel of antibodies would not distinguish a mucinous lung adenocarcinoma from a metastasis that originated in the large intestine. Because of the disparate immunophentype of mucinous BACs, their cell of origin is debated. Being TTF-1 negative would argue against an alveolar cell of origin and support an origin from the bronchial columnar mucin-filled cell of the mid-to-large sized airways.

P. A. Bejarano, MD

Lung Pathology of Severe Acute Respiratory Syndrome (SARS): A Study of 8 Autopsy Cases From Singapore

Franks TJ, Chong PY, Chui P, et al (Armed Forces Inst of Pathology, Washington, DC; Tan Tock Seng Hosp, Singapore; Health Sciences Authority, Singapore)
Hum Pathol 34:743-748, 2003   6–3

Introduction.—Severe acute respiratory syndrome (SARS) is an infection caused by the SARS-related coronavirus. To assess lung pathology in this life-threatening condition, postmortem lung sections were examined in 8 patients who died of SARS during the spring 2003 Singapore outbreak.

Findings.—The predominant pattern of lung injury in every case was diffuse alveolar damage (DAD). Histology differed according to illness duration. Cases of 10 or less days' duration manifested acute-phase DAD, airspace edema, and bronchiolar fibrin. Cases of more than 10 days' duration demonstrated organizing-phase DAD, type II pneumocyte hyperplasia, squamous metaplasia, multinucleated giant cells, and acute bronchopneumonia. In acute-phase DAD, pancytokeratin staining was positive in hyaline membranes along alveolar walls and emphasized the absence of pneumocytes. Multinucleated cells were both type II pneumocytes and macrophages by pancytokeratin, thyroid transcription factor-1, and CD68 staining. SARS-related coronavirus RNA was identified by reverse transcriptase–polymerase chain reaction in 7 of 8 cases in fresh autopsy tissue, and in 8 of 8 cases of formalin-fixed, paraffin-embedded lung tissue, including the 1 negative case in fresh tissue.

Conclusion.—Understanding the pathology of DAD in patients with SARS may provide the basis for therapeutic strategies. Further investigation of the pathogenesis of SARS may uncover new insight into the mechanism of DAD.

▶ SARS appeared first in Guangdong Province, China in mid-November 2002. Since then, outbreaks have been reported around the globe not only by medical authorities but also by the news agencies. The coronavirus that causes SARS is not visualized by light microscopy; thus, no intranuclear or intracytoplasmic inclusions are observed. Although, no cytopathic changes are seen, injury to bronchioles and alveolar epithelium is evident. However, it is not clear whether these histologic findings correspond to the primary injury or represent secondary changes. In SARS, there are multinucleated giant cells formed by pneumocytes that are reactive for keratin, CD68, and thyroid transcription factor-1. However, these types of giant cells are not specific for SARS either. The predominant histologic feature is DAD, but many patients develop superimposed infections in the form of bronchopneumonia. This article had an erratum[1] because the characteristics of 2 patients were mixed up. However, the essence of the article is not altered.

P. A. Bejarano, MD

Reference

1. Erratum. *Hum Pathol* 35:139, 2004.

Prognostic Value of Cytokeratin-Positive Cells in the Bone Marrow and Lymph Nodes of Patients With Resected Nonsmall Cell Lung Cancer: A Multicenter Prospective Study

Yasumoto K, for the Cooperative Project No 24 Group of The Japanese Foundation for Multidisciplinary Treatment of Cancer (Univ of Occupational and Environmental Health, Kitakyushu, Japan; et al)

Ann Thorac Surg 76:194-202, 2003   6–4

Introduction.—About 30% of patients with pathologic stage I non–small cell lung cancer (NSCLC) experience recurrence. This suggests that occult micrometastatic tumor cells not identified by current clinical staging examinations have already spread to distant mesenchymal organs. The prognostic value of cytokeratin-positive (CK+) cells in the bone marrow (BM) and regional lymph nodes (LNs) was examined in resected NSCLC patients from a large population within a multicenter trial.

Methods.—A total of 351 patients with stages I to IIIA NSCLC from 15 Japanese institutions were evaluated. The BM aspirates were stained immunocytochemically with the anticytokeratin antibody, CK2. The hilar and mediastinal LNs of 216 patients with stage I NSCLC were stained immunohistochemically with the anti-CK antibody, AE1/AE3.

Results.—The CK+ cells were identified in 112 (31.9%) of the 351 BM samples. The frequency of CK+ cells demonstrated no differences among pathologic stages. Patients with CK+ cells in the BM had a tendency to experience shorter survival periods, compared with those without CK+ cells ($P = .076$). The presence of CK+ cells in the BM of patients with stage I did not permit the prediction of overall survival; it decreased overall survival significantly in patients with stage II or IIIA disease. The CK+ cells in LNs were identified in 34 (15.7%) of 216 patients with stage I. Patients with CK+ cells in the LNs had poor prognosis by both univariate ($P = .004$) and multivariate analyses ($P = .018$).

Conclusion.—The presence of CK+ cells in the BM was associated with a poor prognosis in patients with stages II to IIIA NSCLC. It did not predict the prognosis of patients with stage I. For stage I NSCLC, the detection of CK+ cells in the LNs suggests a poor prognosis.

▶ It is known that lung cancer can be unpredictable in its behavior. As such, about 30% of patients with stage I NSCLC have a recurrence after complete excision of the tumor. This suggests that circulating malignant cells or micrometastasis are already present at the time of resection. This study analyzes a large number of patients with a median follow-up of 4.02 years. It shows that CK+ cells in the BM reduced the survival significantly in patients with stage II to IIIA without being overtly detrimental in patients thought to be stage I. In patients with stage I, the presence of single CK+ cells in the BM does not necessarily imply systemic malignant disease. A few studies have suggested that these cells are in a nonproliferating or dormant state to explain this paradoxic behavior. On the other hand, in patients who are stage II to IIIA and have isolated CK+ cells in the BM, the latter may represent a sign of a hematogenous spread and systemic dissemination of the tumor. The data obtained on stage I patients with micrometastasis detected by immunohistochemistry may be useful to decide which of these patients should receive postoperative adjuvant chemotherapy.

On a technical note, the authors used different keratins to detect tumor cells in BM (CK2) and LNs (AE1/AE3 cocktail). CK2 detects CK18 in the catalog of human cytokeratins, and the cocktail highlights a broad spectrum of keratins, acidic and basic, that includes number 18 as well.

P. A. Bejarano, MD

Pulmonary Carcinomas With Pleomorphic, Sarcomatoid, or Sarcomatous Elements: A Clinicopathologic and Immunohistochemical Study of 75 Cases
Rossi G, Cavazza A, Sturm N, et al (Univ of Modena and Reggio Emilia, Italy; S Maria Nuova Hosp, Reggio Emilia, Italy; Hosp of Faenza, Ravenna, Italy; et al)
Am J Surg Pathol 27:311-324, 2003   6–5

Background.—The recent World Health Organization (WHO) classification of lung tumors unified the heterogeneous group of non-small-cell lung carcinomas that contain a sarcoma or sarcomalike component under the designation of "carcinomas with pleomorphic, sarcomatoid, or sarcomatous elements" (CPSS). The goals of this study were to analyze the clinical and histologic features of a relatively large series of surgically treated pulmonary CPSS and to investigate the immunohistochemical expression of thyroid transcription factor-1 (TTF-1), surfactant protein-A, cytokeratin 7, and cytokeratin 20 in this group of tumors.

Methods.—The files of 1 French and 1 Italian hospital were searched for surgical cases of pulmonary carcinoma in which a spindle or giant cell component was reported. From a total of 5788 cases of lung carcinoma diagnosed from 1984 to 2001, 75 cases with pleomorphic, sarcomatoid, histologic, or sarcomatous elements were selected for this study. The patients ranged in age from 42 to 81 years, with a mean of 65 years, and the male-to-female ratio was 9.7:1. Nearly all the patients (92%) were smokers. Cough and hemoptysis were the most frequent presenting symptoms. The majority of patients (65%) died from their disease; stage was the only parameter predictive of overall survival.

Results.—Microscopically, 58 cases were classified as pleomorphic carcinoma, 10 as spindle cell carcinoma, 3 as giant cell carcinoma, 3 as carcinosarcoma, and 1 as pulmonary blastoma according to the WHO criteria. Immunohistochemical analysis showed that TTF-1 and cytokeratin 7 were positive in 55% and 70% of the tumors composed exclusively of spindle or giant cells. In contrast, surfactant protein-A was always negative. In the pleomorphic carcinomas with an epithelial component, cytokeratin 7, TTF-1, and surfactant protein-A were positive in the sarcomatoid component in 62.7%, 43.1%, and 5.9% of cases, respectively; however, the same antibodies did not react with the epithelial component of carcinosarcomas. In the blastomas the epithelial part of the tumor was positive for cytokeratin 7 and TTF-1 but negative for surfactant protein-A. Cytokeratin 20 was always negative.

Conclusions.—These findings are supportive of the metaplastic histogenetic theory for this group of tumors and demonstrate that cytokeratin 7 and TTF-1, but not surfactant protein-A, are useful immunohistochemical markers in this setting. These findings also provide confirmation that stage is presently the only significant prognostic parameter, as in conventional non-small-cell lung carcinomas, and that this group of tumors has a worse prognosis than conventional non-small-cell lung carcinoma at surgically curable stage 1. Thus, their segregation as an independent histologic type in the WHO classification appears to be justified.

▶ CPSS is the term given by the WHO to a group of non-small-cell carcinomas of the lung that have histologic features of sarcoma or sarcomalike malignancies. It includes tumors such as pleomorphic carcinoma, spindle cell carcinoma, giant cell carcinoma, carcinosarcoma, and pulmonary blastoma. These tumors are seen predominately in smoking men. This study confirmed the aggressive behavior of these tumors, as the overall median survival was 19 months. For stage I, the survival was 31 months; it was 10.5 and 9 months, respectively, for stages II and III. Antibodies to TTF-1, surfactant protein-A, cytokeratin 7, and cytokeratin 20 have been studied in lung carcinomas. However, this study is one of the first to analyze these antibodies on CPSS. Important is the positive immunoreactivity for TTF-1 and cytokeratin 7 in about half of CPSS because this information can be applied when one is dealing with a spindle cell tumor in the lung that may represent a metastatic sarcoma. Stains for these antibodies would orient toward the possibility of a primary lung carcinoma with metaplastic change. Of course, it is very important to sample such tumors in the lung extensively in an attempt to find the clear-cut epithelial component. Since TTF-1 is much more predominant in adenocarcinoma than squamous cell carcinomas, the immunoreactivity for TTF-1 in a group of CPSS suggests that they had an initial glandular origin.

P. A. Bejarano, MD

Basaloid Carcinoma of the Lung: A Really Dismal Histologic Variant?
Kim DJ, Kim KD, Shin DH, et al (Yonsei Univ, Seoul, South Korea; Ulsan Univ, Seoul, South Korea)
Ann Thorac Surg 76:1833-1837, 2003   6–6

Background.—Basaloid carcinoma of the lung is an uncommon, highly aggressive non-small-cell lung cancer. A 5-year survival rate of only 15% has been reported for basaloid carcinoma of the lung, even in patients with stages I and II disease. It has been suggested that different treatment modalities for basaloid carcinoma should be considered. The prognostic implications of a basaloid carcinoma of the lung were determined.

Methods.—A series of 291 surgically resected tumors were included in the study. These tumors were originally diagnosed as a poorly or undifferentiated carcinoma, a small cell carcinoma, or an atypical carcinoid. Of the 291 tumors, 35 basaloid carcinoma patients were identified and compared with 167 patients with poorly differentiated squamous cell carcinoma (PDSC) on the basis of preoperative clinical data, the procedure performed, and the survival outcome.

Results.—The overall incidence of basaloid carcinoma was 4.8%. The actuarial 5-year survival rate was 40.6% in patients with PDSC and 36.5% in patients with basaloid carcinoma. The actuarial 5-year survival rate for stage I and II patients was 53.9% in the PDSC patients and 57.2% in the basaloid group. There were no differences between the groups in the recurrence rate and the relapse pattern. It was shown on Cox proportional hazards modeling that an age equal to 60 years and an advanced stage were risk factors for postoperative survival in both groups.

Conclusions.—It would appear from these findings that basaloid carcinoma of the lung does not have a worse prognosis than the other non-small-cell lung cancers. Although basaloid carcinoma is a unique histologic entity, it does not require a different treatment modality because its clinical behavior is similar to that of other non-small-cell lung cancers.

▶ Basaloid carcinoma of the lung can be misdiagnosed as small-cell carcinoma in small biopsy tissues. This article addresses the clinical implications of the diagnosis and concludes that the prognosis is not worse than the other non-small-cell carcinomas, and thus the treatment may not be different. While this may be clear for the oncologists, the difficulty for the pathologists is arriving at the correct diagnosis. Basaloid carcinoma of the lung may appear as a solid lobular or anastomic trabecular pattern whose tumor cells are small cuboidal to fusiform with hyperchromatic nuclei and no prominent nucleoli. The cytoplasm is scant, but no nuclear molding is observed. Peripheral palisading and high mitotic rates are seen. Thus, confusion with high-grade neuroendocrine carcinoma (small or large cell) is possible. Immunohistochemistry is very helpful to tell them apart. Basaloid carcinomas are usually negative for TTF-1 and positive for p63. Although in this study the authors did not utilize p63, none of their 35 cases stained positive for TTF-1. This combined immunophenotype favors the view that these tumors are variants of squamous cell carcinomas.

P. A. Bejarano, MD

Prognostic Implications of Neuroendocrine Differentiation and Hormone Production in Patients With Stage I Nonsmall Cell Lung Carcinoma

Pelosi G, Pasini F, Sonzogni A, et al (Univ of Milan, Italy; Univ of Verona, Italy; European Inst of Oncology, Milan, Italy; et al)
Cancer 97:2487-2497, 2003   6–7

Background.—The clinical implications of neuroendocrine differentiation in patients with non–small-cell lung carcinoma (NSCLC) have not been clearly established. Several studies have correlated NSCLC with neuroendocrine differentiation (NSCLC-ND) with shorter survival, more advanced disease stage, and/or increased chemosensitivity. However, other investigators have not shown any correlation between neuroendocrine differentiation and prognosis or susceptibility to therapy, and some have reported better survival rates for patients with NSCLC-ND. Differences in tissue processing, techniques, or markers used for highlighting neuroendocrine differentiation, definitions of positive results, and study population selection may account for these contradictory results. Many of these studies have included patients with more advanced stage lung tumors; however, little is known regarding the prevalence and clinical implications of neuroendocrine differentiation in patients with stage I NSCLC. The prevalence and clinical implications of neuroendocrine differentiation were evaluated in a wide series of patients with stage I NSCLC.

Methods.—A series of 220 consecutive patients with stage I NSCLC who underwent surgical treatment from 1987 to 1993 were evaluated. Light microscopy and immunohistochemical staining for synaptophysin, chromogranin A, and respiratory tract-related hormones were used to identify 28 NSCLC-ND specimens and 11 large-cell neuroendocrine carcinoma (LCNEC) specimens.

Results.—Included in the 28 NSCLC-ND specimens were 15 adenocarcinomas and 13 squamous cell carcinomas. Neoplastic cells with neuroendocrine features never exceeded 20% in the NSCLC-ND specimens, but neoplastic cells amounted to 20% to 90% in LCNEC specimens. Patients with adenocarcinoma but not with squamous cell carcinoma who had more than 5% neuroendocrine-differentiated cells had worse clinical outcomes, including reduced overall survival and disease-free survival rates, than did patients who had ordinary NSCLC. Multivariate analysis showed that neuroendocrine differentiation of more than 5% neoplastic cells in patients with adenocarcinoma was independently predictive of a poorer prognosis. Hormone production was restricted to chromogranin-positive NSCLC-ND but had no effect on the prognosis.

Conclusions.—Stage I adenocarcinomas with 5% or more neuroendocrine tumor cells are clinically aggressive tumors that are similar to LCNECs. Hormone production will identify a more fully developed neuroendocrine phenotype, but it is not relevant to the prognosis. The identification of neuroendocrine-differentiated cells in patients with NSCLC may have clinical relevance.

▶ Neuroendocrine differentiation by immunohistochemical analysis is seen in about 14% of NSCLCs. This may, in part, explain why some patients succumb to their disease more rapidly than others, despite the fact that they have similar clinical stages and histologic features in their tumors to the patients with better outcomes. The more grave prognosis of these tumors may indicate that NSCLC-NDs represent either a distinct clinicopathologic entity or are a transition toward a high-grade neuroendocrine carcinoma. The prognostic impact appears to apply to adenocarcinomas but not to squamous cell carcinomas. Several questions remain after reading articles on this topic. For instance, are we supposed to perform immunohistochemical stains in every adenocarcinoma we encounter in our practices? The authors of this interesting article did not address this issue. The problem is that there are no data on a large number of patients. Pelosi et al ended up with only 15 patients with adenocarcinomas in the final analysis. The initial number of patients with adenocarcinomas was only 88, which is a very small number on which to base a suggestion that we make a change in the way we practice. We need studies with a much larger number of adenocarcinomas that show immunoreactivity of neuroendocrine markers. In addition, what neuroendocrine markers do we have to use to show neuroendocrine differentiation? This article is helpful in that it confirms that markers for chromogranin and synaptophysin are the best compromise between sensitivity and specificity. Other hormones such as gastrin-releasing peptide/bombesin, calcitonin, adrenocorticotropic hormone, α-human chorionic gonadotropin, and serotonin do not have prognostic implications. What is the cutoff of positive cells before qualifying a tumor as having neuroendocrine differentiation? The 5% cutoff point used by the authors was not entirely arbitrary, as this number was the closest to the median distribution among the cases they stained. In addition, they found that greater than 5% immunoreactivity was associated with a poorer patient outcome.

P. A. Bejarano, MD

Histologic Assessment of Non–Small Cell Lung Carcinoma After Neoadjuvant Therapy
Liu-Jarin X, Stoopler MB, Raftopoulos H, et al (Columbia Presbyterian Med Ctr, New York)
Mod Pathol 16:1102-1108, 2003   6–8

Background.—Chemotherapy or chemoradiotherapy is often used in the treatment of stage IIIA non–small-cell lung carcinoma before surgical resection. Among the important aspects of histopathologic review of such tumors after resection are the assessment of tumor regression and the recognition that the pathologic changes are related to prior therapy. A minority of patients have complete responses, and the benefits of therapy may extend to some patients with a small amount of residual tumor. However, the significance of a partial response has not been clarified. In this study, histologic variables for tumor regression were refined, and patterns of tumor reaction to therapy were described.

Methods.—From 1996 to 2000, a retrospective study was conducted of 30 patients with non–small-cell lung carcinoma who received neoadjuvant therapy before definitive surgery. Histologic slides were reviewed on all 30 cases. In 22 cases, biopsy materials before therapy were available for direct histologic comparison. Tumors were divided into different response groups according to the volume of residual tumor. The percentage of residual tumor was estimated by a comparison of the estimated cross-sectional area of the largest residual tumor focus with the estimated cross-sectional area of the inflammatory or fibrous mass. Data regarding the total dose of radiation and the interval between the last radiation treatment and surgery were obtained in 14 of 20 patients who received radiotherapy. The average radiation dose was 4970 ± 260 cGy, and 13 of 14 patients received 5040 cGy; the average interval between the last radiation dose and surgery was 6.1 ± 0.9 weeks. The 30 specimens were graded for tumor regression to identify clinical and histologic variables that correlated with a treatment response.

Results.—No correlation was observed between tumor regression and age, sex, or type of therapy (chemoradiotherapy vs chemotherapy alone). Squamous cell carcinoma showed a significantly higher rate of response than did adenocarcinoma: a significant number of adenocarcinomas were present in the group without a response. A reduction in tumor size on radiologic assessment compared with histologic regression did not show a statistically significant association. However, a positive correlation was observed between the extent of fibrosis and the radiologic estimates of size reduction.

Conclusions.—Tumor regression in non–small-cell lung carcinoma can be classified into 4 subgroups, and this classification will generate responder and nonresponder groups. Radiologic assessments do not correlate with prediction in these groups, but they may correlate with the extent of fibrosis within the tumor.

▶ Neoadjuvant therapy is frequently administered to patients with locally advanced (stage IIIA) lung carcinoma. However, the pathologist is not always informed that the patient underwent treatment before the surgical removal of the tumor. The findings described in this article illustrate the morphological changes that occur in the tumors of patients who received preoperative chemotherapy or chemotherapy combined with radiotherapy. A pathologic response does not correlate with the roentgenographic size of the tumor unless there is fibrosis histologically. Imaging studies showing a size reduction of the tumor when fibrosis is present may be due to retraction. Squamous cell carcinomas have a better response than adenocarcinomas. Overall, there is a trend toward a better survival rate among histologic responders, but the correlation does not seem to be statistically significant. Nonetheless, pathologists may be asked in the future to evaluate changes present in the excised lung specimen due to chemotherapy.

P. A. Bejarano, MD

Kit Expression in Small Cell Carcinomas of the Lung: Effects of Chemotherapy

Rossi G, Cavazza A, Marchioni A, et al (Univ of Modena and Reggio Emilia, Italy; Ospedale degli Infermi, Ravenna, Italy; Ospedale Bellaria, Bologna, Italy)
Mod Pathol 16:1041-1047, 2003   6–9

Background.—Approximately 15% to 20% of all primary lung tumors are small-cell lung carcinomas. Small-cell lung carcinoma is considered to be a systemic disease with a tendency to disseminate early in its natural course, and it is associated with the lowest 5-year survival rate among all lung cancers. It has been established that a significant number of small-cell lung carcinomas show overexpression of the proto-oncogene c-kit product, a tyrosine kinase known as Kit or CD117. There is evidence that would appear to implicate this molecular pathway in the promotion of the neoplastic growth of small-cell lung carcinoma. Whether CD117 expression would be modified by chemotherapy in patients with small-cell carcinoma of the lung who underwent tumor biopsy before first-line chemotherapy and after a relapse was investigated by immunohistochemical analysis.

Methods.—The expression of CD117 of the primary naive tumor (before first-line chemotherapy) was compared with the expression of the same neoplasm after a postchemotherapy relapse in a series of 27 small-cell lung carcinomas. All patients underwent similar chemotherapeutic regimens of cisplatin–carboplatin plus etoposide.

Results.—At diagnosis, 21 of 27 cases (78%) showed strong immunoreactivity for CD117. Among these 21 originally positive tumors, CD117 remained overexpressed in 10 cases after a relapse (48%), whereas the other 11 cases became negative. No originally CD117–negative small-cell carcinomas showed immunoreactivity after chemotherapy. No significant correlation of CD117 expression with overall survival, occurrence of chemoresistance, or clinical response to chemotherapy was found. CD117 expression was also evaluated in a series 46 surgically resected non–small-cell lung carcinomas. CD117 overexpression was observed in 6 of 10 large-cell neuroendocrine carcinomas, but all other histotypes did not result in staining.

Conclusions.—The loss of CD117 expression after chemotherapy in a high proportion of small-cell lung carcinomas may indicate that Kit is likely not representative of the product of a constitutive mutation in this tumor. Oncologists could retest CD117 expression in relapsing small-cell lung carcinoma to establish the best candidates for enrollment in ongoing clinical trials with Kit inhibitors. CD117 may aid in the discrimination of pulmonary high-grade neuroendocrine tumors from other histotypes, but pathologists should be cognizant of the fact that treated small-cell lung carcinomas may remain unstained in a substantial number of cases.

▶ One of the aims of this article was to determine whether the expression of CD117 (c-Kit) in small-cell carcinomas has a prognostic value. It does not, despite that it was seen in 78% of cases. Another goal was to analyze the changes of CD117 expression after chemotherapy. The authors found that many (48%) of small-cell carcinomas lose their immunoreactivity after the administration of cisplatin–carboplatin plus etoposide; thus, these patients are not likely to benefit from treatment with CD117 antagonists, such as imatinib mesylate (Gleevec). However, for the pathologists, this study highlights an important issue in diagnostic immunohistochemical analysis because the authors confirmed that c-Kit helps to distinguish high-grade neuroendocrine carcinomas (ie, small-cell carcinoma and large-cell neuroendocrine carcinoma) from carcinoids and non–small-cell carcinomas. Thus, CD117 could be used when one is dealing with an undifferentiated tumor that may mimic small-cell carcinoma. That is the case with the so-called basaloid squamous cell carcinoma, in which a negative result would be expected for CD117 and thyroid transcription factor-1 but p63 would be positive.

P. A. Bejarano, MD

Combined Status of MUC1 Mucin and Surfactant Apoprotein A Expression Can Predict the Outcome of Patients With Small-Size Lung Adenocarcinoma

Tsutsumida H, Goto M, Kitajima S, et al (Kagoshima Univ, Japan; Natl Minamikyushu Hosp, Kagoshima, Japan)
Histopathology 44:147-155, 2004   6–10

Background.—Despite advances in diagnostic techniques, lung cancer remains a disease of high mortality. These advances have enabled the detection of many asymptomatic, small-size lung cancers, yet many of these small cancers are aggressive. A method for predicting which small-size lung cancers are associated with poorer outcomes was described.

Methods.—Surgical specimens were obtained from 185 patients (72 men and 113 women 43-84 years of age) with primary lung cancer of nonbronchioloalveolar type whose tumors were less than 30 mm in diameter. Specimens were formalin-fixed and paraffin-embedded and stained with hematoxylin and eosin. They were also stained with monoclonal antibodies to mucin MUC1 and surfactant apoprotein A (SP-A) for analysis by immunohistochemistry. Staining results were evaluated semiquantitatively according to a 4-point grade (0 = no staining, 4 = 75%-100% of cells stained positively).

Results.—MUC1 was expressed mainly on the cell surface and in the cytoplasm, whereas SP-A was expressed mainly in the cytoplasm. Most of the cells had grade 4 (74%) or grade 3 (18%) staining for MUC1. Staining for SP-A was more variable, as only 27% of cells had grade 3-4 staining. Neither disease-free survival nor overall survival correlated significantly with either MUC1 or SP-A expression.

However, the relative ratio of MUC1 to SP-A expression was a significant predictor of outcomes. Of the 140 patients (76%) whose MUC1 expression was greater than SP-A expression (MUC1 > SP-A), 31 (24%) had a recurrence. In contrast, of the 45 patients (24%) whose MUC1 expression was less than or equal to that of SP-A (MUC1 ≤ SP-A), only 3 (7%) had recurrence. This between-group difference was significant.

Furthermore, 5-year survival was also significantly lower in the MUC1 > SP-A group (52%) than in the MUC1 ≤ SP-A group (91%). Outcomes in the MUC1 > SP-A group were significantly worse than those in the MUC1 ≤ SP-A group, even in patients with well-differentiated cancer (approximately 96% vs approximately 76%) and in those without lymph node metastases (11% vs 0%).

Conclusion.—A high MUC1/SP-A ratio is associated with significantly poorer outcomes in patients with small-size lung cancer. This holds true even in patients with favorable prognostic characteristics (well-differentiated tumor, no lymph node metastasis). Thus, the proportion of cells staining positively for MUC1 relative to those staining positively for SP-A may be useful in risk stratification of patients with small-size lung cancer.

▶ Small-size carcinomas are being diagnosed more frequently due to the advances in diagnostic medical techniques. In addition, there are many medical centers around the world undergoing studies screening heavy cigarette smokers for the early detection of lung cancer, with the hope that the mortality from this disease decreases as the lesions discovered should apparently be of small size. However, it is known that small-size tumors can behave in an aggressive manner.

The goal of the current study from Japan is to find a way to predict which of these small malignancies will have a poor prognosis. The authors utilized immunohistochemical staining for SP-A and the mucin MUC1. They found that MUC1 expression alone or SP-A expressions alone are not strongly correlated with patient outcome. However, when the combined information of both stains is used, the patients whose tumors showed more cells staining for MUC1 than the ones stained for SP-A had high recurrence rate and poor outcome. On the other hand, patients whose tumors had less number of cells staining for MUC1 than SP-A showed a low recurrence rate and very good outcome.

The poor outcome related to the pattern of MUC1/SP-A staining occurred even in patients who were initially supposed to have favorable features such as well differentiated histology or absence of lymph node metastasis. This study points to the fact that the prognostic information provided by these 2 stains can be used by oncologists to determine appropriate treatment modalities. While work is being performed at the molecular level with arrays to determine prognostic indicators independent of the morphological differentiation, this immunohistochemical study shows a way to more readily assess those indicators.

P. A. Bejarano, MD

The Role of Open-Lung Biopsy in ARDS

Patel SR, Karmpaliotis D, Ayas NT, et al (Massachusetts Gen Hosp, Boston; Univ of British Columbia, Vancouver, Canada)
Chest 125:197-202, 2004   6–11

Background.—Some authorities question the role of open-lung biopsy in acute respiratory distress syndrome (ARDS) because of its potentially high morbidity and low diagnostic yield. This study was done to better define the role of this procedure in ARDS.

Methods and Findings.—A cohort of 57 patients undergoing open-lung biopsy between 1989 and 2000 for evaluation of ARDS was studied. The mean patient age was 53 years. The mean partial pressure of arterial oxygen/ fraction of inspired oxygen ratio was 145 mm Hg at the time of biopsy. Sixty percent of patients had a pathologic diagnosis other than diffuse alveolar damage or fibroproliferation. Infection, alveolar hemorrhage, and bronchiolitis obliterans organizing pneumonia were the most common alternative diagnoses. Alternative diagnoses were present in 60% of immunocompetent and 59% of immunosuppressed hosts.

Biopsy findings resulted in management changes in most patients. Specific treatments were added in 60% of patients, and unnecessary treatments were withdrawn in 37%. Overall, the complication rate was 39%. Major complications occurred in 7%. No deaths were attributed to the procedure.

Conclusion.—Open-lung biopsy in selected patients with clinical ARDS often reveals unsuspected diagnoses and results in treatment changes. This procedure can be performed safely.

▶ The general view is that ARDS is histologically manifested as diffuse alveolar damage (DAD). However, various etiologies can produce DAD and ARDS. In contrast to chronic interstitial pneumonitis where surgically obtained lung biopsy is a recognized important tool for the diagnosis, its role in ARDS is not yet clear. In fact, the frequency of other etiologies causing ARDS with histologic correlation is unknown.

The biopsies in this study revealed a diagnosis other than DAD in about 60% of cases, regardless of the immunocompetent or immunosuppressed state of the patients. These diagnoses included infection (14%), diffuse alveolar hemorrhage (9%), bronchiolitis obliterans organizing pneumonia (9%), bronchiolitis (5%), culture negative pneumonia (3%), drug reaction (3%), lymphoma (3%), and the rest (lymphangitic tumor, organizing pneumonia, desquamative interstitial pneumonia, hypersensitivity pneumonitis, eosinophilic pneumonia, allergic bronchopulmonary aspergillosis, and edema) with 2% each. The etiologies in the cases of hemorrhage included Wegener disease, cryoglobulinemia, paraneoplastic vasculitis, idiopathic vasculitis, and idiopathic thrombocytopenic purpura.

This is the largest series of patients undergoing open-lung biopsy for evaluation of clinical ARDS. It appears that the risk of complications for surgical lung biopsy procedures is outweighed by the benefit of the information obtained with the histologic examination of these tissues. Perhaps pulmonologists may become more confident in recommending open-lung biopsies in causes of ARDS of unknown cases. Thus, the pathologists need to be aware of the variegated histologic changes and diagnostic possibilities that are not limited to DAD.

However, prospective studies are needed in order to validate the results of this retrospective study. Also, a larger number of patients with clinical ARDS undergoing biopsy need to be enrolled because in this study, although the number of patients with clinical ARDS was 1707, only 68 (4%) underwent biopsy, with 57 fulfilling the criteria for inclusion.

P. A. Bejarano, MD

7 Cardiovascular

Iatrogenic Cardiac Papillary Fibroelastoma: A Study of 12 Cases (1990 to 2000)
Kurup AN, Tazelaar HD, Edwards WD, et al (Mayo Clinic, Rochester, Minn; Armed Forces Inst of Pathology, Washington, DC)
Hum Pathol 33:1165-1169, 2002   7–1

Introduction.—Cardiac papillary fibroelastoma (PFE) is a benign tumor of the heart. It is the most frequently observed tumor of cardiac valves and the third most common primary cardiac tumor, after myxoma and fibroma. It is not known whether this rare, slow-growing tumor of the endocardium is a reactive tumoral lesion or a true neoplasm. An anecdotal link between prior cardiac surgery and PFEs has been reported. The frequency and nature of iatrogenic events associated with PFEs were evaluated.

Methods.—Twelve cases of PFEs were seen between 1990 and 2000; 7 specimens were from females and 5 from males. Six lesions developed postoperatively, and 6 developed after thoracic irradiation. Nine Mayo cases represented 18% of all surgically excised PFEs during the evaluation period. The mean age at the time of surgery was 54 years (range, 29-79 years). The mean interval between iatrogenic event and tumor excision was 18 years (range, 9-31 years). The presence of multiple tumors was either verified pathologically (41.7%) or strongly suggested by echocardiography (16.6%) in 58% of cases. Among patients who underwent prior cardiac surgery, PFEs were identified in the chamber closest to the procedure. Similarly, in patients who underwent radiation therapy, tumors developed in the left atrium, in the right ventricle and atrium, and on the tricuspid valve within the radiation field.

Conclusion.—Iatrogenic PFEs may be relatively common manifestations of posttraumatic events, which may be either mechanically induced (ie, cardiac procedures) or radiation induced.

▶ Myxoma, fibroma, and PFE are the 3 most common primary tumors of the heart. However, PFE is the most common tumor of the cardiac valves. The gross appearance is characteristic, resembling a pom-pom or a sea anemone with papillary fronds. PFEs can be asymptomatic, but in general, their excision is advised because they can embolize parts of the tumor or a thrombus to the lung, coronary arteries, or the brain. These lesions have been considered neoplasms, hamartomas, organized thrombi, and endocardial responses to infection or trauma. The current study focuses on the idiopathic PFE, which represents about 18% of all PFEs encountered at the Mayo Clinic in an 11-year period. These patients received radiation, underwent heart surgery, valve replacement, septal myomectomy for hypertrophic cardiomyopathy, or repairs for congenital heart defects, between 9 and 31 years before the discovery of their PFEs. The tumors varied in sizes from 2 to 28 mm. Microscopically, they had a central dense core of elastin and collagen surrounded by a layer of loose myxoid tissue and lined by endothelium contiguous with adjacent endocardium. This article lends support to the view that PFEs are posttraumatic tumors and that patients who undergo some cardiac procedures or receive radiation are at risk for the development of PFEs.

P. A. Bejarano, MD

Surgical Pathology of Subaortic Septal Myectomy Associated With Hypertrophic Cardiopathy: A Study of 204 Cases (1996-2000)
Lamke GT, Allen RD, Edwards WD, et al (Mayo Clinic, Rochester, Minn)
Cardiovasc Pathol 12:149-158, 2003   7–2

Introduction.—The pathology of hypertrophic cardiomyopathy (HCM) has been described in autopsy, surgical, and biopsy specimens, but no single surgical study has systematically examined the microscopic lesions in a large number of cases. Medical records and microscopic slides from 204 Mayo Clinic cases of HCM were reviewed, and microscopic features were compared between patients younger and older than 60 years.

Methods.—Patients included in the review underwent subaortic septal myectomy between January 1, 1996, and December 31, 2000. Demographic features were recorded together with the surgeon's description of the ventricular septum, the degree of left ventricular outflow tract obstruction, functional state of the aortic valve, the angiographic presence of coronary artery disease, and history of previous or concomitant coronary artery bypass surgery. All slides were evaluated for microscopic features of myocytes, interstitium, vessels, and endocardium.

Results.—Data were analyzed for 133 patients younger than 60 years and 71 patients aged 60 years or older. Age at operation for the entire patient group ranged from 1 to 86 years (mean, 48 years). Women made up 53% of the patient group. All patients had obstructive HCM; obstruction was severe in 39%, moderate in 16%, mild in 9%, and undetermined in 36%. Patients 60 years or older were more likely to be women and to have aortic valve disease and severe coronary artery atherosclerosis. Microscopic abnormalities detected included myocyte hypertrophy (100%), endocardial (96%) and myocardial (93%) fibrosis, myocyte disarray (79%) and vacuolization (60%), endocardial inflammation (48%), arterial thickening (46%), dilated venules (28%), and arterial dysplasia (16%). Vacuolization, disarray, and dilated venules were significantly more common in the younger patients, whereas left bundle branch tissue appeared more often in older patients.

Conclusion.—In this series of patients undergoing septal myectomy for HCM, 53% were women and 35% were 60 years or older. Hypertrophy, disarray, fibrosis, inflammation, and vascular alterations were the most frequently observed microscopic features. Disarray was absent, however, in 21% of patients and cannot be used as a morphologic hallmark for HCM in small surgical myectomy specimens. Amyloidosis, previously unreported in HCM, was found in 3 men 65 years or older.

▶ HCM can present with obstruction of the left ventricular outflow. In these cases septal myectomy is performed to relieve the obstruction. Histologic data obtained from autopsy specimens described myocyte hypertrophy, myocyte disarray, endocardial and interstitial fibrosis, and abnormal small arteries in HCM. The current article describes the findings on the largest series of surgical specimens. Hypertrophy is characterized by the presence of enlarged and hyperchromatic nuclei and cell diameter greater than 20 microns. The latter is equivalent to 3 red blood cells. Myocyte disarray is seen as cellular interlacing, whirling, or herringbone patterns. Left bundle branch tissue consists of subendocardial bundles of myocytes that are separated from adjacent myocardium by delicate interstitial connective tissue and often contains large and pale-staining myocytes (Purkinje cells). Among the patients in whom left bundle branch tissue is detected microscopically, more than half develop new conduction deficits postoperatively. Although left bundle branch tissue was observed in only 12% of cases, it is important for pathologists to recognize it in surgical myectomy specimens.

P. A. Bejarano, MD

Cause of Death and Sudden Cardiac Death After Heart Transplantation: An Autopsy Study
Alexander RT, Steenbergen C (Duke Univ, Durham, NC)
Am J Clin Pathol 119:740-748, 2003   7–3

Background.—There are no recent autopsy-based studies examining the causes of death after heart transplantation. One center's autopsy findings in heart transplant patients between 1985 and 2001 were reviewed, with particular attention to patients with sudden cardiac death.

Methods.—Of 325 patients undergoing orthotopic heart transplantation between 1985 and 2001, 97 patients died, and 39 (40%) underwent autopsy. Medical records of these 39 patients were reviewed to determine the primary cause of death and survival time since transplantation.

Results.—The most common indications for heart transplantation were ischemic heart disease (19 patients, or 49%) and idiopathic heart disease (12 patients, or 31%). Survival after transplantation ranged from 0 days to 9.8 years (mean, 2.6 years). Causes of death were complications of transplantation (right-sided heart failure, multisystem organ failure, preservation procurement injury) in 13 cases (33%), infection in 5 cases (13%), complications of noncardiac surgery in 3 cases (8%), acute rejection in 3 cases (8%), malignant neoplasm in 3 cases (8%), graft vascular disease in 3 cases (8%), cardiac arrhythmia in 2 cases (5%), other causes in 4 cases (10%), and unclear causes in 3 patients (8%).

Most patients with complications of transplantation died within 2 months after transplantation, whereas patients with neoplasm or graft vascular disease died more than 2 years after surgery. Seven patients (18%) who were in medically stable condition died after a sudden cardiac arrest; these 7 patients account for 27% of the deaths occurring more than 1 month after transplantation. Two of these patients died of graft vascular disease; both had severe coronary artery fibrointimal hyperplasia and evidence of myocardial ischemia.

Another 2 patients died of cardiac arrhythmias; both had mild atherosclerosis. All 4 of these patients also had cardiac hypertrophy or dilatation. Two sudden deaths were due to acute cellular allograft rejection, and the last patient in this group died of an arrhythmia during an exacerbation of acute renal failure.

Conclusion.—One third of the patients who died after heart transplantation died due to complications of transplantation. About 25% of the patients who survived for more than 1 month after transplantation had sudden cardiac death.

▶ The autopsy rate at Duke University Medical Center in this study was 40% for the 97 patients who died following heart transplantation. Indications for the transplants included ischemic disease (40%), idiopathic disease (31%), congenital disease (8%), viral myocarditis (5%), amyloid changes (3%), valvular disease (3%), restrictive and eosinophilic changes (3%). These numbers are similar to those previously published. Since previous autopsy series were reported more than 10 years ago, this article shows updated data on the findings at autopsy for heart transplant patients.

Apart from the overall complications numbered in this article, this study pays close attention to a subgroup of patients who were in medically stable condition but died in a sudden manner. Two of the latter 7 patients had graft vascular disease. In this complication, the coronary arteries show severe fibrointimal hyperplasia accompanying acute myocardial infarction. Among, the patients who died of other than sudden cardiac death, 2 had malignant tumors and a third one had a presumed tumor as the cause of death. Those tumors were Kaposi sarcoma, large B-cell lymphoma, and pheochromocytoma. The patients who died of acute rejection apparently were noncompliant with the antirejection therapy because of depression.

P. A. Bejarano, MD

Obstruction of St Jude Medical Valves in the Aortic Position: Histology and Immunohistochemistry of Pannus

Teshima H, Hayashida N, Yano H, et al (Kurume Univ, Japan)
J Thorac Cardiovasc Surg 126:401-407, 2003   7–4

Background.—Prosthetic valve dysfunction (PVD) as a result of thrombus or pannus formation is an infrequent but serious complication. Patients with incomplete obstruction of the prosthetic valve may develop acute hemodynamic deterioration, which is a life-threatening condition. Pannus formation in patients who have received prosthetic valve replacement and mitral valve repair has been reported in several clinical and histologic studies. The mechanism of pannus formation in children has been associated with endocardial fibroelastosis and pseudoxanthoma elasticum. The cause of pannus formation is generally recognized as a bioreaction to the prostheses, but the detailed mechanism of its formation has not been fully elucidated. The morphologic, histologic, and immunohistochemical mechanism of pannus formation was investigated with the use of resected pannus tissue from patients with PVD.

Methods.—The study group was composed of 11 patients with PVD in the aortic position who underwent reoperation. Specimens of resected pannus were subjected to histologic staining and immunohistochemical staining.

Results.—Pannus without thrombus was observed in the periannulus of the left ventricular septal side, extending into the pivot guard and interfering with the movement of the straight edge of the leaflet. Histologic staining showed that the specimens were composed mainly of collagen and elastic fibrous tissue, accompanied by endothelial cells, chronic inflammatory cell infiltration, and myofibroblasts. Immunohistochemical analysis showed significant expression of transforming growth factor-beta (TGF-β), TGF-β receptor 1 (TGF-β-R1), CD34, and factor VIII in the endothelial cells of the lumen layer; strong TGF-β-R1, α-smooth muscle actin, desmin, and epithelial membrane antigen in the myofibroblasts of the media layer; and TGF-β, TGF-β-R1, and CD68KP1 in macrophages of the stump lesion.

Conclusions.—Pannus in this population of patients with PVD appeared to originate in the neointima in the periannulus of the left ventricular septum. The structure of the pannus consisted of myofibroblasts and an extracellular matrix such as collagen fiber. Formation of pannus after prosthetic valve replacement may be associated with a process of periannular tissue healing by means of the expression of TGF-β.

▶ Pannus is a fibrocellular expansion consisting of inflammatory cells, granulomatous formation, and fibroblasts. Its presence is more frequently seen in the joints and usually associated with rheumatoid arthritis. In the heart, pannus formation is an infrequent complication in patients who receive valve replacement. The pannus in these situations consists mostly of collagen and elastic fibrous tissue, suggesting that pannus results from an accumulation of extracellular matrix. The strong myofibroblastic TGF-β-R1 expression seen in these cases along with α-smooth muscle actin, suggest that pannus is due to persistent neointimal development by chronic inflammation eliciting proliferation of myofibroblasts and extracellular matrix without thrombus formation. Although infrequent, pannus formation produces a narrowing of the orifice of the aortic prosthetic valve leading to acute hemodynamic alterations and thus it can be life-threatening.

P. A. Bejarano, MD

FK506 vs. Cyclosporin: Pathologic Findings in 1067 Endomyocardial Biopsies
Gajjar NA, Kobashigawa JA, Laks H, et al (Univ of California, Los Angeles)
Cardiovasc Pathol 12:73-76, 2003   7–5

Background.—The Quilty lesion has been of interest and controversy since it was first described in 1981 by Billingham. This lesion is a raised endocardial infiltrate of T and B lymphocytes, plasma cells, macrophages, and sometimes prominent numerous small blood vessels. Quilty A lesions are limited to the endocardium, but Quilty B lesions can extend into the underlying myocardium, where there is often associated myocyte injury. There is still no consensus regarding the pathogenesis of this endocardial/myocardial infiltrate and its significance in the posttransplant cardiac patient, but it would appear that the Quilty B lesion cannot be good for the transplanted heart or the patient. One of the most controversial aspects of the Quilty lesion and the one with the greatest clinical relevance is whether Quilty lesions represent a form of cellular rejection. A statistically significant association has been reported between the presence of Quilty lesions and acute cellular rejection, and that these lesions are predictive of rejection episodes even in the absence of rejection. It has also been speculated that the Quilty lesion results from a toxic effect of cyclosporin on the endocardium, resulting in the inflammatory infiltrates. If the Quilty lesion is somehow related to cyclosporin, then its frequency might be different in patients in whom cyclosporin was not part of the immunosuppression regimen. Tacrolimus (FK506) has been shown to be a safe and effective alternative to cyclosporin as a maintenance immunosuppressive agent after solid organ transplantation. The hypothesis that if the Quilty lesion is related to cyclosporin, then patients treated with tacrolimus might have similar numbers of rejection episodes but fewer Quilty lesions in their endomyocardial biopsies was investigated.

Methods.—A total of 1067 endomyocardial biopsy specimens from 65 patients assigned to FK506 or cyclosporin after heart transplantation were reviewed.

Results.—The number of episodes of rejections was similar in both groups (162 in the FK506 group vs 145 in the cyclosporin group). However, when compared with cyclosporin treatment, FK506 was associated with significantly more Quilty A lesions and fewer Quilty B lesions.

Conclusions.—It would appear from these findings that FK506 can prevent some Quilty A lesions from progressing to Quilty B lesions. This effect of FK506 could be associated with improved long-term graft function because Quilty B lesion is associated with myocyte injury and Quilty A is not.

▶ This study addresses the issue of Quilty effect in cardiac biopsy specimens from transplanted patients. The authors look at the relationship between Quilty effect and the use of 2 antirejection drugs, cyclosporine and FK506. Quilty effect or lesion refers to the presence of a raised endocardial accumulation of T and B lymphocytes, plasma cells, macrophages, and sometimes accompanied by blood vessels. If the lesion is limited to the endocardium, it is called Quilty A, and when it infiltrates the underlying myocardium causing myocyte injury the designation of Quilty B is given. Although it was described more than 20 years ago after the first patient on whom it was observed, it is not clear yet what the mechanism of its genesis or the clinical implications of its presence. It has been postulated that Quilty lesions may be due to cyclosporine toxicity to the endocardium, acute rejection, chronic rejection, posttransplant lymphoproliferative disease, viral infection, and even low levels of cyclosporine leading to localized rejection. To test the view that it is due to cyclosporine, the authors thought that the frequency of Quilty lesions may be different in patients who are not receiving cyclosporine in comparison with those who received this type of antirejection drug. They observed no rejection episode differences between the FK506 and the cyclosporine groups. However, there were more Quilty A lesions in patients receiving FK506 than those on cyclosporine (46% vs 40%, $P < .50$), but less number of Quilty B lesions in these patients (10% vs 18%, $P < .001$). The authors propose that FK506 may prevent some Quilty A lesions from progressing to the more infiltrative Quilty B. However, this is almost speculative because there is no proof yet that Quilty A lesions progress to Quilty B lesions. Although this study does not contribute to clarify the pathogenesis of Quilty lesions, it suggests that the type of immunosuppressive regimen affects them.

P. A. Bejarano, MD

8 Soft Tissue and Bone

Serum Vascular Endothelial Growth Factor as a Tumour Marker in Soft Tissue Sarcoma
Hayes AJ, Mostyn-Jones A, Koban MU, et al (Royal Marsden Hosp, London; Imperial College, London)
Br J Surg 91:242-247, 2004   8–1

Introduction.—The extent of tumor vascularization is a major prognostic indicator in a variety of solid tumors. Vascular endothelial growth factor (VEGF), an important pathologic angiogenic growth factor, is overexpressed in many tumor types and also correlates with prognosis. To assess the value of VEGF as a tumor marker, serum levels of the factor were measured before treatment and during follow-up in patients undergoing primary treatment for suspected soft tissue sarcoma.

Methods.—A total of 165 patients were recruited for the study and had venous blood taken 1 week before surgery, 2 weeks after surgery, and at 3-month intervals thereafter. Serum VEGF was also measured in 15 healthy volunteers. Concentrations of VEGF were determined by an enzyme-linked immunosorbent assay incorporating a polyclonal antibody that detects both $VEGF_{165}$ and $VEGF_{121}$, soluble factors that can be measured easily and accurately by standard immunoassays.

Results.—Twenty-nine of the 133 patients who underwent surgery as primary treatment had a benign lesion and 10 had a nonsarcomatous malignancy, leaving 94 patients eligible for analysis. Thirty-six of their sarcomas were grade 1, 31 were grade 2, and 27 were grade 3. Ten patients were not treated, 10 received cytotoxic chemotherapy, 8 received imatinib, and 3 had radiotherapy. Compared with patients whose lesions were benign and the healthy volunteers, patients with grade 2 and grade 3 sarcomas had significantly elevated pretreatment serum VEGF levels (233 vs 413 and 467 pg/mL, respectively). Posttreatment measurements of VEGF reflected disease status in patients whose tumors had a high level of the angiogenic factor before treatment. Additionally, there was a correlation between VEGF concentration and platelet count in patients with grade 2 and 3 tumors.

Conclusion.—In previous research, intratumoral concentrations of VEGF were shown to have prognostic significance for local recurrence and metastasis of soft tissue sarcoma, regardless of histologic subtype. The findings of this study indicate a correlation between serum VEGF expression and tumor grade and show that VEGF concentrations can reflect response to treatment.

▶ This is an interesting article that deals with what is usually missing in pathology, namely strong clinicopathologic correlation. More often than not, pathology-related articles deal with issues that are of importance only to pathologists—putting us under the gun of criticism of our clinical colleagues that accuse us of making already complex pathology classifications "even more unnecessary complex."

This article reveals in appropriate detail the mechanism of angiogenesis and its role in the development of primary tumor with an emphasis on VEGF. The authors cite an article that measures concentration of VEGF homogenized tumor specimens derived from high-grade tumors. This study, however, deals with concentration of VEGF in the serum of patients with sarcomas.

The authors recruited a significant number of patients to participate in their study (n = 165); they also enlisted the help of 15 healthy volunteers. Importantly, the authors further subclassify patients who underwent chemotherapy and surgery—they even note that 29 patients actually had a benign lesion. Malignant lesions that were surgically treated (the remaining 94 patients) were further broken down into grades 1, 2, and 3.

Astoundingly, median and mean VEGF levels were raised in patients with grade 2 and 3 sarcomas compared with levels identified in the volunteers and patients with benign lesions; this difference could not have been shown for sarcomas or grade 1. Although the authors realize that grade 2 and 3 sarcoma patients also had an increase in platelets that could, potentially, be responsible for an increase in VEGF, platelet count increase was 6-fold less than the percentage increase in mean serum VEGF concentration.

Although not shown in the article, the authors mentioned that there is no statistically significant difference observed in the serum VEGF concentration between the major histologic subtypes; however, it would be of interest to know which histologic subtypes were actually included.

The authors also stated there was a brief increase in serum VEGF about 2 weeks after surgery; it would be of interest to know whether they thought that this could be attributable to the healing process.

As we all know, some of us are using a 3-tier grade scheme for grading of soft tissue sarcomas; others are using either a 2-tier scheme (high-grade, low-grade) or a 4-tier scheme. It would be really interesting to see all the serum levels of VEGF correspond to those. However, the authors themselves note that this is a pilot study; perhaps we could hope for a more comprehensive study that would address those interesting issues? Also, in my opinion, it would be important to know how the serum levels of VEGF would correspond and correlate to the levels of VEGF in the sarcoma itself, as well as how they would compare to the mean size of the neoplasm.

D. M. Jukic, MD, PhD

Myoepithelial Tumors of Soft Tissue: A Clinicopathologic and Immuno-histochemical Study of 101 Cases With Evaluation of Prognostic Parameters
Hornick JL, Fletcher CDM (Harvard Med School, Boston)
Am J Surg Pathol 27:1183-1196, 2003   8–2

Introduction.—Myoepitheliomas and mixed tumors have only recently been recognized to occur mainly in soft tissue. Less than 40 soft tissue myoepithelial tumors have been reported; their characterization has been limited. To further characterize these tumors and examine prognostic parameters, 101 myoepithelial tumors of soft tissue were reviewed.

Methods.—Hematoxylin and eosin sections were reevaluated and immunohistochemistry was performed. Referring physicians provided clinical details.

Results.—The mean age of 53 male and 48 female patients was 38 years (range, 3-83 years). The tumor size ranged from 0.7 to 20 cm (mean, 4.7 cm). Most tumors arose from the extremities and limb girdles. Of these, 41 were from the lower limbs and 35 from the upper limbs. Additionally, 15 arose from the head and neck and 10 from the trunk. Fifty-four tumors were in the subcutis and 37 were in the deep soft tissue (depth not documented in 10). Most cases were grossly well circumscribed; 43 demonstrated microscopically infiltrative margins. On histologic examination, most tumors were lobulated, composed of cords or nests of epithelioid, ovoid, or spindled cells with a variable reticular architecture and a chondromyxoid or collagenous/hyalinized stroma. Eight cases demonstrated a predominantly solid proliferation of spindled or plasmacytoid cells and 17 demonstrated ductular differentiation (mixed tumors). Cartilage was observed in 6 cases, 6 contained bone, and 4 others contained both. Mitosis ranged between 0 and 68/high power fields (mean, 4.7/10 high power fields). Tumors with benign cytomorphology or mild cytologic atypia (low grade) were categorized as myoepithelioma or mixed tumor. Tumors with moderate to severe atypia (high grade) were categorized as myoepithelial carcinoma (epithelioid or spindle cells with vesicular or coarse chromatin, prominent, often large nucleoli, or nuclear pleomorphism) or malignant mixed tumor (cytologically malignant cartilage or bone). Sixty-one cases were either myoepithelial carcinomas or malignant mixed tumors. On immunohistochemistry, all cases with available material were reactive for epithelial markers (keratins or epithelial membrane antigen): 93%, keratins (most frequently AE1/AE3 or PAN-K); 87%, S-100 protein; 86%, calponin; 63%, epithelial membrane antigen; 46%, glial fibrillary acidic protein; 36%, smooth muscle actin; 23%, p63; and 14%, desmin (Table 3). Sixty-four patients had available follow-up data. Among 33 cases with benign or low-grade cytology (mean follow-up, 36 months; range, 4-168 months), 6 (18%) recurred locally. There were no metastases. There was no association between clinical or histologic characteristics and recurrence. Among 31 cytologically malignant cases (mean follow-up, 50 months; range, 4-252 months) 13 (42%) recurred locally and 10 (32%) metastasized; 4 patients died of metastatic tumor.

TABLE 3.—Results of Immunohistochemical Studies on Myoepithelial Tumors of Soft Tissue

Antigen	0	1+	2+	3+	4+	Total+
PAN-K	23	10	13	8	17	48/71 (68%)
AE1/AE3	15	17	10	5	19	51/66 (77%)
CK8/18	20	6	4	4	7	21/41 (51%)
CK14	26	6	4	0	2	12/38 (32%)
EMA	31	7	16	6	23	52/83 (63%)
S-100	13	9	9	9	57	84/97 (87%)
GFAP	47	12	4	9	15	40/87 (46%)
Calponin	7	4	5	5	30	44/51 (86%)
SMA	48	9	7	4	7	27/75 (36%)
Desmin	44	4	2	1	0	7/51 (14%)
p63	51	5	1	2	7	15/66 (23%)

0, No staining; *1+*, <5% tumor cells reactive; *2+*, 5%-25% tumor cells reactive; *3+*, 26%-50% tumor cells reactive; *4+*, >50% tumor cells reactive.

(Courtesy of Hornick JL, Fletcher CDM: Myoepithelial tumors of soft tissue: A clinicopathologic and immunohistochemical study of 101 cases with evaluation of prognostic parameters. *Am J Surg Pathol* 27:1183-1196, 2003.)

Conclusion.—These findings expand the spectrum of myoepithelial tumors of soft tissue to include myoepithelial carcinomas and malignant mixed tumors, which have an aggressive clinical course. Although most morphologically benign or low-grade myoepithelial neoplasms of soft tissue behave benignly, there is an approximately 20% risk for recurrent disease.

▶ We know Christopher Fletcher as one of the most prominent names in the field of soft tissue pathology. Here, his group examines the diagnosis of myoepithelial neoplasms and the relationship of this category to the so-called mixed tumors.

The authors distinctly outline morphologic criteria for diagnosis of myoepithelial neoplasms in the very beginning of the article; they also explain the most common staining patterns and other characteristics. The authors explain in detail their reasoning behind classifying each neoplasm as either benign or malignant; they further discuss proper classification of malignant tumors either as myoepithelial carcinoma or malignant mixed tumors.

Immunohistochemical results, as outlined in Table 3, revealed staining for keratin in 93%; S100 in 87%, and calponin in 86%. However, and as pointed in this article, even an unusual staining pattern was tolerated in the presence of characteristic histopathology.

The article delivers 2 very strong messages. (1) Almost half of soft tissue myoepithelial neoplasms exhibit infiltrating margins; this criterion, in the absence of at least moderate cytologic atypia, is insufficient for classifying them as malignant. (2) Benign myoepithelial neoplasms do possess a risk for recurrence only, while malignant myoepithelial neoplasms exhibit aggressive behavior with metastatic potential.

This is an important take-home message for a practicing pathologist—be careful in classifying a myoepithelial neoplasm as benign—and be equally careful in classifying them as malignant. Just because the malignant diagnosis is less likely (in an already uncommon neoplasia), it is not impossible—and the consequences might be dire. Pathologists are encouraged to read and reread this report frequently, as it also outlines the most common differential diagnoses, thus prompting you to examine these possibilities in a greater detail. This article should also serve as an example of what a review article should look like. I personally think that this article would benefit from inclusion of a greater number of high-power photomicrographs, especially in color. However, this is a drawback of the printed material, and one can't help but wonder whether the publishers of scientific journals wouldn't serve us better by including additional image material on their websites.

D. M. Jukic, MD, PhD

Classification and Subtype Prediction of Adult Soft Tissue Sarcoma by Functional Genomics

Segal NH, Pavlidis P, Antonescu CR, et al (Mem Sloan Kettering Cancer Ctr, New York; Columbia Univ, New York)
Am J Pathol 163:691-700, 2003   8–3

Background.—Soft tissue sarcomas (STSs) are a group of histologically and genetically diverse cancers that account for approximately 1% of all adult malignancies, with an annual incidence of about 8000 cases. There are more than 50 subtypes of STS, all of which are diagnosed by genetic and morphologic criteria. Some STSs may be classified by their recurrent chromosomal translocations or somatic mutation. Pleomorphic tumors are typically characterized by nonrecurrent genetic aberrations and karyotypic heterogeneity, which makes for a diagnostic challenge even for experienced pathologists. The usefulness of gene expression profiling in STS to identify a genomic-based classification system that is useful in diagnosis was evaluated.

Methods.—RNA samples were obtained from 51 pathologically confirmed cases of STS representing 9 different histologic subtypes of adult STS and examined with the Affymetrix U95A GeneChip. Statistical tests were performed on experimental groups that were identified by cluster analysis in an effort to identify discriminating genes that could be subsequently used in a support vector machine algorithm.

Results.—Pleomorphic tumors were found to be heterogeneous. Synovial sarcomas, round-cell/myxoid liposarcomas, clear-cell sarcomas, and gastrointestinal stromal tumors were found to show distinct and homogenous gene expression profiles. One noteworthy finding was that a subset of malignant fibrous histiocytomas, a controversial histologic subtype, was identified as a distinct genomic group. The support vector machine algorithm developed from these findings was supportive of a genomic basis for diagnosis and demonstrated both high sensitivity and specificity.

Conclusions.—These findings support gene expression profiling as a useful tool in the classification and diagnosis of adult STS. The results of this study also indicated a direction for research into potential new therapeutic targets of STS.

▶ The group from Memorial Sloan Kettering Cancer Center, with Senior author Carlos Cordon-Cardo, is undertaking what most of us would think is an impossible feat—they are trying to reclassify STS based on the results of molecular genotyping. However, it seems that they are succeeding.

The group has tested sarcomas from 51 patients, focusing on high-grade lesions; they have used the Affymetrix platform with U95A GeneChip. It is worthwhile mentioning that 9 different histologic subtypes that authors investigated covered approximately 75% of soft tissue cases in the United States (malignant fibrous histiocytomas [MFH], fibrosarcomas, leiomyosarcomas, round-cell liposarcomas, pleomorphic liposarcomas, dedifferentiated liposarcomas, clear-cell sarcomas, synovial sarcomas, and gastrointestinal stromal tumors [GIST]).

There were some interesting results observed: (1) GIST, synovial sarcomas, round-cell liposarcomas, and clear cell sarcomas clustered in distinct groups—as would be expected in tumor groups that harbor distinct genetic change; (2) 5 of 8 fibrosarcomas clustered, as shown in Fig 1, in the close proximity to synovial sarcomas; however, they did not harbor distinct mutations seen in synovial sarcomas (SYT-SSX fusion gene); (3) 5 of 6 leiomyosarcoma specimens clustered together with dedifferentiated liposarcomas—thus being designated "genomic leiomyosarcomas group 1"; and (4) 9 of 11 MFH specimens clustered together with a single fibrosarcoma, thus being designated as a genomic MFH group.

These numbers imply (which the authors also indicate) that genomic profiling might be utilized to explore novel classifications as well as to confirm accepted classification or, indeed, reserve final classification for a genomic analysis only. As the authors imply, the so-called "genomic MFH" might not correspond to the "histologic MFH" group, but again, many people tend to overcall this entity.

Even if somebody's ego would be hurt if his diagnosis of, let's say MFH, gets changed to fibrosarcoma or vice versa, we need to remember a fine red line that the authors also consider in their article: that is, we are here to diagnose the neoplasms so patients get optimal therapy, and not to tend our egos. Thus, it might be that therapy decisions in the field of STS (at least those that are high grade) are better left to genomic pathology—and we better all start freezing (if we are not doing it already) parts of soft tissue tumors to allow for this. Patients will surely demand it in the next decade.

D. M. Jukic, MD, PhD

Altered Expression of Cell Cycle Regulators in Myxofibrosarcoma, With Special Emphasis on Their Prognostic Implications

Oda Y, Takahira T, Kawaguchi K, et al (Kyushu Univ, Fukuoka, Japan)
Hum Pathol 34:1035-1042, 2003

8–4

Background.—The results of several recent studies have cast doubt regarding the cohesive entities of malignant fibrous histiocytoma (MFH), particularly its pleomorphic variant. Some authors, however, have reassessed many pleomorphic sarcomas and have demonstrated that myxoid MFH is a definitive and reproducible tumor type. Myxofibrosarcoma/myxoid MFH has continued to be considered a distinct entity even after the publication of these pleomorphic sarcomas. Several cell cycle–regulated proteins have already been screened by immunohistochemistry in an effort to identify the reliable prognostic indicator of soft tissue sarcomas; however, it is still not known whether the altered expression of these proteins has an effect on patient survival in myxofibrosarcoma. Clinicopathologic prognostic factors in the expression of p53, MDM2, MIB-1 (Ki-67), p21, p27, p16, cyclin A, cyclin D1, and cyclin E were searched for in cases of myxofibrosarcoma.

Methods.—A search was conducted for possible clinicopathologic prognostic factors in 61 cases of myxofibrosarcoma for which follow-up data were available.

Results.—Univariate analysis of these cases showed that large tumor size (≥ 5 cm), deeply situated tumor, and high histologic grade (grade 2 or 3) were indicative of significantly decreased survival. Among 43 cases for which immunohistochemical findings were available for review, high MIB-1 labeling index, high cyclin A labeling index, low p21 labeling index, and reduced abnormal expression of p16 were found to be adverse prognostic factors. Multivariate analysis showed that high mitotic rate, p53 immunoreactivity, high MIB-1 labeling index, low p21 labeling index, and low p27 labeling index were independent poor prognostic factors.

Conclusions.—It would appear from these findings that reduced expression of p21 could be viewed as a new parameter for evaluation in the identification of patients at high risk for myxofibrosarcoma.

▶ The authors give a small introduction in malignant fibrous histiocytoma, the myxoid variant, and myxofibrosarcoma. This group of Japanese authors has defined myxoid MFH myxofibrosarcoma as MFH in which at least 50% of the entire neoplasm reveals a highly vascularized stroma, the distinctive blood vessels, and, of course, myxoid areas. Ninety-three cases were retrieved from the archives, but the authors ended up evaluating 75 of those.

Various cell cycle regulator–related antibodies were used. In addition, the authors have also evaluated other well-known prognostic factors such as size of the neoplasm, location (superficial vs deep), and grade of the neoplasm.

As an interesting addition to the well-known prognostic factors, immunohistochemical expression (reduced) of p16, low p21, and high expression of cyclin A, cyclin D1 did have adverse prognostic value by univariate analysis. It is worth noting that the authors actually counted at least 500 cells in each case.

They conclude that deregulation of p21 might play an important role in the development of myxofibrosarcoma. They do note, however, that this might not be a pivotal event in the development of sarcoma itself; rather, it might be an epiphenomenon and further studies might be needed.

D. M. Jukic, MD, PhD

Gene Expression Patterns and Gene Copy Number Changes in Dermatofibrosarcoma Protuberans

Linn SC, West RB, Pollack JR, et al (Stanford Univ, Calif; Vancouver Gen Hosp, BC, Canada; Univ of Washington, Seattle; et al)
Am J Pathol 163:2383-2395, 2003   8–5

Background.—Dermatofibrosarcoma protuberans (DFSP) is an uncommon soft tissue neoplasm that typically occurs in young adults. Nearly all cases of DFSP have a translocation that involves chromosomes 17 and 22, resulting in fusion of the collagen type 1α1 (*COL1A1*) and platelet-derived growth factor β (*PDGFβ*) genes. The characteristic gene expression profile of DFSP was determined and DNA copy number changes in DFSP characterized by array-based comparative genomic hybridization (array CGH).

Methods.—Fresh-frozen and formalin-fixed, paraffin-embedded samples of DFSP were analyzed by array CGH (4 cases) and DNA microarray analysis of global gene expression (9 cases).

Results.—The 9 DFSPs were easily differentiated from 27 other diverse soft tissue tumors on the basis of their gene expression patterns. Genes characteristically expressed in the DFSPs included *PDGFβ* and its receptor, *PDGFRB*, *APOD*, *MEOX1*, *PLA2R*, and *PRKCA*. Array CGH of DNA extracted either from frozen tumor samples or from paraffin blocks showed equivalent results. Large areas of chromosomes 17q and 22q, which were bonded by *COL1A1* and *PDGFβ*, respectively, were amplified in DFSP. There was a significant increase in the expression of genes in the amplified regions.

Conclusions.—It was established in this genetic profiling study of dermatofibrosarcoma protuberans that DFSP has a distinctive gene expression profile; array can be successfully applied to frozen or formalin-fixed, paraffin-embedded tumor samples; and a characteristic amplification sequence from chromosomes 17q and 22 q, demarcated at the *COL1A1* and *PDGFβ* genes, respectively, was associated with elevated expression of the amplified genes.

▶ This article deals with novel approach to classification of one of the most common soft tissue neoplasms, dermatofibrosarcoma protuberans. As authors themselves point out, the problem with dermatofibrosarcoma protuberans is that it occurs in young adults, has a propensity for aggressive growth, and has a recurrence rate of approximately 20%.

As known from previous studies, highly characteristic translocation is seen between chromosomes 17 and 22; this fuses the *COL1A1* and *PDGFβ* genes.

The authors have used 9 cases of dermatofibrosarcoma protuberans, and 8 of those reacted with marker CD34 by immunohistochemistry.

For comparison, the others have used the 36 soft tissue neoplasms, which included leiomyosarcoma, malignant fibrous histiocytoma, gastrointestinal stromal tumors, synovial sarcomas, and even epithelioid fibrous histiocytoma.

The authors have focused on variation of expression of 4687 genes by microarray studies. It seems that dermatofibrosarcoma protuberans specimens have revealed (in contrast to other sarcomas studied) a cluster of 465 genes whose pattern of expression within this group was highly correlated. In addition, the authors have performed comparative genomic hybridization on the same specimens; the comparison could be performed in 4 cases.

It is refreshing to see that the authors have used gene expression profiles for differential diagnosis of dermatofibrosarcoma protuberans, and not for the sake of performing analysis itself. They have evaluated (by the same methods) other soft tissue neoplasms that could pose diagnostic quandaries. The authors also will plan very clearly that cDNA microarray analysis provides an efficient way to search for new diagnostic markers for routine immunohistochemistry; as we all know, although microarray data analysis is performed at major universities, it is still a highly impractical tool for the practicing pathologist. Rather, one needs to stay abreast of the data obtained by microarray analysis and try to develop and utilize them for future development of highly specific or sensitive immunohistochemical markers.

Although this study might be an overkill for somebody who does not follow microarray literature, it outlines several take-home messages. It accentuates the fact that one could use paraffin-embedded tissue to perform CGH analysis; it also identifies *PDGFβ* as a gene that is consistently elevated in dermatofibrosarcoma protuberans. The authors also go into detail of all the other genes whose expression is elevated in dermatofibrosarcoma protuberans. However, it is an opinion of this editor that this will be hard to fully substantiate for further immunohistochemical studies.

In summary, if you deal with soft tissue pathology or dermatopathology, you might need to follow the progress of this group of authors, as obviously their work on this challenging subject will not stop here.

D. M. Jukic, MD, PhD

***PAX7* Expression in Embryonal Rhabdomyosarcoma Suggests an Origin in Muscle Satellite Cells**
Tiffin N, Williams RD, Shipley J, et al (Inst of Cancer Research, Sutton, Surrey, England)
Br J Cancer 89:327-332, 2003   8–6

Introduction.—Rhabdomyosarcoma (RMS), the most common pediatric soft tissue sarcoma, has 2 main subtypes: the embryonal subtype (ERMS) usually occurs in young children and has a better prognosis; the alveolar subtype (ARMS) is most often seen in adolescents and is frequently metastatic at diagnosis. Comparative genomic hybridization analysis has suggested a biologic basis for this difference in tumor aggressiveness. The ARMS tumors typically exhibit 1 of 2 characteristic translocations that juxtapose *PAX3* or *PAX7* with the forkhead-related *FKHR (FOXO1A)* gene. Polymerase chain reaction was used to quantify the relative levels of chimeric and wild-type *PAX* transcripts in various RMS subtypes.

Methods and Findings.—Thirty-four primary RMS and 3 cell lines were evaluated. Expression levels were quantified relative to expression in the RD cell line (RDCL) for *PAX3* and *PAX7*, the Rh30 cell line for *PAX3-FKHR*, and a primary tumor for *PAX7-FKHR*. *PAX3* levels were compared with relative *PAX3-FKHR* levels, relative *PAX7* levels, and relative *PAX7-FKHR* levels. Upregulation of wild-type *PAX3* was found to be independent of the presence of either fusion gene and thus unlikely to contribute to tumorigenesis. Upregulated *PAX7* expression, which was almost entirely restricted to cases without *PAX3-FKHR* or *PAX7-FKHR* fusion genes, may contribute to tumorigenesis in the absence of chimeric *PAX* transcription factors. Because myogenic satellite cells are known to express *PAX7*, this pattern of *PAX7* expression suggests this cell type as the origin of these tumors. Furthermore, *MET* expression, a marker for the myogenic satellite cell lineage, was detected in all RMS samples expressing wild-type *PAX7*.

Conclusion.—Elevated *PAX3* expression levels were found to be independent of RMS subtype or presence of a *PAX3/7-FKHR* fusion gene. Regardless of subtype or translocation status, *PAX3* expression was detected in 16 of the 34 tumor samples. In ERMS cases, elevated *PAX7* expression and consistent *MET* expression indicate an origin in myogenic satellite cells.

▶ For the pathologists dealing with childhood neoplasms, this article is of utmost interest. Current opinion in pathology is that benign and malignant neoplasms arise from "reserve" or primitive stem cells that then try to recapitulate the morphology of the normal organ.

The authors evaluate the relevance of wild-type *PAX3* and *PAX7* gene expression in various subtypes of RMS. The authors review normal myogenesis and the relation of *PAX3* and chimeric protein *PAX3-FKHR* and its significance as well as *PAX7* and *PAX7-FKHR*. They performed real-time polymerase chain reaction in an attempt to detect levels of those.

The authors evaluated an impressive number of 34 primary RMSs; they also evaluated 3 cell lines. They found that *PAX3* expression is independent of fewer subtype; they further concluded that it was detected in 16 of 34 tumor samples. The authors conclude that it is possible, particularly for the embryonal variety of RMS, that *PAX7* wild-type gene contributes to transformation in the absence of *PAX7-FKHR* fusion product.

PAX7 has been shown to be expressed, in its wild type, in muscle satellite cells; as the authors show, this expression is restricted to RMSs that do not reveal any translocations. This was also consistent with expression of MET in neoplasms with no translocations as well as satellite cells.

The authors will attempt to perform molecular profiling of myogenic genes in satellite cells and rhabdomyosarcomas without fusion product. They hope, by this method, to further strengthen their theory; however, it seems that they've hit the nail on the head. Maybe it is time to reevaluate the classification of poorly differentiated neoplasms and, in fact, leave it for molecular methods. It just might be that classification of neoplasms by those methods will also have therapeutic implications, which is not the case too often these days with current classifications.

D. M. Jukic, MD, PhD

Merkel Cell Carcinoma: A Clinicopathologic Study With Prognostic Implications

Mott RT, Smoller BR, Morgan MB (Univ of South Florida, Tampa; Univ of Arkansas, Little Rock; James A. Haley Veteran's Hosp, Tampa, Fla)
J Cutan Pathol 31:217-223, 2004   8–7

Background.—Merkel cell carcinoma (MCC) is a rare cutaneous neoplasm that presents most often in sun-exposed areas of the head and neck and upper extremities. Many aspects of MCC have not been defined. One of the most important tasks is the identification of prognostic factors that are capable of predicting the biologic behavior of these tumors. A cohort of patients with MCC was evaluated to identify clinical, histopathologic, and immunohistochemical features that are capable of predicting disease outcome.

Methods.—A review was conducted of 25 cases of MCC to evaluate features, including age, sex, race, tumor location, tumor size, depth of invasion, growth pattern, lymphocytic infiltration, mitotic activity, ulceration, necrosis, vascular invasion, and perineural invasion. Neural cell adhesion molecule and cytokeratin-20 expression were examined by immunohistochemical methods.

Results.—Most of the patients (84%) were men, and the average age of the patients was 74 years. Tumors were located on the head (68%) and upper extremities (32%). Overall, 64% of the patients had metastatic disease to regional lymph nodes or distant sites (average follow-up time, 21 months). Local recurrence was also common and occurred in 29% of patients. The overall 1- and 2-year survival rates were 80% and 53%, respectively. Histopathologic findings showed tumors with an average size of 7.2 mm. Common findings were invasion into the subcutaneous adipose tissue, solid growth pattern, tumor necrosis, and vascular and perineurial invasion. Features that had a statistically significant correlation with poor outcome included tumor size 5 mm or greater, invasion into the subcutaneous adipose tissue, diffuse growth pattern, and heavy lymphocytic infiltration. The remaining clinical and histopathologic findings and immunohistochemical results were not correlated with disease outcome. Logistic regression models demonstrate that the depth of invasion and degree of lymphocytic infiltration are strong predictors of disease outcome.

Conclusions.—The importance of identifying clinicopathologic features capable of predicting tumor behavior is underscored by the current controversy regarding the treatment of early-stage MCC. The results of this study led to the identification of several prognostic features in MCC that may be useful in identifying patients in whom more aggressive treatment regimens are required.

▶ MCC is a malignant neoplasm of cutaneous neuroendocrine differentiation that has a grave prognosis and fatal outcome. However (or fortunately), this is a rare neoplasm. This study attempts to identify some of the features that could potentially serve as histologic predictors of prognosis.

The authors investigated 25 cases of MCC; they briefly reviewed known facts about this neoplasm and known immunohistochemical features. It is somewhat disappointing that there is no mention about its other eponym—trabecular cell carcinoma of the skin[1]—as we now suspect that MCC might not even be related to so-called Merkel cells in the epidermis. The authors don't mention whether metastatic small cell carcinoma from the lung was ruled out, which would be a helpful statement, especially with 2 cases in their series that did not stain for cytokeratin-20.

However, this is very valuable study; it is notable that the depth of invasion (level of dermis vs subcutis, akin to Clark's melanoma stages, not an absolute value like Breslow's staging) and the intensity of lymphocytic infiltrate were the most favorable predictors. It would be better if the authors referred to the former value as "level of invasion" rather than depth; in fact, a simple schematic drawing would be great to explain this clearly if it was included.

In conclusion, anyone who deals with routine dermatopathologic specimens would be very clever to read this article in detail and include some of the values reported in here in their report, with the note that this might impart a prognostic value. This is especially important if known that there are more and more centers that practice sentinel node biopsy on MCC.[2]

D. M. Jukic, MD, PhD

References

1. Toker C: Trabecular carcinoma of the skin. *Arch Dermatol* 105:107-110, 1972.
2. Stadelmann WK, Cobbins L, Lentsch EJ. Incidence of nonlocalization of sentinel lymph nodes using preoperative lymphoscintigraphy in 74 consecutive head and neck melanoma and Merkel cell carcinoma patients. *Ann Plast Surg* 52:546-549, 2004.

Nephrogenic Fibrosing Dermopathy: A Novel Cutaneous Fibrosing Disorder in Patients With Renal Failure
Swartz RD, Crofford LJ, Phan SH, et al (Univ of Michigan, Ann Arbor)
Am J Med 114:563-572, 2003   8–8

Background.—Nephrogenic fibrosing dermopathy is a newly recognized cutaneous fibrosing disorder in patients with renal failure. This disorder is characterized by the acute onset of induration involving the upper and lower limbs in patients with acute or chronic renal failure. The etiology, pathogenesis, associated clinical conditions (other than renal failure),and ultimate course of nephrogenic fibrosing dermopathy were defined.

TABLE 1.—Clinical Characteristics of Patients with Nephrogenic Fibrosing Dermopathy at Time of Skin Biopsy

Patient	Age (Years)	Etiology of Renal Failure	Dialysis at Time of Biopsy	Transplant	HLA-A; -B, -C; -DR	Comorbid Diagnoses	Medications
1	75	Atheroembolism	Hemodialysis for 1 month			Aortic aneurysm, peripheral vascular disease	Warfarin, digoxin
2	75	Atheroembolism	None*			Peripheral vascular disease, gout, smoking	Allopurinol, erythropoietin, furosemide, amlodipine, benazepril, metoprolol, trazodone
3	74	Renovascular disease	Hemodialysis for 6 months			Cardiomyopathy, peripheral vascular disease, hypothyroid, myopathy, smoking	Aspirin, furosemide, thyroxine, lisinopril, prednisone
4	77	Hypertension	Peritoneal dialysis for 8 months			Cardiomyopathy, venous thrombophlebitis, amiodarone liver toxicity, myopathy	Aspirin, atenolol, digoxin, megestrol, erythropoietin, tamsulosin, thyroxine, sertraline
5	43	Polycystic disease	Hemodialysis for 40 months	Liver, kidney	(2,11);(44,51);(-,-); (4,8)	Cirrhosis (hepatitis C)	Carbamazepine, cyclosporine, mycophenolate mofetil, erythropoietin, prednisone, metoclopramide
6	58	Membranous nephropathy	Hemodialysis for 3 months			Pulmonary fibrosis, aortic stenosis, cardiomyopathy, gout, arthritis	Allopurinol, aspirin, digoxin, erythropoietin, pravastatin, sertraline
7	46	Focal glomerulonephritis, nephrotic syndrome	None*			None	Prednisone
8	33	Type 2 diabetes	Hemodialysis for 4 months	Kidney	(3,24);(18,-);(-,-); (1,17)	Type 2 diabetes, transplant rejection/ thrombosis	Oral contraceptives, erythropoietin, furosemide, metoprolol, thyroxine
9	51	Chronic glomerulonephritis, cirrhosis	Peritoneal dialysis for 38 months	Kidney	(2,68);(39,50);(6,7); (7,16)	Cirrhosis, hypersplenism, failed kidney transplant	Erythropoietin, gabapentin, omeprazole
10	32	HELLP syndrome (hemolytic anemia, elevated liver enzymes, low platelets)	Hemodialysis for 1 week*			None	None
11	55	Hepatorenal syndrome	Hemodialysis for 1 month	Kidney	(2,23);(7,52);(-,-); (1,8)	Cirrhosis	Warfarin, cyclosporine, erythropoietin, metoprolol, prednisone, trazodone
12	56	Cyclosporine toxicity	Hemodialysis for 11 months	Liver	(2,30);(13,35);(4,-); (4,7)	Cirrhosis (ethanol, hepatitis C), myopathy	Cyclosporine, estrogen, erythropoietin, furosemide, prednisone, omeprazole, sertraline
13	53	Cyclosporine toxicity	Hemodialysis for 3 months	Liver	NA	Cardiomyopathy, biliary disease, gout, myopathy, thymoma	Allopurinol, doxazocin, colchicine, cyclosporine, erythropoietin, glyburide, prednisone, omeprazole

*Not undergoing dialysis at time of disease onset.

Abbreviations: −, Not tested for; *HLA,* human leukocyte antigen; NA, not available.

(Courtesy of Swartz RD, Crofford LJ, Phan SH, et al: Nephrogenic fibrosing dermopathy: A novel cutaneous fibrosing disorder in patients with renal failure. *Am J Med* 114:563-572, 2003, with permission of Excerpta Medica Inc.)

TABLE 2.—Laboratory Values at Time of Skin Biopsy

Patient	Sedimentation Rate	C-Reactive Protein	Parathormone	Calcium-Phosphate Product	Thyrotropin	Serum Iron	Total Iron Binding Capacity	Ferritin	Nuclear Cytoplastmic Antibody
1	3	0.5			2.2	64			—
2		1.1	85	<40	1.7	89	205		—
3	6	2.9		<30	2.5			6	—
4	117	8.1	<60	<40	6.5			124	—
5	14		173	<40	4.1	134	303	450	
6	48	15.8		<30	3.2	72	222	1460	
7		15.8	19	<55	2.2	54	170	1080	—
8	19	0.1	800		0.2	97	190	516	
9		6.4	187	<40		44	332	169	—
10	3	0.1	170		1.2	65	165	13	—
11	15	0.1	75	<40	5	119	153	9000	—
12			18	<50	1.1	81	203	115	
13	22	0.6	190			44	170	2290	

Antinuclear Antibody	SM,Scl 170	Complement 3	Complement 4	Serum Paraprotein	Hepatitic C Antibody	Hepatitis B Antibody	Antiphospholipid Antibody	Cryoglobulin	Other Findings
—	—			Polyclonal	—	+			Eosinophilia
—	—	Normal	Normal	Within normal					Eosinophilia
—		Normal	Normal	Within normal					
1:80 speckled	—	Normal	Normal	Polyclonal				—	Protein C and S
—		Normal	Normal	Elevated alpha	+	—		—	
	—			Antithyroid antibody					
—	—			Polyclonal	—	—	—	—	Rheumatoid factor
1:160 homogenous	—	Normal						—	Rheumatoid factor
—		Low	Normal	Polyclonal	—	—	+	+	
—	—	Low	Normal	Polyclonal	+	—	+	—	
—				Elevated alpha-globlulin	—	—			
				Polyclonal	+				
									Alpha-fetoprotein

Normal levels for select laboratory values: sedimentation rate, <20 mm/h; C-reactive protein, <1.0 mg/dL; parathormone, <75 pg/mL; calcium-phosphate product, <40; thyrotropin, <5.5 mU/L; serum iron, 30-150 µg/dL; total iron binding capacity, 210-400 µg/dL; ferritin, 20-320 ng/mL.

(Courtesy of Swartz RD, Crofford LJ, Phan SH, et al: Nephrogenic fibrosing dermopathy: A novel cutaneous fibrosing disorder in patients with renal failure. *Am J Med* 114:563-572, 2003, with permission of Excerpta Medica Inc.)

Methods.—Clinical and histopathologic data were reviewed in 13 patients from a single institution with the diagnosis of nephrogenic fibrosing dermopathy. Several clinical and laboratory parameters were examined to determine whether any consistently associated with the disease. Biopsy specimens were analyzed to determine whether a pattern existed in the evolution of fibrosis in these patients.

Results.—Renal disease was present in all 13 patients before disease onset; 8 patients were undergoing long-term hemodialysis, 2 were undergoing long-term peritoneal dialysis, and 3 with acute renal failure had never undergone dialysis before the development of dermopathy (Table 1). Most of the patients had other serious underlying medical conditions, and many of the patients were taking erythropoietin, cyclosporine, or both before the onset of disease. No histocompatibility antigens were found in association with nephrogenic fibrosing dermopathy in transplant patients. A variety of laboratory abnormalities were noted, but none was consistently associated with the disease (Table 2). In skin biopsy specimens obtained 7 to 180 days after disease onset, there were histopathologic changes suggestive of a tissue reaction to injury and the development of smooth muscle actin–positive myofibroblasts. There were 2 deaths during the follow-up period in this

TABLE 3.—Clinical Follow-up Since Diagnosis

Patient	Status	Days After Biopsy	Latest Skin Condition	Dialysis Modality Use
1	Surviving	900	Persisting	Chronic hemodialysis
2	Surviving	750	Persisting	None
3	Surviving	90	Persisting	Chronic hemodialysis
4	Died	60	Not applicable	Chronic peritoneal dialysis
5	Surviving	630	Persisting	Chronic hemodialysis
6	Surviving	810	Persisting	Chronic hemodialysis
7	Surviving	720	Partial improvement	None
8	Surviving	330	Persisting	Chronic hemodialysis
9	Surviving	510	Persisting	Chronic peritoneal dialysis
10	Surviving	660	Persisting	Acute hemodialysis*
11	Died	30	Not applicable	Chronic hemodialysis
12	Surviving	360	Persisting	Chronic hemodialysis
13	Surviving	480	Persisting	Chronic hemodialysis

*For 1 week after onset of dermopathy.
(Courtesy of Swartz RD, Crofford LJ, Phan SH, et al: Nephrogenic fibrosing dermopathy: A novel cutaneous fibrosing disorder in patients with renal failure. *Am J Med* 114:563-572, 2003, with permission of Excerpta Medica Inc.)

population, and among the remaining 11 patients there was no substantial improvement in skin condition (Table 3).

Conclusions.—Nephrogenic fibrosing dermopathy is distinguished from other sclerosing or fibrosing skin disorders by distinctive clinical and histopathologic findings that occur in the setting of renal failure. In the 13 patients examined in this study, renal failure was the only risk factor common to all patients; there were no additional clinical risk factors or laboratory findings common to these patients.

▶ Another disease with a long name, or something else? For most of the practicing pathologists, the importance of knowing this entity might be questionable. However, there are more and more patients with renal failure; and rest assured, there are more and more skin biopsies of "unusual lesions" on their extremities that will pose problems for the interpreting pathologist.

As the authors indicate, the histopathologic response and the biopsy features are similar to tissue injury reaction. In short, you will be faced with a tissue biopsy that will look fibrous (increase in connective tissue throughout resembling, but only resembling, morphea); at that point, one has to stop and ask about clinical history. Therefore, do not get tempted to call this biopsy a "scar." Ask for additional clinical history and evaluate the biopsy in depth.

This article is highly valuable; the authors describe 13 new patients with nephrogenic fibrosing dermopathy and painstakingly outline a variety of coexistent clinical and laboratory features, evaluate the biopsies with aid of immunohistochemistry, and draw valuable conclusions. In a nutshell, the authors in this study discuss the differential diagnosis of nephrogenic fibrosing dermopathy: scleromyxedema, scleredema, pretibial myxedema, eosinophilic fasciitis, eosinophilia/myalgia syndrome, Spanish toxic oil syndrome, and scleroderma/morphea, although indeed, histopathologically, the disease expresses similarities with scleromyxedema the most. This disorder is different than calci-phylaxis, although some authors have described disorders with overlap features.[1]

It is evident that, to be able to recognize the entity of nephrogenic fibrosing dermopathy, one needs to rule out all the above; often the differences are subtle. The article stresses clinicopathologic correlation; unusual variants of the above entities might not be distinguishable on the basis of histology alone. The authors admit that both etiology and pathogenesis are unknown (although one of the favored terms of modern medicine, idiopathic, is prob-ably not applicable); indeed, as they note, peculiar clustering of cases at ma-jor medical centers and transplant centers suggests either an infectious or toxic agent. The importance of myofibroblast and tumor growth factor β in wound healing as well as progression of lesions of nephrogenic fibrosing der-mopathy is stressed.

The authors further postulate that continuous proliferation of myofibro-blasts might be responsible for progression of individual lesions; they also sug-gest a possible role of vasculopathy, human leukocyte antigen (in)compatibil-ity, and antiphospholipid antibodies. Some other authors have also suggested role of altered or dysregulated matrix.[2]

In all honesty, this is one of the rare encyclopedic articles I have reviewed in last couple of years; it is really hard to outline it in a short review. My warmest recommendation (to anybody who is reviewing or diagnosing skin biopsies, or will do so in the near future) would be to read this article in detail; otherwise, you run the risk of missing this disease completely.

D. M. Jukic, MD, PhD

References

1. Edsall LC, English JC III, Patterson JW: Calciphylaxis and metastatic calcification associated with nephrogenic fibrosing dermopathy. *J Cutan Pathol* 31:247-253, 2004.
2. Hershko K, Hull C, Ettefagh L, et al: A variant of nephrogenic fibrosing derm-opathy with osteoclast-like giant cells: A syndrome of dysregulated matrix remod-eling? *J Cutan Pathol* 31:262-265, 2004.

9 Female Genital Tract

Frozen Section Examination of the Endocervical Margin of Cervical Conization Specimens
Rouzier R, Feyereisen E, Constancis E, et al (Centre Hospitalier Intercommunal de Créteil, France)
Gynecol Oncol 90:305-309, 2003   9–1

Introduction.—Determination of margin status via frozen section has been reported in breast and prostate carcinomas. There are no known data available regarding cervical cone biopsy specimens. The accuracy of frozen section examination of endocervical margin during cold knife conization was evaluated in a retrospective examination.

Methods.—A total of 310 consecutive patients underwent cervical conization for squamous intraepithelial lesions or stage IA1 cervical cancer between June 1993 and June 2001. Before 1997, the surgical specimens of 149 patients were processed after a standard pathologic procedure (historical group). After 1997, a frozen section of the upper endocervical margin was processed during surgery in 161 patients. In the presence of upper endocervical margin involvement, the surgeon performed a second resection, if possible. Results of frozen section examinations were compared with those of final diagnoses to ascertain sensitivity, specificity, and positive and negative predictive values. The usefulness of this procedure was assessed by comparing positive margin status incidence with that of the historical control group.

Results.—For the diagnosis of intraepithelial neoplasia involving the endocervical margin, the sensitivity, specificity, and positive and negative predictive values of frozen section were 91%, 100%, 100%, and 98%, respectively. Eleven patients had definitive positive endocervical margin in the frozen section group (3 false-negative results, 6 patients without additional resection, and 2 patients with intraepithelial neoplasia involving the upper margin of the additional resection), as did 17 patients in the historical group ($P = .16$) (Table 2).

Conclusion.—Frozen section investigation of the endocervical margin of cervical specimen obtained during cold knife conization is highly accurate.

▶ Cervical conization biopsy specimens can be among the most vexing sent to us in the pathology department. Many pathologists find that multiple levels are required to reconstruct the entire mucosal surface and margins of a very

TABLE 2.—Comparison of Frozen and Final Pathology
of Conization Specimen

	Final Pathology of Endocervical Margin		
	Negative	CIN I	CIN II/CIN III/ IA 1
Frozen section examination			
Negative	128	0	3
CIN I		2	9
CIN II/CIN III/IA 1			19
Historical group	132	2	15

(Courtesy of Rouzier R, Feyereisen E, Constancis E, et al: Frozen section examination of the endocervical margin of cervical conization specimens. *Gynecol Oncol* 90:305-309, 2003. Copyright 2003 by Elsevier Sceince Inc.)

complex 3-dimensional piece of tissue. Although most of us have been asked to do frozen sections to rule out invasive carcinoma before hysterectomy, many of us have little experience with intraoperative frozen sections for evaluation of conization margins. The data in these authors' Table 2 certainly suggest that these frozen sections can be very accurate, and tt is interesting to read about their methods. Apparently, the most proximal portion of the conization, including the margin, was amputated from the main specimen and embedded for frozen section as a donut of tissue similar to the way in which most of us section ureter margins at the time of transitional cell carcinoma resections. Although it is not stated in this article, the usual practice is to begin cutting sections from the nonmargin side of this tissue. Then, if dysplasia or carcinoma were identified, additional sections moving closer and closer to the true resection margin are then prepared. In this study, a frozen section analysis of the cervical cone margin was used to determine whether an additional specimen should be taken from the patient. It is also noteworthy that all these specimens were sharp (cold knife) cones. It seems to me that this procedure would be very difficult to adapt to LEEP cone samples. Whether this will ultimately result in fewer recurrences of cervical intraepithelial neoplasia remains to be seen. One limitation of this study seems to be the use of water-soluble embedding media and toluidine blue stains. Because these preparations are not permanent, coordinated central review of these margin samples would not have been possible as a part of this study. It is unclear how many individuals were involved in preparation and interpretation of these frozen sections or what the reproducibility of their interpretations might have been.

M. W. Stanley, MD

Frozen Section Evaluation of Cervical Cold Knife Cone Specimens Is Accurate in the Diagnosis of Microinvasive Squamous Cell Carcinoma

Giuntoli RI II, Winburn KA, Silverman MB, et al (Thomas Jefferson Univ, Philadelphia; Women's Specialty Ctr, Green Bay, Wis; Kaiser Permanente Med Ctr, San Diego, Calif; et al)
Gynecol Oncol 91:280-284, 2003 9–2

Introduction.—Cold knife conization (CKC) continues to have an important role in the assessment of cervical abnormalities. Pathologic findings from CKC govern subsequent patient management. The accuracy of frozen section assessment of CKC specimens in the diagnosis of microvascular squamous cell carcinoma (SCC) was evaluated.

Methods.—The 1986 through 1998 International Classification of Disease ninth revision (ICD-9) codes for invasive and microvascular carcinoma of the cervix were reviewed and identified 110 potential research subjects. For the diagnosis of microinvasion, Society of Gynecologic Gynecologists criteria were used: depth of invasion of 3 mm or less and the absence of lymph-vascular space involvement. A total of 27 patients met all criteria, including frozen section diagnosis of SCC on a cervical CKC specimen. A pathologist who was blinded to patient diagnosis reassessed histologic findings, including grade, depth of invasion, and cell type.

Results.—Median age at the time of diagnosis was 41 years and median follow-up was 3.6 years. The median time for pathologic examination was 28 minutes (15-44 minutes). The independent pathologic review of the permanent sections verified the diagnosis of microinvasion in 100% (27/27) of the cohort (Table 2). There were no cervical SCC recurrences. The disease-specific survival was 100% at 10 years.

Conclusion.—Frozen section is reliable in the assessment of CKC specimens with microinvasive SCC. This may provide a simplified approach in

TABLE 2.—Comparison of Pathologic Evaluations of 17 CKC Specimens by Frozen Section, Permanent Section, and Retrospective Blinded Review

Characteristic	Frozen Section	Permanent	Reevaluation
Invasion range in mm	0.3-3.0	1.0-3.0	0.3-3.0
	No. (%)	No. (%)	No. (%)
Microinvasive SCC	27 (100)	27 (100)	27 (100)
LVI	0 (0)	0 (0)	0 (0)
Any positive margin	13 (48)	13 (48)	13 (48)
Microinvasive positive margin	3 (11)	3 (11)	3 (11)
Grade			
1	N/A	0 (0)	0 (0)
2	N/A	25 (93)	25 (93)
3	N/A	2 (7)	2 (7)

Abbreviations: LVI, Lymph vascular space invasion; *SCC,* squamous cell carcinoma; *re-evaluation,* all specimens subjected to blinded retrospective review by a single pathologist.

(Courtesy of Giuntoli RL II, Winburn KA, Silverman MB, et al: Frozen section evaluation of cervical cold knife cone specimens is accurate in the diagnosis of microinvasive squamous cell carcinoma. *Gynecol Oncol* 91:280-284, 2003. Copyright 2003 by Elsevier Science Inc.)

some cases. The accuracy of these findings cannot be assumed to apply to adenocarcinoma or adenosquamous carcinoma of the cervix. The use of CKC in this cohort did not impact disease-free survival.

▶ This article looks at issues similar to those discussed in the last article (Abstract 9–1). Both use frozen section analysis applied to CKC specimens. However, the focus in this article is not evaluation of margins for resections of intraepithelial neoplasia, but is for identification of microinvasive SCC of the uterine cervix. It should be noted that in this Mayo Clinic study, the technique and instruments of frozen section preparation are not those used in most other pathology laboratories. The degree to which these results can be generalized to the rest of us remains to be seen. Furthermore, review of the actual toluidine blue-stained frozen section material would not have been possible in this study design. Also, in literature reviewed by the authors, problems with some previous evaluations of microinvasion by frozen section are described.

M. W. Stanley, MD

Evaluation of MIB-1-Positive Cell Clusters as a Diagnostic Marker for Cervical Intraepithelial Neoplasia
Kruse A-J, Baak JPA, Helliesen T, et al (Rogaland Central Hosp, Stavanger, Norway; Vrije Universiteit, Amsterdam)
Am J Surg Pathol 26:1501-1507, 2002   9–3

Introduction.—Earlier reports have demonstrated that MIB-1 immunostaining can be valuable as an adjunct to histopathologic routine evaluation in distinguishing cervical intraepithelial neoplasia (CIN) from non-neoplastic lesions that may mimic CIN. Seventy-seven consecutive cervical specimens routinely diagnosed (Dx_orig) as CIN 1 (Fig 2) or 2, or no-CIN, were re-examined to determine whether the application of the MIB-1-positive cell cluster (ie, a cluster of at least 2 stained nearby nuclei in the upper two thirds of the epithelial thickness) aids in the distinction between histologic low-grade CIN lesions and normal, metaplastic, and reactive cervical epithelia.

Methods.—All 77 specimens were independently revised by 2 expert gynecopathologists. Both MIB-1 staining and oncogenic human papillomavirus (HPV) evaluation (via polymerase chain reaction) were conducted. Independent diagnoses (plus oncogenic HPV status, in the event of a disagreement between reviewers) were used to determine a final diagnosis (Dx_final); these were compared with MIB-C.

Results.—Four (15%) of Dx_final = normal were HPV positive. Agreement between reviewers was 94% (72/77). Thirty (39%) discrepancies were observed between Dx_orig and Dx_final (23 = 30% downgrades; 7 = 9% upgrades). The 23 downgrades were HPV negative and the 7 upgrades were

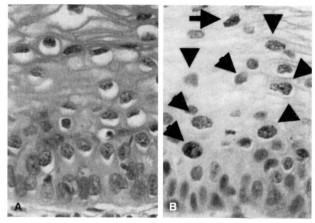

FIGURE 2.—Example of a CIN 1 lesion (**A**) (hematoxylin and eosin) with (**B**) MIB-1-positive cell clusters (*arrows*). (Courtesy of Kruse A-J, Baak JPA, Helliesen T, et al: Evaluation of MIB-1-positive cell clusters as a diagnostic marker for cervical intraepithelial neoplasia. *Am J Surg Pathol* 26:1501-1507, 2002.)

HPV positive. The overall agreement between Dx-orig and MIB-C was 73%; agreement for Dx_final was 99%. Sensitivity, specificity, and positive and negative predictive values for MIB-C were very high and there were no false-negative results (Table 5).

Discussion/Conclusion.—Tangential cutting of MIB-1-positive parabasal cells and inflammatory cells can be falsely overdiagnosed as MIB-C (Fig 3). One single false-positive result of the 48 non-CIN cases (an immature squamous metaplasia) demonstrated a special, easily recognizable MIB-1 pattern (Fig 5), which was different from CIN (the MIB-1 staining in the nuclei was not diffuse as in CIN) and was clumped. Positive nuclei are somewhat less

TABLE 5.—Correlation Between the Final Diagnosis and the MIB-1 Positive Cell Cluster

Final Diagnosis	MIB-1-Positive Cell Cluster		Total
	Negative	Positive	
No-CIN	47	1	48
CIN	0	29	29
Total	47	30	77

Overall agreement = (47 + 29)/77 × 100 = 99%.
Sensitivity (no-CIN vs CIN) = 29 (29 + 0) × 100 = 100%.
Specificity (no-CIN vs CIN) = 47 (47 + 1) × 100 = 98%.
Positive predictive value (no-CIN vs CIN) = 29 (29 + 1) × 100 = 97%.
Negative predictive value (no-CIN vs CIN) = 47 (47 + 0) × 100 = 100%.
(Courtesy of Kruse A-J, Baak JPA, Helliesen T, et al: Evaluation of MIB-1-positive cell clusters as a diagnostic marker for cervical intraepithelial neoplasia. *Am J Surg Pathol* 26:1501-1507, 2002.)

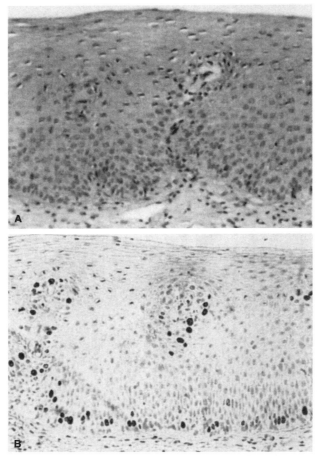

FIGURE 3.—Tangentially cut epithelium: (**A**) Hematoxylin and eosin. (**B**) MIB-1, with many MIB-1-positive cell clusters in the "upper two thirds" of the epithelium. This is clearly a false-positive result. Tangential cutting is evident in such a case by intraepithelial stroma with or without capillaries and/or remarkable concentric parabasal cells in the higher parts of the epithelium. (Courtesy of Kruse A-J, Baak JPA, Helliesen T, et al: Evaluation of MIB-1-positive cell clusters as a diagnostic marker for cervical intraepithelial neoplasia. *Am J Surg Pathol* 26:1501-1507, 2002.)

densely packed, compared with CIN. When tangentially cut parabasal cells and inflammatory cells are meticulously excluded, MIB-C is a strong diagnostic adjunct in distinguishing CIN from normal or benign squamoepithelial lesions.

▶ If we are to use MIB-1 immunostaining as a potential marker of CIN, it is essential that the definition of positivity be as uniform as possible. Both in this article and in the literature cited, a MIB-1 positive cluster was carefully defined as 2 or more nearby positively staining cells located in the upper two thirds of the epithelial thickness. Immunostaining confined to the lower levels of the

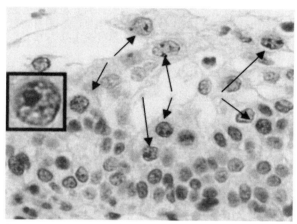

FIGURE 5.—Immature squamous metaplasia can be MIB-1 cluster positive. This false-positive case showed a special, easily recognizable MIB-1 staining pattern, different from CIN, as the MIB-1 staining in the nuclei is not diffuse (as in CIN) but clumped (inset, nucleus at higher magnification). Moreover, positive nuclei (*arrows*) are somewhat less densely packed than in CIN. (Courtesy of Kruse A-J, Baak JPA, Helliesen T, et al: Evaluation of MIB-1-positive cell clusters as a diagnostic marker for cervical intraepithelial neoplasia. *Am J Surg Pathol* 26:1501-1507, 2002.)

epithelium is not sufficient. Furthermore, the authors carefully describe and illustrate false-positive staining in which positive cell clusters that appear to be high in the epithelium are actually very close to tangentially sectioned connected tissue extensions, thus representing a part of the parabasal epithelial cell compartment. Improved recognition of low-grade squamous intraepithelial lesions is desirable. However, the distinction of some such cases from what the authors refer to as atypical immature squamous metaplasia remains difficult, even when special testing is brought to bear on the material. Furthermore, current trends in clinical management seem to emphasize the importance of high-grade lesions and downplay the importance of low-grade lesions. So far, this mindset seems to have impacted the practice of gynecologic cytopathology more than surgical pathology.

M. W. Stanley, MD

Multiple High Risk HPV Infections Are Common in Cervical Neoplasia and Young Women in a Cervical Screening Population

Cuschieri KS, Cubie HA, Whitley MW, et al (Royal Infirmary of Edinburgh, Scotland)

J Clin Pathol 57:68-72, 2004   9–4

Introduction.—Accumulating evidence indicates that persistent infection with the same high-risk human papillomavirus (HR-HPV) type may place patients at greater risk of progression of cervical neoplasia. The degree and importance of multiple HR-HPV infections in the progression of cervical neoplasia and its management remains unknown. If HPV testing is to be included with cervical screening programs, the significance of multiple HPV infections needs to be determined. The diversity of multiple HPV types was evaluated in a routine cervical screening population; associations with cervical neoplasia were examined.

Methods.—The overall HPV prevalence, type specific prevalence, and extent of multiple infections were examined in residual material from 3444 liquid-based cytology samples via real-time GP5+/GP6+ polymerase chain reaction for screening and linear array assay for genotyping. The HPV status was assessed in relation to age and concurrent cytologic evidence of dyskaryosis.

Results.—Of the 3444 samples tested, 705 (20%) were HPV positive. About 10% exhibited some degree of cytologic neoplastic abnormality, including 3.3% borderline dyskaryosis, 3.7% mild dyskaryosis, and 2.7% high-grade dyskaryosis. The HPV type diversity was broad and multiple HPV infections eventuated in half of the HPV positive samples. Younger women were significantly more likely to experience multiple HR-HPV infections. Infections with multiple HR-HPV types were detected in 3.4% of samples negative for neoplasia, and in 33.3%, 41.8%, and 40.4% of samples with borderline, mild, or high-grade dyskaryosis, respectively (Table 2). Single HR-HPV infections were identified in 4.9%, 38.6%, 45.0%, and 51.1% of negative, mild, or high-grade dyskaryosis samples, respectively (Fig 1).

Conclusion.—Multiple HR-HPV infections were most prevalent in young women. Multiple HR-HPV infections were not more common in high-grade versus low-grade cervical neoplasia, reflecting common sexual transmission

TABLE 2.—Prevalence of Multiple HPV Infections According to Cytologic Grade of Dyskaryosis and Age

	Multiple HPV Infection	Total Single HR-HPV +ve	Total Multiple HR-HPV +ve
Dyskaryosis			
Negative	139 (4.5)	152 (5.0)	105 (3.4)
Borderline	50 (43.8)	44 (38.6)	38 (33.3)
Mild	73 (56.6)	58 (44.9)	54 (41.8)
High grade	43 (45.7)	48 (51.1)	38 (40.4)
U/S	1 (5.5)	2	1 (5.5)
Age			
<25	186 (25.3)	113 (15.4)	147 (20.0)
25-35	78 (8.3)	97 (10.4)	61 (6.5)
35-45	28 (3.1)	61 (6.8)	19 (2.1)
45-55	11 (1.8)	26 (4.3)	7 (1.2)
>55	3 (1.1)	7 (2.5)	2 (0.7)
Total	306	304	236

Values are numbers of samples and percentages in parenthesis. Multiple HPV infection, sample tested positive for > HPV type by LA assay. Total single HR-HPV +ve, sample tested positive for a single HR-HPV infection, either alone or with other LR-HPV types present. Total multiple HR-HPV +ve samples tested positive for >1 HR-HPV type (sample could have combined LR-HPV types also).

Abbreviations: HPV, Human papillomavirus; *HR*, high risk; *LA*, linear array; *LR*, low risk; *U/S*, unsatisfactory.

(Courtesy of Cushieri KS, Cubie HA, Whitley MW, et al: Multiple high risk HPV infections are common in cervical neoplasia and young women in a cervical screening population. *J Clin Pathol* 57:68-72, 2004. With permission from the BMJ Publishing Group.)

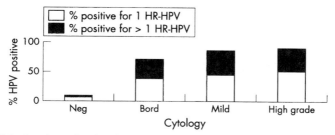

FIGURE 1.—Prevalence of single and multiple high-risk human papillomavirus (HR-HPV) infections associated with concurrent cytologic grade of dyskaryosis. *Abbreviations: Neg*, Negative for dyskaryosis; *Bord*, borderline dyskaryosis; *Mild*, mild dyskaryosis; *High-grade*, moderate or severe dyskaryosis or suspected invasion. (Courtesy of Cushieri KS, Cubie HA, Whitley MW, et al: Multiple high risk HPV infections are common in cervical neoplasia and young women in a cervical screening population. *J Clin Pathol* 57:68-72, 2004.)

of multiple HR-HPV. Prospective cohort investigations linking sequential loss or gain of HPV types with cytologic analysis are needed to evaluate the impact of multiple HR-HPV infections on neoplastic progression.

▶ The results of this study are not surprising. However, their clinical implications remain to be evaluated. The relevant importance to cervical carcinogenesis of multiple HR HPV types versus persistent infection with 1 or a few types is unknown at this time. Another issue from this study is the fact that the methods used to identify HPV in these samples (polymerase chain reaction) is a much more sensitive detection method than that used in most routine clinical work. As with other studies, a certain rate of HPV positivity was detected in patients without evidence of disease. In this regard, identification of HPV-26 only in cytologically abnormal samples is very interesting and strongly supports its suggested role as a carcinogenic virus type.

M. W. Stanley, MD

Prognostic Value and Reproducibility of Koilocytosis in Cervical Intraepithelial Neoplasia
Kruse A-J, Baak JPA, Helliesen T, et al (Rogaland Central Hosp, Stavanger, Norway; Vrije Universiteit, Amsterdam; Duke Univ, Durham, NC)
Int J Gynecol Pathol 22:236-239, 2003   9–5

Introduction.—Virus-induced warts in the skin usually exhibit prominent perinuclear vacuolization and atypical nuclei. Similar changes in cervical cells are known as koilocytotic atypia, a finding seen both in cytologic smears and histologic biopsies with dysplasia and invasive carcinoma. The influence of koilocytosis on the progression of cervical intraepithelial neoplasia (CIN) to a higher grade during follow-up was examined in cervical specimens with CIN 1 and 2.

Methods.—In adequate, consecutive, biopsy specimens of 103 CIN 1 and 2 patients, the CIN grade and presence or absence of koilocytosis were evaluated. Patients underwent colposcopy and cytology according to proto-

TABLE 2.—Progression Rates in CIN 1 and CIN 2 Groups With and Without Koilocytosis

| | CIN 1 | | CIN 2 | | |
	KC Negative	KC Positive	KC Negative	KC Positive	Total
No progression	8 (73%)	18 (100%)	14 (65%)	42 (9%)	82 (80%)
Progression	3 (27%)	0 (0%)	8 (35%)	10 (21)	21 (20%)
Subtotal	11 (38%)	18 (62%)	22 (30%)	52 (70%)	
Total	29 (28%)		74 (72%)		103 (100%)

Abbreviation: KC, Koilocytosis.
(Courtesy of Kruse A-J, Baak JPA, Helliesen T, et al: Prognostic value of reproducibility of koilocytosis in cervical intraepithelial neoplasia. *Int J Gynecol Pathol* 22:236-239, 2003.)

col. When recurrent CIN was suspected with either of the methods, a re-biopsy was obtained. Progression of CIN was defined as an increase in grade by at least 1. Univariate analysis was used for the overall cohort and in the CIN 1 and 2 subgroups separately. Koilocytosis was assessed by an experienced gynecologic pathologist using strict criteria. Interobserver reproducibility of koilocytosis was evaluated via the Kappa test.

Results.—Koilocytosis was observed in 70 (68%) specimens (18/29, 62% of CIN 1 cases; 52/74, 70% of CIN 2 cases). Twenty-one of 103 (20%) dysplasias progressed, 10 (48%) of which exhibited koilocytosis. Koilocytosis was observed more often (60/82; 73%) in cases that demonstrated no progression. Patients with koilocytosis had a significantly lower likelihood of progression ($P = .02$). In the CIN 1 group, progression with and without koilocytosis was 27% and 0%, respectively ($P = .03$). In the CIN 2 group, a similar trend was observed; only 19% (10/52) of CIN 2 cases with koilocytosis progressed; 36% (8/22) of lesions lacking koilocytosis progressed, which was a difference just below significance ($P = .06$) (Table 2). In agreement with earlier trials, interobserver diagnosis of koilocytosis was poorly reproducible.

Conclusion.—The presence of koilocytosis is linked with a lack of progression in CIN 1 lesions; reproducibility of koilocytosis evaluation is not optimal. Other more objective and better reproducible criteria are needed to extract the potentially important prognostic information contained in the microscopic image of CIN 1 and 2 lesions.

▶ As emphasized in recently revised Papanicolaou (Pap) test diagnostic terminology, current clinical practices emphasize identification and treatment of high-grade dysplasias and place relatively less emphasis on the importance of low-grade lesions. Thus, it would be highly desirable to have some means of predicting which low-grade lesions are likely to progress and which are not. These authors evaluate the potential use of koilocyte identification in this regard, and the results are not surprising. One difficulty inherent in studies such as this is the definition of progression. Given the enormous problem and unknowable extent of sampling error in cervical cytology and biopsies, the possibility that a higher-grade lesion was missed on initial studies and then more successfully targeted on subsequent biopsies, always exists. Thus, a description of progression rates is offered by these authors and reviewed in the literature cited must always be viewed with some skepticism. The suggestion that koilocytosis indicates lower-grade lesions that are not likely to progress is interesting and of potential clinical use. An additional difficulty in reading this literature is the extremely subjective nature of histologic diagnoses of low-grade dysplasia. It is ironic that these lesions are among the most straightforward in Pap test diagnosis but subject to considerable uncertainty in biopsy specimens. Paralleling this is the authors' description of poor reproducibility in recognition of koilocytes. Some evidence suggests that development of readily identifiable koilocytes is likely to be associated with low-risk HPV types. The extent of which identification of koilocytosis will ultimately be shown to indicate a low-risk of progression deserves further study. The authors' comments regarding the potential use of Ki-67 analyses are also important, as emphasized by other articles in this series.

M. W. Stanley, MD

Measurement of Brn-3a Levels in Pap Smears Provides a Novel Diagnostic Marker for the Detection of Cervical Neoplasia

Sindos M, Ndisang D, Pisal N, et al (Univ College London; Whittington Hosp, London)
Gynecol Oncol 90:366-371, 2003   9–6

Introduction.—It has been shown that Brn-3a cellular transcription factor activates transcription of the human papillomavirus (HPV) E6 and E7 oncogenes in human cervical cells. The Brn-3a levels are greatly elevated in biopsies from women with high-grade cervical neoplasia. The association between Brn-3a levels in Papanicolaou (Pap) smears and the histologic diagnosis was assessed, along with whether Brn-3a levels can be used in combination with Pap smears to predict the presence of cervical intraepithelial lesions.

Methods.—A total of 238 women referred with abnormal Pap smears underwent a diagnostic colposcopy, repeat in-study Pap smear, colposcopically directed biopsy, and evaluation of Brn-3a and HPV-16 E6 messenger RNA

TABLE 1.—Brn-3a and E6 Levels in Pap Smears from Patients Categorized on the Basis of the Histologic Diagnosis

			Mean Value	
Category	Count	Percentage	Brn-3a	E6
Negative	74	31%	0.201	0.125
LGSIL (HPV–CIN1)	83	35%	0.259	0.231
HGSIL (CIN2–CIN3)	79	33%	0.438	0.358
Cancer	2	1%	0.575	0.475
Total	238	100%	—	—

(Courtesy of Sindos M, Ndisang D, Pisal N, et al: Measurement of Brn-3a levels in Pap smears provides a novel diagnostic marker for the detection of cervical neoplasia. *Gynecol Oncol* 90:366-371, 2003. Copyright 2003 by Elsevier Science Inc.)

TABLE 4.—Prediction of Histologic Diagnosis by Smear Alone or by Smear Analysis and Measurement of Brn-3a Level

Histological Diagnosis	Total No. of Patients	In-Study Smear Availability	Smear Correct	Smear Positive but Discordant With Histology	Totally Missed by Pap Smear (Negatives + Inadequates)	Detected by Pap Smear as Lesion of any Degree	Combined Pap Smear and Brn-3a
LGSIL	83	71	39 (55%)	8 (11.2%)	24 (19+5) (33.8%) Brn-3a − 6 + 18	47 (66.2%)	65 (91.6%)
HGSIL/cancer	81	67	46 (68.7%)	14 (20.9%)	7 (5+2) (10.4%) Brn-3a − 2 + 5	60 (89.6%)	65 (97%)
Total (LGSIL, HGSIL/cancer)	164	138	85 (61.6%)	22 (15.9%)	31 (24+7) (22.5%)	107 (77.5%)	130 (94.2%)

(Courtesy of Sindos M, Ndisang D, Pisal N, et al: Measurement of Brn-3a levels in Pap smears provides a novel diagnostic marker for the detection of cervical neoplasia. *Gynecol Oncol* 90:366-371, 2003. Copyright 2003 by Elsevier Science Inc.)

TABLE 4.—Sensitivity, Specificity, Positive (PPV) and Negative (NPV) Predictive Value for Different Screening Techniques

	Conventional Cytology	LBC	HPV Testing by PCR	HPV Testing by HCII	0.2 ASCUS	0.2 HSIL	0.4 ASCUS	0.4 HSIL
Sensitivity	52.0 to 68.0	61.3 to 87.0	88.2 to 91.0	73.3 to 100	68.0	90.0	51.0	75.0
Specificity	52.8 to 95.0	82.4 to 93.0	78.8	62.3 to 87.3	61.0	61.0	73.0	73.0
PPV	23.5 to 60.	15.7	ND	14.2 to 88.3	87.1	66.7	88.5	71.4
NPV	43.8 to 99.3	99.8	ND	62.3 to 100	32.6	87.5	27.9	77.3

Data from the literature are given in percentages. Complementary diagnostic indices are given for 2 thresholds of Ki-67 immunochemistry in 2 different diagnostic circumstances. 0.2/0.4 ASCUS/HSIL represents a threshold of 0.2/0.4 Ki-67 immunopositive cells/1000 cells for the diagnosis of ASCUS/HSIL.

Abbreviations: ASCUS, Atypical squamous cells of undetermined significance; *HCII,* Hybrid Capture II (Digene); *HPV,* human papillomavirus; *HSIL,* high-grade squamous intraepithelial lesion; *LBC,* liquid-based cytology; *ND,* no data; *PCR,* polymerase chain reaction.

(Reprinted with permission by BMJ Publishing Group from Sahebali S, Depuydt CE, Seegers K, et al: Ki-67 immunocytochemistry in liquid based cervical cytology: Useful as an adjunctive tool? *J Clin Pathol* 56:681-686, 2003.)

Results.—Comparison of the number of Ki-67 immunoreactive cells per 1000 cells in the different cytologic groups revealed that the high-grade squamous intrapeithelial lesion (HSIL) group produced a significantly higher mean count compared with the other groups (Fig 2). The number of Ki-67 immunoreactive cells per 1000 cells was significantly higher in HPV-16 positive samples compared with samples containing infections with other high-risk types (Fig 3). Receiver operating characteristic curves showed a test accuracy (area under the curve) of 0.68, 0.72, and 0.86 for atypical squamous cells of undetermined significance (ASCUS), low-grade squamous intraepithelial lesions (LSIL), and HSIL, respectively. The thresholds for 95% sensitivity were 0.07, 0.08, and 0.15 Ki-67 immunopositive cells per 1000 cells for ASCUS, LSIL, and HSIL, respectively. For 95% specificity, the threshold was 1.9 Ki-67 immunopositive cells per 1000 cells (Table 4).

Conclusion.—It appears that Ki-67 immunocytochemistry can be applied to liquid-based cytology. The accuracy and diagnostic indices of the test are good versus those of other methods. As part of a panel of screening procedures, it could be used as an adjunct to liquid-based cytology to detect HSIL, and as a surrogate marker of HPV-16 infection.

▶ An earlier article in this series reviewed application of Ki-67 (monoclonal antibody MIB-1) studies in evaluation of cervical biopsy specimens. These authors focus on similar analyses in Papanicolaou (Pap) test samples. This progression is a natural one, and it is likely that some measure of epithelial cell proliferative activity will be included in Pap testing in the future. This article makes a number of methodologic steps forward that will probably serve as models for future studies. First, these authors use Bethesda System (2001) recommendations for determination of the number of cells under evaluation. Although these are not standardized and not yet a part of routine clinical practice for many laboratories, they probably represent the best cell enumeration method that does not rely on image analysis techniques. Furthermore, the authors' expression of Ki-67 labeling as the number of positive cells per 1000 cells evaluated is sensible and easy to grasp. An interesting feature that this article has in common with the previous article in this series is the suggestion that this testing method might be used to improve Pap test diagnosis and that some false-negative cases might be identified by ancillary testing. Another potential advantage is resolution of classical problems in cytology such as lowering the number of patients with ASCUS and distinguishing atrophy from proliferative lesions.

M. W. Stanley, MD

The Proto-Oncogene c-kit Is Expressed in Leiomyosarcomas of the Uterus

Wang L, Felix JC, Lee JL, et al (Univ of Southern California, Los Angeles)
Gynecol Oncol 90:402-406, 2003   9–8

Introduction.—The proto-oncogene c-kit, the cellular homologue of the oncogene v-kit of HZ4 feline sarcoma virus, encodes for a 145-kD transmembrane tyrosine kinase receptor. Interaction with its ligand, stem cell factor, is crucial to the development of hematopoietic stem cells, mast cells, gametocytes, melanocytes, and interstitial cells of Cajal. C-kit expression has been observed in several different neoplasms, including mastocytosis/mast cells leukemia, acute myeloblastic leukemia, seminoma/dysgerminoma, and gastrointestinal stromal cells. The c-kit expression was examined in uterine endometrial stromal sarcomas, leiomyomas, and leiomyosarcomas with the use of immunohistochemistry.

Methods.—Archival tissue from 38 patients with uterine mesenchymal tumors (16 leiomyosarcomas, 8 leiomyomas, 11 low-grade endometrial stromal sarcomas, and 3 high-grade endometrial stromal sarcomas) was stained with the use of polyclonal antibody for c-kit. A modified avidin biotin (ABC) immunoperoxidase technique was used for antibody identification. Individual tumors were regarded as positive if more than 10% of the cells of the neoplasm exhibited immunoreactive staining. Staining intensity was graded 1+ to 3+ and distribution was graded as focal (10% to 30% of the cells), intermediate (30% to 60% of the cells) or diffuse (>60% of the cells).

Results.—C-kit was positive in 12 of 16 (75%) leiomyosarcomas. Staining was 3+ and diffuse in most of the positive tumors. There was no c-kit expression in any of the 8 leiomyosarcomas. Two of the 3 high-grade endometrial stromal sarcomas expressed c-kit positivity; staining was diffuse and 3+ in both tumors. Expression of c-kit was seen in 3 of 11 low-grade endometrial stromal sarcomas (Table 1).

Conclusion.—C-kit is expressed in both uterine leiomyosarcomas and endometrial stroma sarcomas. Adjunctive diagnostic testing with the use of

TABLE 1.—Summary of C-kit Expression in the Different Uterine Mesenchymal Tumors Showing Distribution and Intensity of the Observed Immunostaining

Tumor Type	*n*	Positive (%)	Focal	Intermediate	Diffuse	1+	2+	3+
				Distribution			Intensity	
Leiomyoma	8	0 (0%)	0	0	0	0	0	0
Leiomyosarcoma	16	12 (75%)	0	3	9	0	1	11
LGESS	11	3 (28%)	0	1	2	0	2	1
HGESS	3	2 (67%)	0	0	2	0	0	2

Abbreviations: LGESS, Low-grade endometrial stroma sarcoma; *HGESS*, high-grade endometrial stroma sarcoma.
(Courtesy of Wang L, Felix JC, Lee JL, et al: The proto-oncogene c-kit is expressed in leiomyosarcomas of the uterus. *Gynecol Oncol* 90:402-406, 2003. Copyright 2003 by Elsevier Science Inc.)

c-kit may be helpful in distinguishing leiomyosarcomas from benign leiomyomas in uterine tumors with uncharacteristic features.

▶ As noted elsewhere in these commentaries, the number of neoplasms in which c-kit expression as assessed by immunostaining for CD117 continues to grow. This article essentially describes a pilot study, and the selection of cases is certainly very sensible. Given our longstanding difficulties in confident distinction between some examples of stromal sarcoma and some examples of smooth muscle tumors in the uterine corpus, the overlap between these 2 groups in c-kit expression is very interesting. However, the result in this study with the most obvious potential clinical implication is the difference in c-kit expression between leiomyosarcomas and leiomyomas. In most such studies, clear-cut examples of these entities would have been selected. Given the striking nature of these results, it would be fascinating to see CD117 immunostaining applied to a greater number of smooth muscle tumors. Furthermore, investigation of atypical cases or those in which an assignment of biologic potential is difficult would be interesting. One could also envision a survey of other soft tissue tumors in an effort to determine other areas of potential use for this procedure. It is also reasonable to envision fast-tract trials of new drugs with tyrosine kinase inhibitory activity for patients with metastatic uterine sarcomas. The authors of this study are careful to emphasize the details of immunohistochemical technique. On the basis of their review of earlier studies, it seems that antigen retrieval may be a necessary part of such procedures.

M. W. Stanley, MD

Clinicopathological Analysis of *c-kit* Expression in Carcinosarcomas and Leiomyosarcomas of the Uterine Corpus
Winter WE III, Seidman JD, Krivak TC, et al (Walter Reed Army Med Ctr, Washington, DC; Washington Hosp Ctr, DC; Natl Cancer Inst, Rockville, Md)
Gynecol Oncol 91:3-8, 2003   9–9

Introduction.—Given the histologic similarities between uterine leiomyosacromas and gastrointestinal stromal tumors (GIST) and the presence of KIT in normal uterine tissue, it is possible that uterine sarcomas may have the same c-kit expression pattern as those of GIST. Tumor specimens were examined for c-kit expression in uterine sarcomas, including carcinosarcomas, leiomyosarcomas, and endometrial stroma sarcomas. The link between c-kit expression and clinicopathologic factors, including clinical outcome, was examined.

Methods.—Immunohistochemical staining was conducted on formalin-fixed paraffin-embedded tissue blocks with the use of a polyclonal anti-KIT-antibody. Twenty-one, 17, and 1, respectively, carcinosarcomas, leiomyosarcomas, and endometrial stromal sarcoma were examined. The KIT-positive tumors were defined as tumors that exhibit immunopositivity in 30% or more of the tumor cells examined; KIT-negative lesions were considered to exhibit immunopositivity in less than 30% of the tumor cells. Two

TABLE 1.—Association Between Tumor Histology and *C-kit* Expression*

Tumor Histology	Total	KIT Positive (%)	*P* Value
Carcinosarcoma	21	9 (43)	0.029†
Homologous	13	4 (31)	
Heterologous	7	4 (57)	
Leiomyosarcomas	17	1 (6)	
Endometrial stromal sarcoma	1	0 (0)	
Total	39	10 (26)	

*Based on all evaluable formalin-fixed, paraffin-embedded tumor specimens.

†Pearson's χ^2 comparing expression among the carcinosarcomas, leiomyosarcomas, and endometrial stroma sarcoma.

(Courtesy of Winter WE III, Seidman JD, Krivak TC, et al: Clinicopathological analysis of *c-kit* expression in carcinosarcomas and leiomyosarcomas of the uterine corpus. *Gynecol Oncol* 91:3-8, 2003. Copyright 2003 by Elsevier Science Inc.)

reviewers independently score the slides as positive or negative. Staining was repeated on all specimens, which were independently scored. A third staining was performed in the presence of a mismatch. The carcinosarcomas were catalogued according to whether the sarcomatous and/or carcinomatous elements expressed c-kit. Clinical data were documented for patients with uterine carcinosarcomas. The link between clinicopathologic characteristics and c-kit expression were compared via univariate and multivariate analyses. Progression-free and overall survival were calculated.

Results.—Nine of 21 (43%) carcinosarcomas exhibited immunopositivity for the KIT receptor; staining was relatively weak. One of 17 (6%) leiomyosarcomas exhibited KIT immunopositivity (P = .029) (Table 1). The solitary endometrial stromal sarcoma did not exhibit significant KIT positivity. Most of the KIT-positive carcinosarcomas (6/9; 67%) exhibited KIT presence in the sarcomatous portion compared with the carcinomatous portion (4/9; 44%). No clinical characteristic had a statistically significant link with c-kit expression. The lack of c-kit expression was the only factor significantly correlated with disease recurrence in both univariate and multivariate analyses (P < .05); there seemed to be a trend toward a low stage associated with kit positivity. Median progression-free interval among KIT-

TABLE 3.—Disease Recurrence by *C-kit* Expression*

Disease Status	Total	KIT Positive (%)	*P* Value
Disease free	8	6 (67)	0.019†
Recurrence	12	2 (18)	
Regional	2	1 (50)	0.350‡
Distant	8	1 (13)	
Persistent	2	0 (0)	

*Median follow-up 15 ± 10.2 months (range, 1-35).

†Pearson's α^2 test.

‡Fisher exact test.

(Courtesy of Winter WE III, Seidman JD, Krivak TC, et al: Clinicopathological analysis of *c-kit* expression in carcinosarcomas and leiomyosarcomas of the uterine corpus. *Gynecol Oncol* 91:3-8, 2003. Copyright 2003 by Elsevier Science Inc.)

negative participants was 8 months; this had not been reached for the KIT-positive cohort after a median follow-up of 15 months ($P = .0462$) (Table 3).

Conclusion.—A significant proportion of carcinosarcomas of the uterine corpus exhibit immunoreactivity for c-kit. Patients with KIT-positive carcinosarcomas may experience improved progression-free survival versus those with KIT-negative tumors.

▶ In view of the previous article in this series, the most striking conclusion by the authors of the current article is that leiomyosarcomas do not show immunoreactive c-kit expression. Such a striking difference regarding what would be a clinically useful diagnostic maneuver compels us to compare the methods section of these 2 articles. Both groups of investigators used a polyclonal antibody. Some differences are noted in the antigen retrieval methods, and this may be a point that merits clarification in future articles. Another point is interpretation of positive results. Both studies used a semiquantitative assessment of the fraction of total tumor cells positive for c-kit immunostaining. In the previous study showing positive staining for many leiomyosarcomas, tumors showing only 10% positive staining were interpreted as positive, whereas in the current study many leiomyosarcomas were negative, based on a requirement that 30% of cells show positive staining. Although neither method of interpretation was precise, this might account for some differences in final results. Thus, as the c-kit immunostaining literature continues to explode, some agreement regarding methods and interpretation will probably be required if we are to see meaningful results emerge. As we have suggested elsewhere, c-kit immunoreactivity shines a fascinating light on certain aspects of tumor biology. However, the most compelling reason for "getting it right" is that pharmacologic agents active against tumors with this abnormal molecular phenotype are now clinically available. It does not matter what the stain shows if the patients do not respond.

M. W. Stanley, MD

Benign Cystic Mesothelioma of the Peritoneum: A Clinicopathologic Study of 17 Cases and Immunohistochemical Analysis of Estrogen and Progesterone Receptor Status
Sawh RN, Malpica A, Deavers MT, et al (Univ of Texas, Houston)
Hum Pathol 34:369-374, 2003   9–10

Introduction.—Benign cystic mesothelioma (BCM) is a rare lesion of the peritoneum that occurs primarily in women of reproductive age. Most patients are managed via surgical resection. Yet, the high rate of cyst recurrence has led to the use of hormonal therapy in isolated cases in an attempt to manage cyst size and relieve local symptoms. Until now, estrogen receptor (ER) and progesterone receptor (PR) status has not been examined. Reported is the experience with 17 cases (13 women; 4 men) of BCM evaluated during a 19-year period, including an immunohistochemical analysis of ER and PR status in 14 cases.

TABLE 2.—Histopathologic Findings and Immunohistochemical Results in Patients With Benign Cystic Mesothelioma

	Histopathologic Feature			Immunohistochemistry		
Case	Squamous Metaplasia	Adenomatoid Areas	Mural Proliferation	Calretinin	ER	PR
1	+	−	+	+	−	−
2	+	−	−	ND	ND	ND
3	+	−	+	+	−	−
4	+	−	−	+	−	−
5	+	+	−	+	−	−
6	+	−	−	ND	ND	ND
7	+	−	−	+	+	−
8	+	+	−	ND	ND	ND
9	+	−	+	+	−	−
10	+	−	−	+	−	−
11	+	−	−	+	+	+
12	+	−	−	+	−	−
13	+	−	−	+	−	+
14	+	−	−	+	−	−
15	−	−	−	+	−	−
16	+	−	−	+	−	−
17	+	−	−	+	−	−

Abbreviations: ND, Not done; +, present/positive; −, absent/negative.
(Courtesy of Sawh RN, Malpica A, Deavers MT, et al: Benign cystic mesothelioma of the peritoneum: A clinicopathologic study of 17 cases and immunohistochemical analysis of estrogen and progesterone receptor status. *Hum Pathol* 34:369-374, 2003.)

Findings.—All lesions demonstrated typical morphologic characteristics of BCM. Calretinin immunostaining was positive in all 14 cases (Table 2). Five patients had either 1 or 2 tumor recurrences. There were no deaths caused by the disease. One case each, respectively, was diffusely positive for ER only, focally positive for PR only, or focally positive for both ER and PR.

Conclusion.—Immunohistochemical identification of female sex hormone receptors in BCM is rare, yet the focal presence of ER and/or PR in some lesions provides weak biologic support for their use as a therapeutic option.

▶ This fairly large series of an uncommon entity confirms much of what we have previously thought to be true about BCM. Perhaps the most useful part of this study is the detailed description of differential diagnostic considerations. The evaluation of ER and PR protein is an interesting feature of this study. The results suggest that a minority of patients will benefit from hormonal manipulation, but that these should be identified. Such evaluations may be useful in the clinically very difficult situation of patients with symptomatic recurrence of this benign but frequently bulky tumor.

M. W. Stanley, MD

Ovarian Endometrioid Tumors of Low Malignant Potential: A Clinico-pathologic Study of 30 Cases With Comparison to Well-Differentiated Endometrioid Adenocarcinoma

Roth LM, Emerson RE, Ulbright TM (Indiana Univ, Indianapolis)
Am J Surg Pathol 27:1253-1259, 2003   9–11

Introduction.—There is no agreement concerning the criteria for diagnosis of ovarian endometrioid tumor of low malignant potential (ETLMP). Criteria that would help define these tumors were examined and their behavior was compared with that of well-differentiated endometrioid adenocarcinoma.

Methods.—Thirty cases of ovarian ETLMP were compared with 32 cases of well-differentiated endometrioid adenocarcinoma. The ETLMPs were distinguished from well-differentiated endometrioid adenocarcinomas by the absence of destructive stromal invasion, glandular confluence, or stromal disappearance. Intraepithelial carcinoma in a low malignant potential tumor was defined as areas demonstrating grade 3 nuclei, sometimes linked

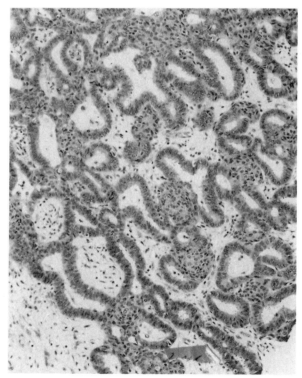

FIGURE 1.—ETLMP showing numerous squamous morules. Although they connect glands, this does not constitute confluence. (Courtesy of Roth LM, Emerson RE, Ulbright TM: Ovarian endometrioid tumors of low malignant potential: A clinicopathologic study of 30 cases with comparison to well-differentiated endometrioid adenocarcinoma. *Am J Surg Pathol* 27:1253-1259, 2003.)

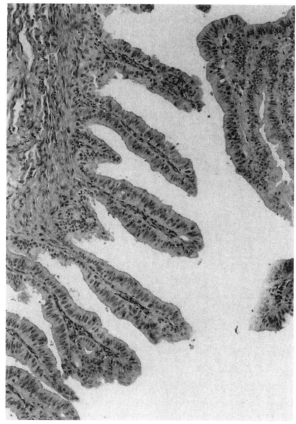

FIGURE 3.—ETLMP showing prominent villoglandular architecture and grade 1 nuclei. (Courtesy of Roth LM, Emerson RE, Ulbright TM: Ovarian endometrioid tumors of low malignant potential: A clinico-pathologic study of 30 cases with comparison to well-differentiated endometrioid adenocarcinoma. *Am J Surg Pathol* 27:1253-1259, 2003.)

with an intracystic villoglandular or cribriform pattern. Microinvasion in an ETLMP was considered to be 1 or more areas of invasion with an area of 10 mm² or less. Because a cribriform pattern may be observed in purely intraglandular proliferations, the latter was not regarded as evidence of invasion.

Results.—Mean age of patients with ETLMP was 54.9 years (range, 28-86 years). One patient (3%) with ETLMP had other than stage I disease at the time of diagnosis. The mean age of patients with well-differentiated endometrial carcinoma was 51.1 years (range, 26-87 years). Three patients (9%) had stage II disease at the time of diagnosis. Among cases of ETLMP, an adenomatous pattern was observed in 47%, squamous differentiation in 47% (Fig 1), intraepithelial carcinoma in 7%, and stromal microinvasion in 7%. Eleven (37%) tumors were entirely (Fig 3) or partially villoglandular. Desmoplasia was observed in 1 case and was related to a focus of microin-

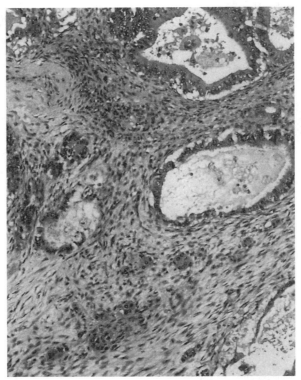

FIGURE 6.—ETLMP with foci of stromal microinvasion. Note small cords of cells representing micro-invasion between larger glands of low malignant potential tumor. (Courtesy of Roth LM, Emerson RE, Ulbright TM: Ovarian endometrioid tumors of low malignant potential: A clinicopathologic study of 30 cases with comparison to well-differentiated endometrioid adenocarcinoma. *Am J Surg Pathol* 27:1253-1259, 2003.)

vasion (Fig 6). None of these findings appeared to affect the prognosis because all patients with ETLMP were free of recurrent disease or metastasis. By contrast, 20% of patients with well-differentiated endometrioid adenocarcinoma followed for more than 6 months had recurrent disease develop.

Conclusion.—The prognosis of ETLMP, when defined by the described criteria, is favorable and superior to that of well-differentiated endometrial adenocarcinoma.

▶ These authors attempt to bring standardization to diagnosis of ETLMPs. Although clinically very important, the distinction of these tumors from well-differentiated endometrioid carcinomas of the ovary is likely to remain difficult for those of us who rarely encounter such lesions. Invasion is a useful criteria and is described in this article as an irregular pattern of stromal penetration, glandular confluence, and disappearance (overgrowth) of stroma. In combination with higher-grade nuclei, these features indicate an invasive carcinoma rather than a tumor of low malignant potential.

M. W. Stanley, MD

---

p16 Immunoreactivity May Assist in the Distinction Between Endometrial and Endocervical Adenocarcinoma
McCluggage WG, Jenkins D (Queens Med Ctr, Nottingham, England)
Int J Gynecol Pathol 22:231-235, 2003   9–12

Introduction.—The distinction between an endometrial and an endocervical origin of an adenocarcinoma may be challenging, particularly with small biopsy specimens or when tumor is present in both endometrial and cervical specimens. Earlier trials have examined the value of antibodies, including carcinoembryonic antigen, estrogen receptor, and vimentin, in establishing this distinction. The value of p16 immunohistochemistry for distinguishing between an endometrial and an endocervical origin for adenocarcinoma was assessed.

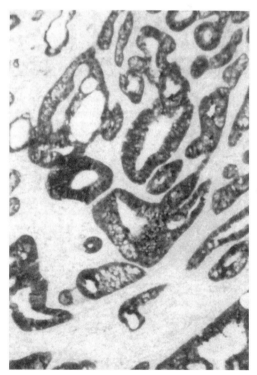

FIGURE 1.—Cervical adenocarcinoma with strong, diffuse p16 immunoreactivity of 100% of tumor cells. (Courtesy of McCluggage WG, Jenkins D: p16 immunoreactivity may assist in the distinction between endometrial and endocervical adenocarcinoma. *Int J Gynecol Pathol* 22:231-235, 2003.)

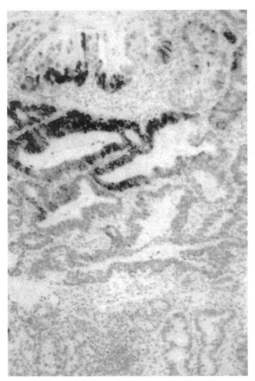

FIGURE 2.—Focal positivity with p16 in an endometrial endometrioid adenocarcinoma. (Courtesy of McCluggage WG, Jenkins D: p16 immunoreactivity may assist in the distinction between endometrial and endocervical adenocarcinoma. *Int J Gynecol Pathol* 22:231-235, 2003.)

Methods.—Twenty-nine consecutive cases of primary endometrial and 23 cases of endocervical adenocarcinoma were retrieved for examination. The cases were scored with a 0 to 5 scale, depending on the percentage of positive tumor cells: 0 for negative or occasional cells positive, 1 for less than 5% cells positive, 2 for 5% to 20% cells positive, 3 for 21% to 50% cells positive, 4 for 51% to 99% cells positive, and 5 for 100% cells positive. A score of 5 was given to 22 (96%) of 23 endocervical adenocarcinomas; 1 had a score of 1. The scores of 0 to 5 among endometrial adenocarcinomas were, respectively, 1, 7, 4, 9, and 3.

Conclusion.—Many of the primary endocervical adenocarcinomas were characterized by strong, diffuse positivity of 100% of cells with p16 (Fig 1). The endometrial adenocarcinomas were usually positive. Positivity was typically focal and often involved less than 50% of cells (Fig 2). The occasional endometrial adenocarcinomas displayed 100% positivity. Diffuse, strong positivity with p16 indicates an endocervical versus an endometrial origin of an adenocarcinoma. In the presence of morphologic doubt, this antibody may be useful as part of a panel for determining the origin of an adenocarcinoma. Diffuse, strong positivity with p16 in endocervical adenocarcinomas may be caused by inactivation of the retinoblastoma protein by the E7 human papillomavirus oncoprotein, which acts as a p16 transcript repressor.

▶ Whether for reasons of tumor morphology or tumor location, it can be very difficult to distinguish endocervical from endometrial adenocarcinomas with certainty. The results of p16 immunoreactivity in distinguishing these 2 tumors as reported by these authors shows very limited success. The tumor that shows little or only focal staining is more likely to be endometrial than endocervical. Somewhat more confusing is the fact that many endometrial adenocarcinomas can show appreciable staining. The molecular reasons for this are unclear given what we know about the relative frequencies of human papillomavirus involvement in endometrial and endocervical adenocarcinomas. The degree to which this situation can be improved by adding p16 to a panel of other immunostains remains to be demonstrated. In some institutions, the distinction between endometrial and endocervical adenocarcinomas forms the basis for differences in surgical or even postoperative therapy. Given the difficulty of this differential diagnosis as reflected in this study, one wonders how meaningful such distinctions are in any but the most morphologically and anatomically unequivocal of cases.

M. W. Stanley, MD

The Distinction Between Primary and Metastatic Mucinous Carcinomas of the Ovary: Gross and Histologic Findings in 50 Cases

Lee KR, Young RH (Harvard Med School, Boston)
Am J Surg Pathol 27:281-292, 2003   9–13

Introduction.—The problem of distinguishing primary ovarian tumors from metastatic tumors that may have spread to the ovaries from diverse sites is well described. The gross and routine microscopic characteristics of 25 stage I primary mucinous ovarian carcinomas without clinical evidence of recurrence and 25 mucinous carcinomas metastatic to the ovaries were compared.

Findings.—Characteristics that were common and strongly favored metastatic mucinous ovarian carcinomas were bilaterality, microscopic surface involvement by epithelial cells (surface implants), and an infiltrative pattern of stromal invasion. Characteristics that were less common, yet present exclusively or nearly exclusively in metastatic carcinomas, were a nodular invasive pattern, ovarian hilar involvement, single cell invasion, signet-ring cells, vascular invasion, and microscopic surface mucin. Features common in, and that strongly favored primary ovarian carcinoma, were an "expansile" pattern of invasion (Fig 11) and a complex papillary pattern (Fig 12). Features less common yet favored a primary tumor were size greater than 10 cm, a smooth external surface, benign-appearing and borderline-appearing areas, microscopic cystic glands, and necrotic luminal debris. Findings that did not distinguish any of these tumors were a cystic gross appearance; gross solid,

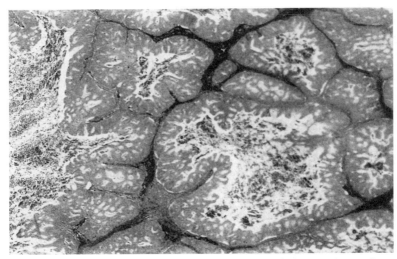

FIGURE 11.—Primary mucinous carcinoma of ovary. Large, sharply demarcated areas of expansile growth are seen. (Courtesy of Lee KR, Young RH: The distinction between primary and metastatic mucinous carcinomas of the ovary: Gross and histologic findings in 50 cases. *Am J Surg Pathol* 27:281-292, 2003. Copyright 2003, with permission from Excerpta Medica Inc.)

papillary, necrotic, or hemorrhagic areas; nature of cyst contents (mucinous vs nonmucinous); stromal mucin (pseudomyxoma ovarii); cribriform, villous, or solid growth patterns; focal area resembling typical colonic carcinoma; goblet cells; or tumor grade (Table 1).

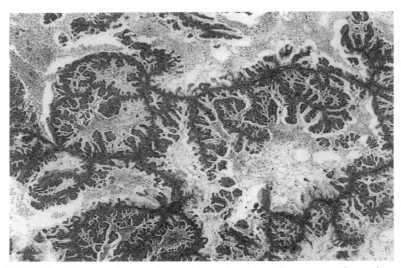

FIGURE 12.—Primary mucinous carcinoma of ovary. Complex papillary pattern with central necrotic luminal debris. (Courtesy of Lee KR, Young RH: The distinction between primary and metastatic mucinous carcinomas of the ovary: Gross and histologic findings in 50 cases. *Am J Surg Pathol* 27:281-292, 2003. Copyright 2003, with permission from Excerpta Medica Inc.)

TABLE 1.—Differential Diagnostic Findings of Primary and Metastatic Mucinous Carcinomas

	Percent of Tumors With Finding		
	Primary (n = 25)	Metastatic (n = 43)	*P* Value
Findings favoring metastasis			
Bilateral tumors	0	75	<.0001
Microscopic surface involvement by epithelial cells	0	79	<.0001
Hilar involvement	4	31	.0105
Nodular growth pattern	0	42	.0003
Infiltrative invasive pattern	16	91	<.0001
Small glands/tubules	12	94	<.0001
Single cells	8	42	.005
Signet ring cells	0	27	.032
Findings favoring primary			
Size >10 cm	88	48	.007
Grossly smooth surface	80	38	.005
Benign-appearing areas	76	36	.008
Borderline-appearing areas (with atypia)	57	31	.035
Borderline with intraepithelial carcinoma	60	30	.046
Expansile invasive pattern	88	18	<.0001
Microscopic cysts (>2 mm)	84	40	.002
Complex papillae	60	8	.0004
Necrotic luminal debris	44	14	.019
Nondiscriminatory findings			
Grossly cystic tumor	88	90	.877
Gross solid areas	76	72	.868
Gross papillary areas	24	8	.139
Gross necrotic areas	14	4	.801
Gross hemorrhagic areas	8	22	.168
Mucoid cyst contents	68	57	.600
Serous cyst contents	0	0	—
Microscopic surface mucin	0	8	.350
Stromal mucin extravasation	12	32	.088
Cribriform growth pattern	28	8	.112
Villous papillary growth pattern	24	23	.902
Solid growth pattern	4	5	.987
Colonic carcinoma-like appearance	14	12	.901
Vascular invasion	0	5	.522
Goblet cells	48	47	.852
Grade 1 or 2	96	95	.680

(Courtesy of Lee KR, Young RH: The distinction between primary and metastatic mucinous carcinomas of the ovary: Gross and histologic findings in 50 cases. *Am J Surg Pathol* 27:281-292, 2003. Copyright 2003, with permission from Excerpta Medica Inc.)

Conclusion.—Primary and metastatic mucinous ovarian tumors can be distinguished from each other in many instances based solely on their conventional histopathologic findings. Careful gross examination is important, with particular attention paid to the external surface of the ovarian tumor(s) to identify abnormalities that have the characteristics of surface implants on microscopic evaluation.

▶ This paper addresses a problem that is not infrequent and may be extremely difficult to resolve, especially in those cases where the possibility of ovarian metastases from an occult primary located in some other site must be considered. A number of features are described by these authors that are useful in distinguishing a primary from metastatic mucinous carcinomas involving the ovary. A number of these are already familiar to us. For me, the surprising part of this detailed study was the number of factors that are not predictive of either type of tumor origin. As summarized in an article cited by these authors, the extent to which one encounters metastatic carcinomas of the ovary depends in part on referral patterns and the nature of patients seen in a given institution. The authors' observation that metastatic tumors are more likely to simulate endometrioid carcinoma of the ovary than primary mucinous carcinoma is helpful. Metastatic colonic carcinoma seems to be a major offender in this category. Fortunately, there are immunohistochemical ways to improve the diagnostic certainty. Another useful point to keep in mind is that very large mucinous tumors of the ovary are more likely to be primary than metastatic. This feature is especially useful in the case of unilateral lesions, which are also more likely to be primary. These authors also discuss at length the fact that both primary and metastatic mucinous carcinomas involving the ovary can show very bland foci. Furthermore, the presence of such elements may be problematic at the time of frozen section. Other helpful features are involvement of the ovarian hilus and vascular invasion, both of which favor metastatic origin.

M. W. Stanley, MD

Pathologic Evaluation of Inguinal Sentinel Lymph Nodes in Vulvar Cancer Patients: A Comparison of Immunohistochemical Staining Versus Ultrastaging With Hematoxylin and Eosin Staining
Moore RG, Granai CO, Gajewski W, et al (Brown Univ, Providence, RI)
Gynecol Oncol 91:378-382, 2003   9–14

Introduction.—The pathologic examination of the sentinel lymph node (SLN) has evolved from routine assessment with bisection of the lymph node to ultrastaging with serial sections stained with hematoxylin and eosin (H&E). Some investigators have added immunohistochemical staining (IHC) of the SLN to aid in identifying micrometastatic disease. The value of IHC staining in addition to ultrastaging has yet to be defined and was examined in SLNs determined to be negative for metastatic disease by ultrastaging with H&E staining.

Methods.—Twenty-nine patients who had undergone an inguinal SLN dissection for squamous cell carcinoma of the vulva were evaluated. All SLNs determined to be negative for metastatic disease based on ultrastaging with H&E staining were reassessed by pancytokeratin antibody (AE1/AE3) IHC staining to identify micrometastasis.

Results.—Of 29 patients evaluated, 19 had inguinal dissections negative for metastatic disease, 2 had bilateral inguinal metastasis, and 8 had unilateral inguinal metastasis. Forty-two dissections with SLN biopsies were performed: 12 groins were positive for metastatic disease and 30 were negative on ultrastaging with H&E staining. A total of 107 SLNs (2.5 SLN/groin) were harvested. Of these, 18 SLNs contained metastatic disease detected by

TABLE 1.—Results of 107 SLNs Stained with H&E and IHC

107 SLN	H&E Staining Results	AE1/AE3 IHC Staining Results
89 negative for metastasis	Negative	Negative
16 macrometastasis (3 to 15 mm)	Positive	Not performed
2 micrometastasis (0.2 and 0.3 mm)	Positive	Positive

(Courtesy of Moore RG, Granai CO, Gajewski W, et al: Pathologic evaluation of inguinal sentinel lymph nodes in vulvar cancer patients: A comparison of immunohistochemical staining versus ultrastaging with hematoxylin and eosin staining. *Gynecol Oncol* 91:378-382, 2003. Copyright 2003 by Elsevier Science Inc.)

ultrastaging and staining with H&E. Two SLNs had micrometastasis of less than 0.3 mm; 16 contained metastasis greater than 2 mm. Eighty-nine SLNs negative for metastasis on ultrastaging with H&E staining were also negative for micrometastasis on examination with pancytokeratin antibody AE1/AE3 IHC staining (Table 1).

Conclusion.—The addition of IHC staining to ultrastaging with H&E staining in the pathologic assessment of inguinal SLN does not enhance the identification of micrometastasis in patients with primary squamous cell carcinoma of the vulva.

▶ Here is yet another tumor in which the desire to limit the complications of extensive lymph node dissection may be leading to more extensive use of SNL procedures. It is important to note that these authors have employed a protocol for extensive sampling of an SNL with multiple levels throughout the entire thickness of the lymph node. One important conclusion of this study is that the addition of immunohistochemistry for cytokeratins did not improve detection of metastases. However, it is important to note that, at least as I read the methods section, these were based on permanent section evaluations and not on intraoperative frozen section study of SLNs. Thus, by its nature, this report describes a preliminary study. It is difficult to correlate the SLN findings with the histology of non-SLN based on the information provided in this article. The implication is that when only micrometastases are present, the non-SLNs are very unlikely to contain metastatic disease. The degree to which this observation stands up and the extent to which SLN biopsy becomes the standard of care in patients undergoing resections of vulvar malignancies remain to be seen.

M. W. Stanley, MD

Sarcoma-Like Mural Nodules in Mucinous Cystic Tumors of the Ovary Revisited: A Clinicopathologic Analysis of 10 Additional Cases
Bagué S, Rodríguez IM, Prat J (Autonomous Univ, Barcelona)
Am J Surg Pathol 26:1467-1476, 2002   9–15

Introduction.—Sarcomalike mural nodules (SLMNs) have been observed in benign, borderline, and malignant mucinous cystic tumors of the ovary.

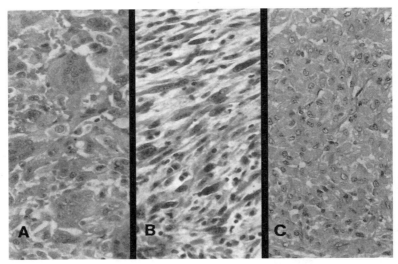

FIGURE 2.—Histologic types of SLMNs. **A,** Pleomorphic and epulislike type contains numerous multinucleated giant cells and scattered mononucleated cells. **B,** Pleomorphic and spindle cell type shows atypical spindle cells and inflammatory cells. **C,** Giant cell histiocytic type is predominantly composed of large mononucleated cells. (Courtesy of Bagué S, Rodríguez IM, Prat J: Sarcoma-like mural nodules in mucinous cystic tumors of the ovary revisited. *Am J Surg Pathol* 26:1467-1476, 2002.)

The indolent clinicopathologic characteristics of SLMNs and their favorable outcome in many patients with prolonged follow-up suggest they represent a reactive phenomenon without neoplasia. Their exact nature is unknown. Reported are 10 additional cases in which the nodules arose in association with mucinous cystic tumors of the ovary.

Findings.—The nodules were evaluated by conventional and immunohistochemical techniques. The SLMNs were observed predominantly in middle-aged women, were multiple and sharply demarcated from adjacent mucinous tumor, were small in size, and displayed a heterogeneous cell population. Three histologic types of SLMNs were observed (Fig 2). Some of the nodules contained scattered gland structures or isolated nests of epithelial cells that may have resulted from entrapment of the mucinous epithelial component (Fig 5). Distinction of these lesions from true sarcomatous nodules and foci of anaplastic carcinoma is important because of the worse prognosis of the 2 latter tumors versus the favorable behavior of the SLMNs. Six of 8 patients with available follow-up information were alive and clinically free of recurrent disease at a mean follow-up of 12 years. One patient died of thyroid carcinoma and 1 of breast carcinoma.

Conclusion.—SLMNs may represent a reactive and self-limited phenomenon within a neoplasia. Their coexpression of vimentin and cytokeratins is concordant with an origin from submesothelial mesenchymal cells, which undergo partial transformation into epithelial cells.

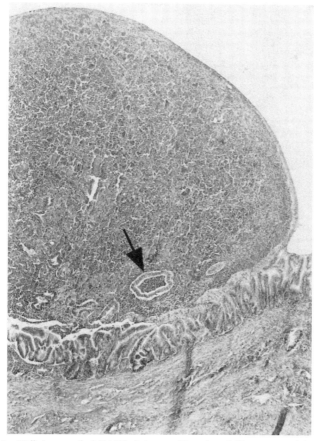

FIGURE 5.—Well-circumscribed SLMN of pleomorphic and epulislike type containing scattered entrapped mucinous glands (*arrow*) (case 2). (Courtesy of Bagué S, Rodríguez IM, Prat J: Sarcoma-like mural nodules in mucinous cystic tumors of the ovary revisited. *Am J Surg Pathol* 26:1467-1476, 2002.)

▶ These authors begin by providing a useful review of mural nodules in mucinous ovarian tumors. The clinical and morphologic differences between true sarcomatous nodules and SLMNs can be very helpful at the time of initial evaluation. The authors go on to illustrate giant cell and spindle cell types of SLMN. The latter seems to have an almost nodular fasciitislike appearance based on the authors' illustrations. The prolonged survival typical of SLMNs contrasts with the much more aggressive behavior of mucinous tumors showing mural nodules with features of true sarcoma or anaplastic carcinoma. Immunohistochemically, the frequent staining for vimentin and CD68 in these pseudosarcomatous cases, coupled with negative staining for cytokeratins and anaplastic lymphoma kinase, help underscore their benign nature.

The authors' suggestion that occasional cytokeratin-positive cells represent entrapped mucinous epithelial cells seems very reasonable. The authors seem to conclude by saying that most of these features are secondary to the finding of circumscription and a lack of invasion. The latter morphologic features are strong evidence that the process involved is benign and represents an SLMN rather than a truly sarcomatous mural nodule.

M. W. Stanley, MD

SCC Antigen in the Serum as an Independent Prognostic Factor in Operable Squamous Cell Carcinoma of the Cervix
Strauss H-G, Laban C, Lautenschläger C, et al (Martin-Luther Univ Halle-Wittenberg, Germany)
Eur J Cancer 38:1987-1991, 2002   9–16

Introduction.—Squamous cell cancer (SCC) antigen is a glycoprotein that has 2 almost identical structural variants: SCC AI and SCC A2. Both are coded on chromosome 18q21.3 and are identifiable in the cytosol of squamous epithelia. In routine clinical use, both structural variants are identified indiscriminately by an enzyme immunoassay. The SCC antigen level of the serum, depending on disease stage, is elevated in 37% to 90% of all SCCs. The preoperative significance of an elevated SCC antigen level is unknown, as is whether it could be an independent prognostic factor in cervical carcinoma. The prognostic significance of SCC antigen tumor marker in the serum was retrospectively examined in operable SCC of the cervix for International Federation of Gynecology and Obstetrics (FIGO) stages IA2 to IIB.

Methods.—A total of 129 patients who had undergone a radical hysterectomy for SCC of the uterine cervix between 1991 and 2000 were evaluated. The SCC antigen (Ag) was determined by IMx SCC-Ag microparticle enzyme immunoassay. A step-by-step multivariate analysis based on the Cox proportional hazard regression model was used to determine the prognostic value of SCC antigen in the serum.

Results.—The 5-year survival rate was 93.0% for the 129 patients evaluated. The recurrence rate was highest among patients with FIGO-stage IIB disease. Using a cutoff value of 3.0 ng/mL (Table 1), preoperative SCC antigen was identified in the serum as an independent factor in SCC of the cervix for both recurrence-free and overall survival ($P = .003$ and $.0078$, respectively). The value of the SCC antigen tumor marker correlated with the prognosis in operable cases of SCC of the cervix. This was independent of tumor size, pelvic nodal status, cervical stromal infiltration, parametrial spread, and tumor grading.

Conclusion.—A preoperative increase in SCC antigen levels in the serum in patients with SCC of the cervix allows the selection of operable patients with a less favorable prognosis. These patients may need adjuvant therapy.

TABLE 1.—Tumor Characteristics of SCC of the Uterine Cervix in the Study Population (n = 129)

FIGO Stages	Total No. of Patients (n)	Pelvic Nodal Infiltration (n)			Grading (n)				Cervical Stroma Infiltration (n)		SCC Value (n)	
		No	1 Lymph Node	>1 Lymph Node	G1	G2	G3	GX[a]	Inner Third	>Inner Third	≤3.0 ng/ml	>3.0 ng/ml
IA2	1	1	0	0	0	0	0	1	1	0	1	0
IB1	87	76	4	7	1	29	45	12	66	21	82	5
IB2	8	6	1	1	0	1	7	0	2	6	5	3
IIA	9	5	1	3	0	2	7	0	3	6	4	5
IIB	24	10	4	10	0	6	18	0	5	19	8	16

Abbreviation: GX, Grading not determined.
(Courtesy of Strauss H-G, Laban C, Lautenschläger C, et al: SCC antigen in the serum as an independent prognostic factor in operable squamous cell carcinoma of the cervix. *Eur J Cancer* 38:1987-1991, 2002, with permission of Elsevier Science.)

Unusual Epithelial and Stromal Changes in Myoinvasive Endometrioid Adenocarcinoma: A Study of Their Frequency, Associated Diagnostic Problems, and Prognostic Significance

Murray SK, Young RH, Scully RE (QEII Health Sciences Ctr, Halifax, Nova Scotia, Canada; Harvard Med School, Boston)
Int J Gynecol Pathol 22:324-333, 2003   9–17

Introduction.—When myoinvasive glands of endometrioid carcinomas evoke a prominent fibromyxoid stromal reaction, they periodically undergo distinct changes characterized by outpouchings from typical neoplastic glands that become detached and are frequently lined by flattened epithe-

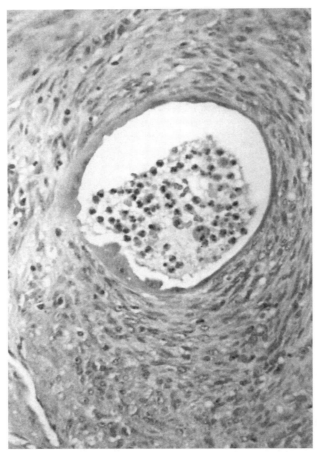

FIGURE 4.—Typical microcystic gland lined largely by flattened epithelium, but at 1 pole a few cells had abundant cytoplasm that was eosinophilic. Gland is collared by cellular fibroblastic stroma. (Courtesy of Murray SK, Young RH, Scully RE: Unusual epithelial and stromal changes in myoinvasive endometrioid adenocarcinoma: A study of their frequency, associated diagnostic problems, and prognostic significance. *Int J Gynecol Pathol* 22:324-333, 2003.)

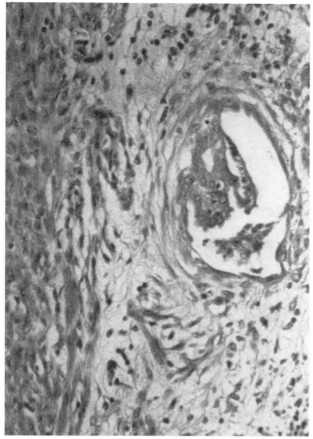

FIGURE 5.—Microcystic gland with intraluminal tuft of cells. Note myxoid appearance of stoma, which was basophilic. (Courtesy of Murray SK, Young RH, Scully RE: Unusual epithelial and stromal changes in myoinvasive endometrioid adenocarcinoma: A study of their frequency, associated diagnostic problems, and prognostic significance. *Int J Gynecol Pathol* 22:324-333, 2003.)

lium (Fig 4). Sometimes they appear as microcysts (Fig 5). These glands infrequently become elongated or undergo fragmentation into small solid clusters or single cells. This constellation of changes has been coined MELF (microcystic, elongated, fragmented). The prognostic significance of these stromal and glandular characteristics and their relations with each other and with other histopathologic and clinical prognostic factors were examined in 115 unselected myoinvasive endometrial endometrioid carcinomas.

Methods.—Histologic slides and medical records were reviewed to gather data concerning age, recurrence or metastases, survival, stromal reaction pattern (fibromyxoid, lymphocytic, or absent), presence of MELF, FIGO grade, depth of myometrial invasion, vascular invasion, squamous differentiation, and presence or absence of necrosis.

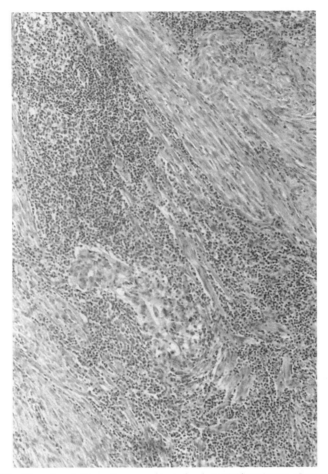

FIGURE 8.—Heavy lymphatic reaction around typical endometrioid carcinoma. (Courtesy of Murray SK, Young RH, Scully RE: Unusual epithelial and stromal changes in myoinvasive endometrioid adenocarcinoma: A study of their frequency, associated diagnostic problems, and prognostic significance. *Int J Gynecol Pathol* 22:324-333, 2003.)

Results.—Factors linked with an unfavorable outcome (recurrence or death) included fibromyxoid stromal reaction, age older than 70 years, advanced disease stage, vascular invasion, FIGO grade, depth of myoinvasion, and the presence of tumor necrosis. The presence of a host lymphocytic reaction was correlated with a favorable outcome (Fig 8). Stage and age greater than 70 years were independent prognostic factors, as determined by a multivariate logistic regression model. The MELF changes were linked with the presence of a host stromal reaction (most strongly with a fibromyxoid reaction) and vascular invasion. Within the group associated with a fibromyxoid reaction, patients displaying MELF had better survival (Table 2).

TABLE 2.—Proportion With Unfavorable Outcome (Recurrence or Death) for Each Histopathologic Factor Except MELF

	Alive [No. (%)]	Unfavorable [No. (%)]	P Value	Multivariate Analysis
Stromal reaction				
Fibromyxoid	29 (55.8)	23 (44.2)	p (F/L) = 0.009	0.29
Lymphocytic	26 (83.9)	5 (16.1)	p (F/N) = 0.038	
No reaction	25 (78.1)	7 (21.9)	p (L/N) = 0.561	
FIGO stage				
I/II	74 (73.3)	27 (26.7)	0.013	0.045
III/IV	6 (54.5)	5 (45.5)		
VI				
Absent	64 (76.2)	20 (23.8)	0.011	0.92
Present	16 (51.6)	15 (48.4)		
FIGO grade				
1	38 (71.7)	15 (28.3)	p (G1/G2) = 0.433	0.36
2	30 (78.9)	8 (21.1)	p (G1/G3) = 0.065	
3	12 (50)	12 (50)	p (G2/G3) = 0.018	
Depth of invasion*				
<½	55 (79.7)	14 (20.3)	0.008	0.411
≥½	19 (59.4)	13 (40.6)		
Necrosis				
Absent	74 (73.3)	27 (26.7)	0.032	0.54
Present	6 (42.9)	8 (57.1)		
Age				
>70	20 (51.3)	19 (48.7)	0.003	0.02
≤70	60 (78.9)	16 (21.1)		

Abbreviations: F/L, Comparison of fibromyxoid and lymphocytic; F/N, comparison of fibromyxoid and no reaction; L/N, comparison of lymphocytic and no reaction; G1/G2, comparison of grade 1 and grade 2; G1/G3, comparison of grade 1 and grade 3; G2/G3, comparison of grade 2 and grade 3.
*Excludes cases not confined to uterus.
(Courtesy of Murray SK, Young RH, Scully RE: Unusual epithelial and stromal changes in myoinvasive endometrioid adenocarcinoma: A study of their frequency, associated diagnostic problems, and prognostic significance. *Int J Gynecol Pathol* 22:324-333, 2003.)

Conclusion.—A fibromyxoid reaction in cases of endometrioid carcinoma is linked with a higher incidence of death or recurrence and is often accompanied by distinctive morphologic changes (MELF) in myoinvasive glands and lymphatic or blood vessel invasion. MELF is linked with a fibromyxoid reaction yet is not independently correlated with an adverse effect on prognosis. A lymphatic stromal reaction is linked with a favorable effect on prognosis; it is less frequently accompanied by MELF changes.

A Panel of Immunohistochemical Stains Assists in the Distinction Between Ovarian and Renal Clear Cell Carcinoma

Cameron RI, Ashe P, O'Rourke DM, et al (Belfast City Hosp Trust, Northern Ireland)
Int J Gynecol Pathol 22:272-276, 2003   9–18

Introduction.—Diagnostic problems occasionally arise when a renal clear cell carcinoma (CCC) metastasizes to the ovary or vice versa, or where disseminated CCC is found with an uncertain primary site. A previous study that investigated the ability of a panel of antibodies to distinguish between

TABLE 2.—Staining Properties of Ovarian CCCs (n = 14)

Antibody	0	1+	2+	3+
		Score		
CD10	14	0	0	0
CK7	0	0	2	12
CK20	14	0	0	0
RCC	12	1	1	0
ER	12	0	1	1
Vimentin	8	2	2	2

Abbreviation: RCC, Renal cell carcinoma.
(Courtesy of Cameron RI, Ashe P, O'Rourke DM, et al: A panel of immunohisto-chemical stains assists in the distinction between ovarian and renal cell carcinoma. *Int J Gynecol Pathol* 22:272-276, 2003.)

primary renal and ovarian CCCs found considerable overlap in their immunoprofile. A different panel of markers was evaluated in this study.

Methods.—Pathology department files yielded 14 consecutive ovarian and 14 consecutive renal CCCs. No cases consisted of simultaneous ovarian and renal involvement. All original hematoxylin and eosin–stained slides were reviewed. The panel was composed of cytokeratin (CK)7 and 20, vimentin, estrogen receptor (ER), CD10, and renal cell carcinoma (RCC) marker. Cases were scored by 2 pathologists who used a double-headed microscope and evaluated the percentage of positive cells. Positive and negative controls were included in immunohistochemical studies.

Results.—There was staining of all positive controls, but none of negative controls. In general, ovarian CCCs (Table 2) were diffusely positive with CK7 (14 of 14) and negative with CD10, CK20, ER, and RCC marker. Renal CCCs (Table 3) were generally diffusely positive with CD10 (14 of 14) and RCC marker (14 of 14) and negative with CK7, CK20, and ER.

Conclusion.—This panel of markers reveals that ovarian and renal CCCs each have a characteristic immunophenotype. Primary ovarian CCCs are characterized by CK7 positivity and primary renal CCCs by CD10 and RCC marker positivity. A panel that includes CK7, CD10, and RCC marker can distinguish between primary CCC of the ovary and kidney and is a useful adjunct to histologic examination.

TABLE 3.—Staining Properties of Renal CCC (n = 14)

Antibody	0	1+	2+	3+
		Score		
CD10	0	1	2	11
CK7	12	0	1	1
CK20	13	1	0	0
RCC	0	0	2	12
ER	14	0	0	0
Vimentin	7	0	2	5

Abbreviation: RCC, Renal cell carcinoma.
(Courtesy of Cameron RI, Ashe P, O'Rourke DM, et al: A panel of immunohisto-chemical stains assists in the distinction between ovarian and renal cell carcinoma. *Int J Gynecol Pathol* 22:272-276, 2003.)

▶ One of the themes we have followed through the last several years of these commentaries is the increasing role of immunostains for CD10 in nonhemato-poietic tissues. These authors review its distribution in normal tissues and in various neoplasms. This information forms the basis for the authors' motivation to include this marker in the current immunostain panel. The other new member of this panel is the renal cell carcinoma marker (RCC). In concert with CK7, these 2 recently described markers form a panel that is useful in addressing the differential diagnostic problem discussed in this article. The lack of utility for ER protein staining is also interesting. Although this has not been tested with sufficient rigor, this study tempts us to suggest that a renal origin for metastatic CCC could be established from other body sites as well. This might be especially useful if this immunostain panel can be applied to paraffin-embedded cell block sections from needle aspirations of lesions thought clinically to represent metastatic renal cell carcinoma. It might also find utility in metastases of CCCs of uncertain origin.

M. W. Stanley, MD

10 Urinary Bladder and Male Genital Tract

Use of Interphase Fluorescence In Situ Hybridization in Prostate Needle Biopsy Specimens With Isolated High-Grade Prostatic Intraepithelial Neoplasia as a Predictor of Prostate Adenocarcinoma on Follow-up Biopsy
Bastacky S, Cieply K, Sherer C, et al (Univ of Pittsburgh, Pa; Johns Hopkins Univ, Baltimore, Md)
Hum Pathol 35:281-289, 2004   10–1

Background.—The frequency of isolated high-grade prostatic intraepithelial neoplasia (HGPIN) without invasive carcinoma in sextant prostate needle biopsy specimens has been estimated to be 1% to 16.5% in men screened for prostate cancer. The identification of HGPIN on needle biopsy has been reported to be associated with an increased risk of prostate carcinoma on follow-up biopsy, with the likelihood of identifying an invasive prostate adenocarcinoma on immediate repeat biopsy increasing by between 22.6% and 79%. Higher detection rates have been reported in older studies and in studies with longer follow-up intervals. It was determined whether paraffin-section fluorescence in situ hybridization (FISH) of specific chromosome/oncogene copy number abnormalities (CNAs) in biopsy specimens with isolated HGPIN increases the predictive value for prostate carcinoma on repeat biopsy.

Methods.—Cases were seperated into the following 3 groups: controls (n = 8) and sextant biopsy specimens with isolated HGPIN without prostate carcinoma (n = 11, group A) and with prostate carcinoma (n = 14, group B) on follow-up biopsy. Dual-color FISH was performed for assessment of *c-myc*, *HER-2/neu*, chromosome region 7q31 (D7S486), and corresponding chromosome centromeres. An amplification ratio for each marker centromere was derived for each biopsy specimen, and the percentage of cells with marker amplification, hyperdiploidy, and monosomy was also calculated for each marker. A composite score for each biopsy specimen was calculated on the basis of these parameters, with a possible range of 0 to 15.

Results.—Composite scores of 4 or higher for the 3 groups were 0% in controls, 12% in group A, and 57% for group B, differences that were statistically significant. The specific chromosomal oncogene CNAs were 18%

189

in group A and 43% for group B for chromosome 7/7q31; 36% in group A and 69% in group B for chromosome 8/*c-myc*; and 100% for group A and 93% for group B for chromosome 17/*HER-2/neu*.

Conclusions.—Chromosome/oncogene CNAs were uncommon in control patients but occurred with increasing frequency and magnitude in patients with isolated HGPIN without and with follow-up prostate carcinoma. CNAs in HGPIN were mainly of the low to intermediate level and showed intercellular heterogeneity. Patients with HGPIN without prostate carcinoma were more likely to have a low composite score, but a subset of patients with follow-up prostate carcinoma had a low composite score, which suggests (1) the presence of mutational pathways independent of chromosomes 7, 8, and 17 and *HER-2/neu*, *c-myc*, and chromosome region 7q31 CNAs; (2) prostate carcinoma derived from an independent, unsampled focus of HGPIN; or (3) prostate carcinoma not derived from HGPIN.

▶ HGPIN identified alone on needle biopsy confers an increased risk of prostate carcinoma on subsequent follow-up biopsies. This study evaluated the utility of FISH for 3 markers (*c-myc*, *HER-2/neu*, and chromosome region 7q31). Assessment of amplification ratio was evaluated in the areas of HGPIN. A composite score of 4 or greater was significantly associated with subsequent detection of prostate cancer on follow-up biopsy. This provides a new technology that might guide the subsequent clinical approach to a diagnosis of HGPIN on prostate needle biopsy.

R. Dhir, MD

Effect of Subclinical Prostatic Inflammation on Serum PSA Levels in Men With Clinically Undetectable Prostate Cancer
Kwak C, Ku JH, Kim T, et al (Seoul Natl Univ, Korea)
Urology 62:854-859, 2003   10–2

Background.—Prostate-specific antigen (PSA) is widely used as a serum marker for the early detection and monitoring of prostate cancer. However, PSA is not a cancer-specific serum marker, and serum PSA concentrations may be affected by a variety of physiologic and benign pathologic processes. The relationship between serum PSA and subclinical prostatic inflammation has continued to be an important question, and patients with elevated PSA levels or an abnormal digital rectal examination but negative biopsy findings pose a problem in prostate cancer screening programs. Whether subclinical prostatic inflammation might influence serum PSA levels in men with clinically undetectable prostate cancer was determined.

Methods.—A total of 461 patients who underwent prostate biopsy at one hospital were studied from January 1996 to December 1999. Of these patients, 125 without detectable prostate cancer or a history of symptom of prostatitis, with serum PSA levels of less than 20 ng/mL, and without other specified exclusion criteria were included in the study. Inflammation observed at biopsy was scored for the extent of inflammation and inflammatory aggressiveness, and the effects of these morphologic aspects of serum PSA levels were examined.

Results.—The extent of inflammation tended to increase with increasing prostate volume. Patients with a PSA greater than 2.5 ng/mL had a greater extent and aggressiveness of inflammation than those with PSA levels of 2.5 ng/mL or less. However, no statistically significant differences were noted in terms of the extent of inflammation or inflammatory aggressiveness between patients with PSA levels greater than 4.0 ng/ml and those with PSA levels of 4.0 ng/mL or lower. In addition, the extent of inflammation did not explain PSA levels greater than 2.5 or 4.0 ng/mL by multivariate analysis.

Conclusions.—Subclinical prostatic inflammation is not the cause of a serum PSA level greater than 4.0 ng/mL in men who do not have clinically detectable prostate cancer.

▶ Prostatic inflammation is frequently found in biopsies of older individuals. Current thinking favors contribution of this subclinical inflammation to increased serum PSA levels in men in whom prostate cancer is not identified on biopsies dictated by elevated PSA levels. This study of 461 patients did not show any correlation of the extent and severity of inflammation with PSA elevations. These findings suggest that subclinical prostatic inflammation might not play a significant contributing role in instances of elevated serum PSA levels, especially when PSA levels are greater than 4 ng/mL.

R. Dhir, MD

Diagnostic Potential of Prostate-Specific Antigen Expressing Epithelial Cells in Blood of Prostate Cancer Patients

Gao C-L, Rawal SK, Sun L, et al (Uniformed Service Univ of the Health Science, Bethesda, Md; Armed Forces Inst of Pathology, Washington, DC; Walter Reed Army Med Ctr, Washington, DC)
Clin Cancer Res 9:2545-2550, 2003   10–3

Introduction.—Serum prostate specific antigen (PSA) screening has revolutionized early detection of prostate cancer (CaP). Yet the high false-positive rate of this test has led to unnecessary biopsies and is of concern. The development of CaP-specific diagnostic and prognostic markers is important. The identification of circulating PSA-expressing cells (CPECs) in the blood and bone marrow of patients with CaP has potential in both molecular diagnosis and prognosis. Reported were data demonstrating the presence of CPECs in a high proportion of patients with CaP, along with the diagnostic potential of the ERT–polymerase chain reaction (PCR)/PSA for CaP.

Methods.—Epithelial cells from peripheral blood of patients who underwent radical prostatectomy or prostate biopsy were isolated with the use of antiepithelial cell antibody and Ber-EP4-coated magnetic beads and total RNA specimens from these cells were investigated for PSA expression by reverse transcriptase–PCR.

Results.—The peripheral blood specimens of 108 of 135 (80.0%) patients with CaP tested positive in the ERT-PCR/PSA assay and were virtually negative (97.8%) in 45 control men. In a blinded investigation, 84 patients who underwent biopsy for suspicion of CaP were evaluated by ERT-PCR/PSA assay. Eighteen of 22 (81.8%) patients with biopsy-verified CaP tested positive; 54 of 62 (87.1%) patients who were biopsy negative for CaP were also negative by this assay.

Conclusion.—Most patients with clinically organ-confined CaP have CPECs. Strong concordance between biopsy results and the ERT-PCR/PSA assay (sensitivity, 81.8%; specificity, 87.1%) indicates a potentially new diagnostic application of the ERT-PCR/PSA assay in the diagnosis of CaP.

▶ There have been isolated reports of identification of CPECs in the blood. This article uses an ERT-PCR-PSA assay to identify epithelial cells enriched from peripheral blood. This study evaluated 135 patients with CaP. Eighty percent demonstrated positivity for this assay. Forty-five control individuals showed a false-positive rate of 2.2%. A subsequent validation set using 84 patients showed a high incidence (81.8%) of positivity rate. However, the false-positive rate was approximately 13%. Although the data are statistically significant, the false-positive rate precludes immediate adoption of this technology. This technique can be useful when combined with conventional biopsy methodology.

R. Dhir, MD

Can Prostate Specific Antigen Derivatives and Pathological Parameters Predict Significant Change in Expectant Management Criteria for Prostate Cancer?
Khan MA, Carter HB, Epstein JI, et al (Johns Hopkins Univ, Baltimore, Md and Quakertown, Pa)
J Urol 170:2274-2278, 2003   10–4

Introduction.—Localized prostate cancer exhibits extraordinary heterogeneity as it relates to the natural disease history in racially divergent populations. Prostate cancer may be present histologically in about 30% of all men older than 50 years, yet the lifetime risk of clinically important disease development is below 12%. Some of these men will experience disease progression with time and need definitive therapy. A group of men with low-volume prostate cancer who were managed expectantly were assessed. Univariate and multivariate independent variables most helpful in predicting cases that demonstrate tumor burden progression were determined, based on pathologic findings on follow-up biopsy.

Methods.—Initial and repeat biopsy information, along with transrectal US measurements of gland volume, total prostate specific antigen (PSA), percentage free PSA (%fPSA), and total PSA velocity were assessed in 78 men, 45 from a prior investigation, in whom disease was being managed expectantly. Univariate and multivariate logistic regression analyses were used to

cer occurs in 7% to 43% of prostate malignancies. Men with direct transmural invasion of the prostate by bladder TCC have a worse outcome than those whose bladder TCC is present with prostate carcinoma yet has no sign of direct infiltration. The extent to which extension from TCC into the prostate impacts survival was examined. Also evaluated was whether prostatic stromal invasion occurring by direct extension through the bladder wall differs from stromal invasion arising intraurethrally.

Methods.—Seventy-six men who underwent radical cystectomy for TCC also had prostate involvement. Patients were placed in either group 1 (primary bladder tumor extending transmurally through the bladder wall to invade the prostate) or group 2 (prostate involvement arising from within the prostatic urethra). There were 18 and 58 patients, respectively. In the latter group, the extent of prostate invasion was classified as urethral mucosal involvement, ductal/acinar involvement, or stromal invasion.

Results.—The 5-year overall survival and recurrence-free rates, respectively, were 22% and 28% for group 1 and 43% and 45% for group 2. For group 2 patients, the survival rates were similar in patients with prostatic urethral and ductal tumors (without stromal invasion). The 5-year overall survival rates with and without stromal invasion were 49% and 25%, respectively ($P = .024$).

Prostate involvement reduced survival, which varied according to primary bladder stages (Pis, P1, P2a/b, and P3a/b; $P = .004$) or superficial (Pis, Pa, and P1) disease and muscle invasive (P2a/b and P3/b; $P = .045$), disease in 2 groups. For both groups, patients with positive lymph nodes had poorer outcome. The 5-year overall survival rate in 19 men with positive lymph nodes was 13%; it was 44% in the 57 patients with negative lymph nodes ($P = .034$). The major prognostic factors were age, extent of prostate invasion, and lymph node involvement.

▶ Extension of urothelial carcinoma into the prostate is not an infrequent occurrence in diagnostic pathology. This extension can occur either directly or through an intraurethral route. Direct extension through the bladder wall into the prostate had much worse outcomes as compared to spread to the prostate via the intraurethral route. This provides a direct evidence that these 2 are distinct clinical pathologic entities. There might be a need to modify the staging criteria to incorporate these results. It is also important to highlight this fact in a diagnostic report communicating much poorer outcomes in urothelial carcinomas extending to the prostate via direct extension.

R. Dhir, MD

Hereditary Prostate Cancer in African American Families: Linkage Analysis Using Markers That Map to Five Candidate Suceptibility Loci
Brown WM, Lange EM, Chen H, et al (Wake Forest Univ, Winston-Salem, NC; Univ of Michigan, Ann Arbor; Ann Arbor Dept of Veterans Affairs, Mich; et al)
Br J Cancer 90:510-514, 2004   10–7

Introduction.—African American men have the highest rate of prostate cancer in the world. This may be due to a combination of dietary, environmental, and genetic factors. A set of multiplex prostate cancer families were evaluated for linkage to 5 previously reported prostate susceptibility loci: HPC1 at 1q24-25, PCAP at 1q42.2, CAPB at 1p36, HPC20 on chromosome 20, and HPCX at Xq27-28. Multipoint mode-of inheritance–free linkage analyses were conducted with the use of GENEHUNTER software.

Results.—A total of 126 men, including 89 with prostate cancer, were genotyped. Some evidence of prostate cancer linkage was mapped to HPCI for all families with a maximum NPL Z score of 1.12 near marker DIS413 ($P =$ .13). Increased evidence of linkage was identified in the 24 families with prostate cancer diagnosis before age 65 years and in the 20 families with male-to-male transmission. Some evidence of prostate cancer linkage was also seen at markers mapping to PCAP, HPC20, and HPCX.

Conclusion.—Continued collection and analysis of African American prostate cancer families with provide improved understanding of inherited susceptibility in this high-risk group.

▶ Molecular techniques have contributed by identifying genes and markers of value in diagnosis and prediction of outcomes. These technologies are applied to prostate cancer in this particular study assessing familial prostate cancer in a cohort of African American men. The results provide evidence of certain hot spots, which could provide additional information regarding genes of interest for prostate cancer. These studies are important as they provide new insight into molecular mechanisms leading to prostate carcinogenesis.

R. Dhir, MD

Multiplex Biomarker Approach for Determining Risk of Prostate-Specific Antigen-Defined Recurrence of Prostate Cancer
Rhodes DR, Sanda MG, Otte AP, et al (Univ of Michigan, Ann Arbor; Univ of Amsterdam; Harvard Med School, Boston)
J Natl Cancer Inst 95:661-668, 2003   10–8

Introduction.—Molecular signatures in cancer tissue may be helpful in diagnosis. They are correlated with survival. Results from high-density tissue microarrays were used to define combinations of candidate biomarkers linked to the incidence of prostate cancer progression after radical prostatectomy that could identify patients at high risk for recurrent disease.

Methods.—Fourteen candidate biomarkers for prostate cancer for which antibodies are obtainable included hepsin, pim-1, E-cadherin (ECAD; cell adhesion molecule), α-methylacyl-coenzyme A racemase, and EZH2 (enhancer of zeste homolog 2, a transcriptional repressor). The tissue microarrays containing over 2000 tumor samples from 259 patients who underwent radical prostatectomy for localized prostate cancer were evaluated by means of these antibodies.

Immunohistochemistry results were assessed in conjunction with clinical parameters linked with prostate cancer progression, including tumor stage, Gleason score, and prostate-specific antigen (PSA) level. Recurrent disease was defined as a postoperative PSA level of over 0.2 ng/mL.

Results.—Moderate or strong expression of EZH2 coupled with at most moderate expression of ECAD (ie, a positive EZH2:ECAD status) was the biomarker combination most strongly linked with recurrent prostate cancer. The EZH2:ECAD status was statistically significantly correlated with prostate cancer recurrence in a training set of 103 patients (relative risk [RR], 2.52, 95% confidence interval [CI], 1.09-5.81; $P = .21$), in a validation set of 80 patients (RR, 3.72; 95% CI, 1.27-10.91; $P = .009$), and in the combined set of 183 patients (RR, 2.96; 95% CI, 1.56-5.61; $P < .001$). The EZH2:ECAD status was statistically significantly linked with disease recurrence, even after adjustment for clinical parameters, including tumor stage, Gleason score, and PSA level (hazard ratio = 3.19; 95% CI, 1.50-6.77; $P = .003$).

Conclusion.—Patient EZH2:ECAD status was statistically significantly correlated with prostate cancer recurrence after prostatectomy and may be helpful in defining high-risk patients.

▶ A variety of ongoing research projects have focused on trying to identify molecular signatures in cancer tissue useful for diagnosis and associated with survival. This article validates markers using a paraffin tissue microarray approach and immunohistochemistry. The results of this study indicate that assessment of EZH2 (a transcriptional repressor) and ECAD could provide a significant mechanism for identifying prostate cancer with a risk for disease occurrence. This study shows that increased EZH2 expression combined with minimal ECAD expression was significantly associated with prostate cancer recurrence. The markers were studied using a training set and subsequently validated with a validation set.

This study provides an interesting approach to prostate cancer evaluation. Subsequent studies should focus on using this panel as a potential mechanism of assessing prostate needle biopsies to guide therapeutic decisions. Since many prostate cancers are indolent and incidental, results from studies like this could potentially provide markers useful for predicting patients suitable for "watchful waiting."

R. Dhir, MD

Soy Isoflavones Do Not Modulate Prostate-Specific Antigen Concentrations in Older Men in a Randomized Controlled Trial

Adams KF, Chen C, Newton KM, et al (Fred Hutchinson Cancer Research Ctr, Seattle; Univ of Washington, Seattle; Group Health Cooperative, Seattle)
Cancer Epidemiol Biomarkers Prev 13:644-648, 2004   10–9

Introduction.—Mortality rates for prostate cancer are low in Asia and are high in the West. The high level of soy consumption in Asia may have a role in the lower rates in Asia. Soy isoflavones diminish prostate tumor growth in many, yet not all, animal models. The effect of 12-months of soy isoflavone supplementation on serum prostate-specific antigen (PSA) concentration was evaluated in healthy older men in a double-blind, parallel-arm, randomized trial, the Soy Isoflavone Prevention Trial.

Methods.—Eighty-one participants were randomly assigned to consumption of either a soy protein providing 83 mg/d of isoflavones (+ISO) or a similar drink with isoflavones removed (−ISO). Serum PSA was determined at 0 and 12 months by a commercial radioimmunometric assay.

Results.—Serum PSA concentrations rose in both groups during the 12-month intervention; the changes were similar. The geometric mean PSA concentration rose 0.5% more in the +ISO group versus the −ISO group ($P =$ .94; 95% confidence interval, −17.3 to 22.2). The proportion of participants with a serum PSA velocity over 1 ng/mL/y was similar in the +ISO and −ISO groups (17.6% vs 12.8%; $P =$ .54).

Conclusion.—There was no evidence that a 12-month 83 mg/d isoflavone treatment modifies serum PSA concentration or velocity in apparently healthy men aged 50 to 80 years.

▶ There has been a significant interest over the past few years regarding the role of soy proteins in prevention of prostate cancer. This study evaluated serum PSA levels over a period of time and the potential impact of soy administration on PSA levels. This study of 81 men demonstrated no significant differences between the treated and nontreated groups regarding impact on serum PSA levels by administration of soy proteins.

This study demonstrates that soy protein administration has no affect on circulating PSA, an intermediate marker of tumor growth. However, it is possible that soy proteins might affect earliest stages in the cancer process or have other affects on tumor growth not reflected in PSA levels. This article suggests the need for other surrogate markers to assess the effect of dietary intervention for prostate cancer progression detection.

R. Dhir, MD

Role of Intraoperative Biopsies During Radical Retropubic Prostatectomy

Lepor H, Kaci L (New York Univ)
Urology 63:499-502, 2004

10–10

Introduction.—Intraoperative biopsy represents a potential strategy to reduce positive surgical margins and enhance the likelihood of totally eradicating and curing prostate cancer after radical prostatectomy. An experience with intraoperative biopsy was reviewed to ascertain its role in lowering the positive surgical margin rate.

Methods.—Radical retropubic prostatectomy was performed by a single surgeon between October 2000 and August 2002 in 500 men with clinically localized adenocarcinoma of the prostate. A 2- to 3-mm circumferential biopsy specimen was routinely acquired from the apical and bladder neck soft tissue margin. The samples were submitted for frozen section evaluation. In selective cases with suspected capsular incision, a biopsy specimen was sent from what was considered to be the contiguous neurovascular bundle/lateral pedicle.

Results.—Prostate cancer was identified in 4.5%, 0.8%, and 1.6% of the intraoperative biopsies of the apical, bladder neck, and neurovascular bundle/lateral pedicle soft tissue margins, respectively. Patient age, Gleason score, perineural invasion on diagnostic prostate biopsy, and clinical stage were not correlated with prostate cancer at the apical soft tissue margin. The sensitivity, specificity, positive predictive value, negative predictive value, and accuracy of the surgical biopsy specimens to predict cancer in the apical soft tissue margin were 57.5%, 98.2%, 62%, 97.7%, and 96%, respectively. Intraoperative biopsy of the apical soft tissue margin decreased the positive margin rate by 3.8%.

Conclusion.—The yield of the intraoperative biopsy of the bladder neck and neurovascular bundle/lateral pedicle is too low to support its use in routine surgical practice. It is recommended that biopsy of the apical soft tissue be performed routinely to decrease the incidence of positive surgical margins.

▶ The finding of a positive surgical margin at pathologic examination of a radical prostatectomy specimen is associated with an increased risk of biochemical disease recurrence. Widespread prostate-specific antigen screening over the last 20 years has contributed to a dramatic decrease in positive margins, primarily because of detection of cancer at a much earlier stage. In addition, this article describes a novel methodology for intraoperative assessment to minimize positive margins. The recommended protocol is to routinely evaluate the apical and bladder neck soft tissue margins and perform frozen sections. Apical soft tissue frozen sections seem justified, based on this study of 500 radical prostatectomy specimens.

R. Dhir, MD

Basal Cell Cocktail (34βE12 + p63) Improves the Detection of Prostate Basal Cells

Zhou M, Shah R, Shen R, et al (Univ of Michigan, Ann Arbor)
Am J Surg Pathol 27:365-371, 2003   10–11

Introduction.—Antibodies against high molecular weight cytokeratin (34βE12) and p63 are commonly used basal cell markers to help in the diagnosis of prostate cancer (Pca). The absence of a basal cell marker in an atypical lesion histologically suspicious for cancer is supportive of a diagnosis of Pca. The absence of basal cells using basal cell immunohistochemistry is not always conclusive for Pca. Some benign prostatic lesions may have inconspicuous or a lack of basal cell lining focally.

Technical factors may make identification of basal cells difficult. Improving the sensitivity of current basal cell markers is important if these tests are being used in making diagnostic decisions in conjunction with standard histology. The influence of inclusion of both 34βE12 and p63 in the same immunohistochemistry reaction (basal cell cocktail) for detection of prostatic basal cells was examined.

Methods.—A total of 1350 glands from 9 transurethral resectioned prostate specimens with benign prostatic hypertrophy were used to assess the immunostaining intensity and pattern of 34βE12, p63, and the basal cell cocktail. Basal cell marker expression, basal cell staining intensity, and aberrant expression of 34βE12 and p63 in clinically localized and poorly differentiated Pca were evaluated.

Results.—The prostate glands in the transition zone had variable basal cell staining intensity and pattern with 34βE12, p63, or the cocktail. Histologic examination showed that benign glands lacked basal cell lining in 2%, 6%, and 2% of glands with cocktail, 34βE12, and p63 staining, respectively. The staining variance for the cocktail was significantly smaller, compared to 34βE12 (0.0100 vs 0.1559; $P = .0008$) and was smaller than for p63 (0.011 vs 0.0345; $P = .099$; not significant).

The basal cell cocktail stained the basal cell layers more intensely than did 34βE12 or p63 alone, with complete and partial strong basal cell staining in 93% and 1% of benign glands, respectively, vs 55% and 4% with 34βE12 and 81% and 1% with p63. Both complete and partial weak staining was observed in 0% and 0% of benign glands with basal cell cocktail vs 8% and 7% with 34βE12 and 4% and 1% with p63 ($P = .007$ and .014 for cocktail vs 34βE12 and cocktail vs p63, respectively).

Positive 34βE12 staining and positive p63 staining were observed in 2.8% and 0.3% of clinically localized Pca, respectively. Five (22%) of metastatic Pca were positive for 23βE12; none had p63 expression. Staining patterns were identical for the basal cell cocktail and 34βE12.

Conclusion.—Immunohistochemistry of the prostate glands from the transition zone is susceptible to staining variability that results in commonly variable and occasionally negative basal cells staining in histologically benign glands. Variability was highest in 34βE12 and lowest in the basal cell cocktail. The basal cell cocktail increases the sensitivity of basal cell detection and also decreases the staining variability, making basal cell staining more consistent. The basal cell cocktail is recommended in the routine Pca diagnostic workup.

▶ Diagnosis of Pca can sometimes be challenging. It is essential to document the absence of basal cells prior to making this diagnosis in subtle cases. Immunohistochemical stains developed for basal cells have provided an important tool in making the diagnosis of Pca. Two markers commonly used are antibodies against high molecular weight cytokeratin (34βE12) and p63. The high molecular weight cytokeratin is a cytoplasmic marker while p63 is a nuclear marker. This article describes results using a basal cell cocktail combining both 34βE12 and p63. The overall results indicate better capability of basal cell detection and subsequently avoiding making a false positive diagnosis of Pca. The results of the study are clinically useful and should be evaluated for broader application in diagnostic pathology.

R. Dhir, MD

Detection of Clinically Significant, Occult Prostate Cancer Metastases in Lymph Nodes Using a Splice Variant-Specific RT-PCR Assay for Human Glandular Kallikrein
Shariat SF, Kattan MW, Erdamar S, et al (Baylor College of Medicine, Houston; Mem Sloan-Kettering Cancer Ctr, New York)
J Clin Oncol 21:1223-1231, 2003   10–12

Background.—Most patients with prostate cancer confined to the organ are free from biochemical progression in the long term after radical prostatectomy. However, patients with locally advanced prostate cancer with extraprostatic extension or seminal vesicle involvement have an increased risk for disease progression. Detection of human glandular kallikrein 2 (hK2) mRNA expression in archival lymph nodes was compared with disease progression, the development of prostate cancer metastases, and mortality in patients having radical prostatectomy for locally advanced nonmetastatic prostate cancer.

Methods.—One hundred ninety-nine patients with pT3N0 prostate cancer were studied. One hundred fifty had extraprostatic extension only, and 49 had seminal vesicle involvement. Total RNA extracted from fixed, paraffin-embedded, histopathologically normal pelvic lymph nodes removed at radical prostatectomy was analyzed for hK2-expressing cells by means of a novel reverse transcriptase–polymerase chain reaction (RT-PCR)/hK2 assay.

Findings.—Results were positive in 20% of patients, negative in 40%, and equivocal in 40%. Patients' RT-PCR/hK2 status did not correlate with any pathologic characteristics. Postoperative multivariate models indicated that the RT-PCR/hK2 result correlated with progression of prostate cancer, development of distant metastases, and prostate cancern–specific survival.

Among patients with biochemical progression, RT-PCR/hK2 status predicted failure to respond to salvage radiotherapy.

Conclusion.—In patients with histopathologically normal lymph nodes, RT-PCR/hK2 can detect biologically and clinically significant occult prostate cancer metastases. In patients with locally advanced prostate cancer, RT-PCR/hK2 correlates strongly with disease progression, failure after salvage radiotherapy, development of clinically evident metastases, and prostate cancer–specific mortality after surgery.

▶ This study evaluates molecular detection of hK2 mRNA expression. The authors extracted total RNA from paraffin-embedded tissue samples from radical prostatectomy specimens. One hundred ninety-nine cases were evaluated and assessed using RT-PCR for hK2 status. This study demonstrates that hK2 can be detected even in histopathologically normal lymph nodes. Expression of hK2 was associated with prostate cancer progression, development of distant metastases, and prostate cancer–specific survival. Expression of hK2 in patients experiencing biochemical progression was a predictor of failure to respond to salvage radiotherapy. This article documents the utility of hK2 as an adjunct to currently known markers of aggressive prostate cancer.

R. Dhir, MD

DNA Stability and Serum Selenium Levels in a High-Risk Group for Prostate Cancer
Karunasinghe N, Ryan J, Tuckey J, et al (Univ of Auckland, New Zealand; Auckland Hosp, New Zealand; Waikato Hosp, Hamilton, New Zealand; et al)
Cancer Epidemiol Biomarkers Prev 13:391-397, 2004   10–13

Background.—Selenium, an essential micronutrient, is a component of a number of proteins involved in the maintenance of genomic stability. Levels of this micronutrient are low in the New Zealand diet. Recommended daily allowances are set on saturation levels for glutathione peroxidase, a key enzyme in surveillance against oxidative stress. It is assumed that this level will be adequate for other key selenoenzymes. The New Zealand Negative Biopsy Trial was initiated to determine the efficacy of supplementing persons at high risk of prostate cancer with a yeast-based tablet with or without selenium for an extended period. Data from this study were analyzed to investigate whether selenium levels in this population are sufficient to maintain genomic stability.

Methods and Findings.—Forty-three men participated in the study. Age at study entry ranged from 50 to 75 years. Blood leukocytes were harvested from these volunteers, and the single-cell gel electrophoresis assay was used to study DNA damage. Before randomization to supplementation with or without selenium, the mean serum selenium levels of these men was 97.8 ng/mL, which is low by international standards. In the half of the participants with values below this mean, lower serum selenium levels were significantly, inversely correlated with overall accumulated DNA damage.

Conclusion.—Selenium intake in half of this population is marginal for adequate repair of DNA damage, which increases susceptibility to cancer and other degenerative diseases. These data also raise the question as to whether glutathione peroxidase saturation levels are appropriate indicators of optimal selenium levels in a given population.

► Selenium is a component of a number of proteins that have been shown to be significant in maintaining genomic stability. This article is based on a "negative biopsy trial" performed in New Zealand. This study assessed DNA stability and its possible correlation with serum selenium levels. The patient population was a high-risk group for development of prostate cancer.

This study demonstrated an overall increase in accumulated DNA damage and an inverse relationship of DNA damage with selenium levels. Lower selenium levels were associated with increased DNA damage. The overall baseline selenium levels were also lower than international standards. This study provides an interesting insight into additional dietary factors that may play a role in prostate cancer development. It reinforces the need to evaluate dietary patterns and modify them to provide a better chance to lower the incidence of prostate cancer.

R. Dhir, MD

Can the Number of Cores With High-Grade Prostate Intraepithelial Neoplasia Predict Cancer in Men Who Undergo Repeat Biopsy?

Naya Y, Ayala AG, Tamboli P, et al (Univ of Texas, Houston)
Urology 63:503-508, 2004   10–14

Background.—High-grade prostate intraepithelial neoplasia (PIN) consists of a proliferation of epithelial cells within preexisting ducts, ductules, and acini. These cells exhibit nuclear and nucleolar features of malignant cells. High-grade PIN is believed to be a precursor of adenocarcinoma of the prostate. This study investigated whether the presence of or number of cores containing high-grade PIN in men undergoing initial extended multisite biopsy can predict which patients would subsequently be found to have prostate cancer on repeat biopsies.

Methods.—One thousand eighty-six men underwent initial prostate biopsy between June 1997 and January 2003 for early detection of prostate cancer. An extended multisite biopsy scheme was used. Of this cohort, 175 men without cancer had 1 to 3 repeat biopsies, with a median 3 months between biopsies. Forty-seven of these patients had high-grade PIN on the initial biopsy.

Findings.—The initial extended biopsy identified cancer in 33.8% of the original cohort of 1086 men. High-grade PIN was identified in 20.8%. Patients found to have cancer on the initial biopsy had a 29.7% incidence of high-grade PIN only. The finding of high-grade PIN correlated with concurrent prostate cancer at the initial biopsy. Cancer was identified on repeat biopsy in 18.3% of the 175 men. In the group of 47 with high-grade PIN, 10.6% were found to have cancer on repeat biopsy.

The number of biopsy specimens positive for high-grade PIN on the initial biopsy was unrelated to the likelihood of finding prostate cancer on repeat biopsy. In a multivariate logistic regression analysis, neither the presence of high-grade PIN nor the number of cores containing high-grade PIN on initial biopsy predicted the finding of prostate cancer on repeat biopsy.

Conclusion.—The number of cores positive for high-grade PIN does not appear to predict cancer on repeat biopsy. Thus, patients found to have high-grade PIN may not need immediate repeat biopsy. The benefits of delaying repeat biopsy have yet to be defined.

▶ A frequent problem encountered in evaluating biopsy specimens for detection of prostate cancer is the presence of high-grade PIN only, without concurrent detection of prostate cancer. The current clinical approach consists of a rebiopsy for these patients since the presence of high-grade PIN is considered a histologic surrogate indicator of possible coexistence of invasive prostatic cancer. This study evaluated the potential correlation between initial detection of high-grade PIN and subsequent detection of invasive prostatic carcinoma.

Assessment of data from 1086 patients shows a very high correlation between high-grade PIN and concurrent prostate carcinoma at the initial biopsy. However, statistical analysis shows that presence of high-grade PIN only at the initial biopsy did not serve as a predictor for subsequent detection of prostate carcinoma on a repeat biopsy. In addition, the number of cores containing high-grade PIN also did not have any predictive value in identifying patients with a higher risk of detection of prostate carcinoma on a repeat biopsy.

R. Dhir, MD

Evolution of the Presentation and Pathologic and Biochemical Outcomes After Radical Prostatectomy for Patients With Clinically Localized Prostate Cancer Diagnosed During the PSA Era
Ung JO, Richie JP, Chen M-H, et al (Brigham and Women's Hosp, Boston; Worcester Polytechnic Inst, Mass; Harvard Med School, Boston)
Urology 60:458-463, 2002   10–15

Background.—The increase in the incidence of prostate cancer is due partly to the use of serum prostate-specific antigen (PSA) testing. The evolution of the clinical presentation and pathologic and biochemical outcomes were investigated among patients with clinically localized prostate cancer treated with radical prostatectomy in the PSA era.

Methods.—The cohort study consisted of 1059 consecutive men undergoing radical prostatectomy between January 1989 and December 2000. Three intervals were studied: 1989 to 1992, 1993 to 1996, and 1997 to 2000. Proportions of patients in each time period were compared as to PSA level, biopsy Gleason score, clinical T stage, percentage of positive biopsy cores, age, risk group, pathologic T stage. Gleason score, margin status, and lymph node status. Actual PSA recurrence-free survival rates at 2 years were established for patients with a minimal 24-month follow-up, stratified by interval and preoperative risk group.

Findings.—Preoperative characteristics shifted significantly over time, with patients being younger and with nonpalpable disease, lower PSA levels, fewer percentages of positive biopsies, and lower preoperative risk group classification. Pathologically, there was a significant downward stage migration toward organ-confined disease and improvement in surgical margin status. Actual 2-year PSA recurrence-free survival rates improved over time, from 60% in the earliest period to 78% and 82%.

Conclusion.—The introduction of serum PSA testing has been accompanied by an evolution toward lower pathologic stage and grade at diagnosis and improved PSA outcomes. Serum PSA screening appears to increase the proportion of patients who are potentially curable after radical prostatectomy.

▶ This article discusses in detail the changing patterns of prostate cancer. Introduction of serum PSA as a screening tool has significantly impacted the clinical profile of prostate cancer. This article further reinforces the fact that recent years have seen a shift toward a lower pathologic stage and grade of prostate cancer and associated better outcomes, especially as measured by using PSA failure as a clinical end point. This study assessed the results from 1059 consecutive men treated surgically from January 1989 through December 2000. These findings further provide evidence that serum PSA screening has impacted prostate cancer by increasing the proportion of patients potentially curable after a radical prostatectomy procedure.

R. Dhir, MD

11 Kidney

Evaluation of a Protocol for Examining Nephrectomy Specimens With Renal Cell Carcinoma
Griffiths DFR, Nind N, O'Brien CJ, et al (Univ of Wales, Cardiff; Princess of Wales Hosp, Bridgend, Wales; Morriston Hosp, Swansea, Wales; et al)
J Clin Pathol 56:374-377, 2003   11–1

Introduction.—About two thirds of renal cell carcinomas (RCCs) are localized at the time of diagnosis. Despite apparent complete tumor excision, 40% of patients have metastases and die of disease. Prediction of the patients who will relapse is challenging and depends upon pathologic assessment of the surgically resected RCC specimen, for which there is no generally accepted or validated approach. The practicality of use and the effectiveness of a standard protocol for evaluating nephrectomy specimens for RCC was assessed, with emphasis on detection of vascular invasion.

Methods.—A standardized protocol created to identify the major prognostic determinants was used to evaluate 79 consecutive tumors submitted to 4 histopathology departments. The incidence of detected vascular invasion was compared with that of a historical series of tumors.

Results.—The protocol was easy to follow and seemed to enhance the incidence of identified vascular invasion (40/69 cases vs 69/176 cases in the historical series; $P = .059$).

Conclusion.—If pathologic prognostic determinants are to be used in the clinical management of RCC, it is crucial that they be identified and documented consistently. The protocol described offers a method for examining nephrectomy specimens that can be used in routine practice and are likely to reliably identify recognized prognostic variables.

▶ RCCs are an important cause of cancer-related deaths. Pathologic assessment of the resected specimen is an important component of defining parameters related to bad outcomes. It is therefore important to have a standard protocol for examining nephrectomy specimens. The major reason is the importance of identifying vascular invasion. This article describes a method that appears practical and easy to implement. Incorporating this into standard pathology practice would help in increasing detection of vascular invasion. The article compares results using conventional protocols. It is therefore recommended that this protocol be assessed by practicing pathologists and incorporated into routine diagnostic workup if thought to be appropriate.

R. Dhir, MD

Malignant Papillary Renal Tumors With Extensive Clear Cell Change: A Molecular Analysis by Microsatellite Analysis and Fluorescence In Situ Hybridization
Salama ME, Worsham MJ, DePeralta-Venturina M (Henry Ford Hosp, Detroit)
Arch Pathol Lab Med 127:1176-1181, 2003   11–2

Introduction.—The histologic subtyping of renal cell carcinomas (RCCs) is based on the cytoarchitectural pattern and on distinct cytogenetic abnormalities. Some renal tumors exhibit overlapping morphological characteristics, making histologic subtyping challenging. One such group of tumors is papillary renal neoplasms with extensive clear cell change. Because histologic subtyping is of prognostic value, it is important that malignant epithelial renal tumors be subtyped precisely. Whether these tumors should be classified as papillary RCC or conventional/(clear cell) RCC (CRCC) is not known. Molecular techniques, particularly fluorescence in situ hybridization (FISH) and microsatellite analysis (eg, the detection of loss of heterozygosity and microsatellite instability), were performed to ascertain the genetic alterations in 7 malignant renal tumors with papillary architecture and extensive clear cell change.

Methods.—Seven RCCs from 6 patients that demonstrated more than 75% papillary architecture and over 75% clear cell change were evaluated. Tumor size ranged between 2.5 and 7.0 cm (mean, 4.7 cm). All were confined to the kidney (stage I). DNA was extracted from formalin-fixed paraffin-embedded tissue and FISH was performed using Chromosome In Situ Kits (Vysis, Downers Grove, Ill) for centromere probes for chromosomes 7 and 17.

For loss of heterozygosity, microsatellite analysis via labeled primers for 4 markers in the 3p13 through 3p24.2 region was utilized. The amplified polymerase chain reaction products were evaluated with an automated DNA sequencer. When compared with normal DNA, loss of heterozygosity in tumor was identified as a loss of 1 allele; microsatellite instability was the addition of an extra allele.

Results.—Loss of heterozygosity in at least 1 of the markers spanning 3p13 through 3p24.2 was identified in 6 of 7 specimens (86%), of which 1 also demonstrated concomitant microsatellite instability. FISH did not identify trisomy for either chromosome 7 or 17. Rather, monosomy 7 was seen in 4 of 6 tumors (67%). Monosomy was seen in all tumors (100%).

Conclusion.—Because malignant papillary renal tumors with extensive clear cell changes demonstrate molecular changes identical to CRCC, this tumor subgroup may need to be classified as CRCC. Molecular studies are important in refining light-microscopic criteria for accurate histologic subtyping of RCCs.

▶ Classification of renal cell tumors has evolved over the last decade, with significant input from cytogenetics and molecular diagnostics. The current trend is to use FISH and evaluation of the 3p von-Hippel Lindau locus to try to delineate CRCCs from chromophobe and papillary renal carcinomas. This study evaluates a morphologically challenging area of tumors with a papillary renal neoplasm with extensive clear cell change. Histology is limited by not being able to distinguish the 2. Immunohistochemical assessment does not really provide any significant tools for discrimination.

This study utilized the FISH assays for chromosomes 7 and 17 and loss of heterozygosity for the 3p region adjacent to the *VHL* gene. The results suggest most papillary tumors with very prominent clear cell change represent CRCCs. This is an interesting and important finding since clinical outcomes are different between these 2 groups. This study further highlights the utility of molecular studies in aiding and refining light microscopic diagnoses.

R. Dhir, MD

Detection of Bladder Cancer in Urine by a Tumor Suppressor Gene Hypermethylation Panel
Dulaimi E, Uzzo RG, Greenberg RE, et al (Fox Chase Cancer Ctr, Philadelphia)
Clin Cancer Res 10:1887-1893, 2004   11–3

Introduction.—Bladder cancer is potentially curable in most patients. The prognosis for patients with advanced disease at the time of diagnosis continues to be poor. Current noninvasive tests, including cytology, lack adequate sensitivity to identify low-grade, low-stage tumors. The silencing of tumor suppressor genes—including $p16^{INK4a}$, VHL, and the mismatch repair gene hMLH1—has demonstrated that promoter hypermethylation is a common mechanism for tumor suppressor inactivation in human cancers. It is also a promising new target for molecular identification in body fluids, including urine.

Methylation-specific polymerase chain reaction (MSP) can detect the presence or absence of methylation of a gene locus at a sensitivity level of up to 1 methylated allele in 1000 unmethylated alleles, which is appropriate for detecting cancer cell DNA in a body fluid. The hypermethylation status of APC, RASSFIA, and $p14^{ARF}$ was examined in paired bladder tumor and urine DNA samples, along with normal and benign disease controls.

Methods.—The incidence of hypermethylation of the Rb tumor suppressor gene by bisulfite sequencing and of the $p16^{INK4a}$, $p14^{ARF}$, APC, and RASSFIA tumor suppressor genes by MSP in 45 bladder cancers was examined. A panel optimal for diagnostic coveraged composed of the APC, RASSFIA, and $p14^{ARF}$ tumor suppressor genes was constructed. This panel was evaluated for identification of hypermethylation in matched sediment DNA from urine tested before surgery from the same 45 patients with bladder cancer (2 Tis, 16 Ta, 10 T1, and 17 T2-4), along with normal and benign control DNAs.

Results.—Hypermethylation of at least 1 of 3 suppressor genes (*APC*, *RASSFIA*, and *p14^ARF*) was detected in all 45 tumor DNAs (100% diagnostic coverage). Gene hypermethylation was identified in the matched DNA urine from 39 of 45 patients (87% sensitivity), including 16 patients with negative cytology.

No hypermethylation of *APC*, *RASSFIA*, or *p14^ARF* was seen in normal transitional cell DNAs or in urine DNAs from normal, healthy persons and patients with inflammatory urinary disease (cystitis). An unmethylated gene in the tumor DNA was also determined to be unmethylated in the matched urine DNA (100% specificity).

Conclusion.—Promoter hypermethylation of tumor suppressor genes is frequently observed in bladder cancer. It was detected in all grades and stages of tumors. Hypermethylation was identified in the urine DNA from 87% of patients, including patients with early stage disease amenable to cure. Early detection of bladder cancer may be enhanced by MSP noninvasive urine testing.

▶ Urothelial carcinoma of the bladder is potentially curable in a majority of patients diagnosed at an early stage of the disease. However, this early detection is significantly hampered by reliance on clinical manifestations leading onto detection of the disease. There has been a significant push over the last few years to come up with molecular methods for earlier detection of urothelial carcinomas.

This article addresses one such approach focusing on methylation of tumor suppressor genes known to be silenced during the development of many common human cancers. The results of this study suggest that the use of methylation-specific polymerase chain reaction (MSP) focused on 3 tumor suppressor genes (*APC*, *RASSFIA*, and *p14^ARF*) can provide significant insight into early detection. This approach is very interesting and needs further validation prior to introduction into the clinical arena.

R. Dhir, MD

Correlation of Ki-67 and Gelsolin Expression to Clinical Outcome in Renal Clear Cell Carcinoma
Vasapää H, Bui M, Huang Y, et al (Univ of California, Los Angeles; Univ of Helsinki)
Urology 61:845-850, 2003   11–4

Introduction.—Ki-67 is a nuclear antigen that is present in all cycling human cells. It is a marker of active cell proliferation. Immunohistochemical staining of Ki-67 produces an index that estimates the growth fraction of a population of cells. The expression levels of Ki-67 and gelsolin, an actin-binding protein, were examined in renal cell carcinoma (RCC). Their prognostic value in association with other clinicopathologic factors was examined by tissue microarray technology.

Methods.—A renal cancer tissue microarray was used to correlate the expression of Ki-67 and gelsolin with grade, stage, and survival in patients with clear cell RCC.

Results.—Cox multivarite regression analysis revealed that stage pT was the most important predictor of cancer-specific survival ($P < .0001$), followed by Ki-67 ($P = .0216$). Univariate analysis showed that increased Ki-67 expression predicted poor cancer-specific survival ($P = .0006$) when a cutoff value for Ki-67 staining was applied. In patients with grade 2 tumors, increased Ki-67 expression and reduced gelsolin expression in the same tumor indicated poor cancer-specific survival ($P = .0507$).

Conclusion.—It appears that Ki-67 is a prognostic biomarker for RCC and indicates that gelsolin may have a role in renal carcinogenesis.

► RCC is an important cause of cancer-related mortality and morbidity. This article evaluates 2 markers and their role in predicting prognosis for RCC. Ki-67 is a well-known nuclear antigen, related to cell proliferation. Gelsolin is a member of the actin-binding protein family and has been linked to carcinogenesis of several organs. The results of this study of 355 RCCs primarily reiterates the importance of stage. The pathologic stage was the most significant predictor of cancer-specific survival. However, increased expression of Ki-67 and decreased expression of gelsolin did provide additional information. These markers are of interest, especially when combined with pathologic and clinical data.

R. Dhir, MD

Human DNA Topoisomerase-IIα Expression as a Prognostic Factor for Transitional Cell Carcinoma of the Urinary Bladder

Koren R, Kugel V, Dekel Y, et al (Rabin Med Ctr, Petah Tikva, Israel; Tel Aviv Univ, Israel)
BJU Int 91:489-492, 2003

11–5

Introduction.—DNA topoisomerase II-α (TII-α) is an important nuclear enzyme involved in vital cellular functions, including DNA replication, transcription, recombination, and mitosis. It is a marker of cell proliferation in both normal and neoplastic tissues that has been evaluated in various solid tumors, including breast cancer, testicular teratoma, and transitional cell carcinoma. Several data indicate that the sensitivity of a cell to TII-α–targeted drugs is directly proportional to the amount of cellular TII-α. The correlation of TII-α expression with grade, stage, and survival was evaluated in urothelial neoplasms.

Methods.—Histologic sections from 57 urothelial neoplasms underwent immunohistochemical staining for TII-α expression. The percentage of positive cells in the area of greatest staining was documented as the TII-α index.

Results.—DNA topoisomerase II-α nuclear staining was positive in 56 of the 57 samples. The mean TII-α index was 10.7 for urothelial neoplasms of low malignant potential (grade 1), 15.5 for low-grade (grade 2), and 42.1 for high-grade urothelial carcinoma (grade 3). The mean TII-α index was 10.7

for stage pTa, 26.3 for stage pT1, and 44 for stage pT2. The TII-α index was significant for predicting death from cancer and was independent of the stage or grade of the disease (P = .010; hazard ratio, 1.1).

Conclusion.—A higher TII-α index indicates a greater probability of disease and lower overall survival. Thus, TII-α expression has prognostic value in patients with bladder carcinoma.

▶ Urothelial carcinomas of the urinary bladder account for significant morbidity and mortality. Currently, no definite markers are available to help predict clinical outcomes. This article assesses human DNA TII-α expression in urothelial carcinomas of the urinary bladder. The current results seem to indicate a strong association between a high TII-α expression index and death from urothelial carcinoma. This marker seems to pick up cases with a greater probability of recurrence of disease and lower overall survival. This prognostic marker could provide an additional handle for predicating outcomes. This could also lead to more aggressive clinical intervention in patients with high levels of TII-α expression.

R. Dhir, MD

The Role of Calretinin, Inhibin, Melan-A, BCL-2, and C-kit in Differentiating Adrenal Cortical and Medullary Tumors: An Immunohistochemical Study

Zhang PJ, Genega EM, Tomaszewski JE, et al (Univ of Pennsylvania, Philadelphia)

Mod Pathol 16:591-597, 2003   11–6

Introduction.—The morphological distinction between adrenal cortical and medullary tumors can be challenging. Inhibin, melan-A, and BCL-2 have been shown to be useful markers for adrenal cortical tumors. A high level of calretinin expression has been detected in the normal adrenal cortex but not the medulla. C-kit expression has been reported in the adrenal medulla and in pheochromocytoma; it has not been assessed in adrenal cortical tumors. The immunoreactivity of calretinin, c-kit, inhibin, melan-A, and BCL-2 was examined in a series of adrenal tumors and paraganglioma in routine surgical specimens.

Methods.—Twenty-eight adrenal cortical tumors (12 carcinomas, 16 adenomas), 20 pheochromocytomas, and 20 extra-adrenal paragangliomas were analyzed for calretinin, inhibin, melan-A, BCL-2, and c-kit expression by standard immunohistochemical assays on paraffin sections.

Results.—The percentage of immunoreactivity in adrenal cortical tumors was as follows: calretinin, 96%; melan-A, 89%; inhibin, 92%; BCL-2, 20%; and c-kit, 5%. Normal adrenal medulla did not stain for c-kit; it was positive for BCL-2. Among pheochromocytomas, 85% stained for BCL-2 and none for calretinin (with the exception of the ganglioneuromatous areas in 5 composite pheochromocytomas). Extra-adrenal paragangliomas exhibited reactivity with calretinin in 25% of cases, melan-A in 5%, inhibin in 16%, BCL-2 in 38%, and c-kit in 8%.

Conclusion.—Calretinin is the most sensitive of the evaluated adrenal markers. Calretinin, along with melan-A and inhibin, is a very specific marker for differentiating cortical from medullary adrenal tumors. Calretinin may be used to verify a composite pheochromocytoma. It appears that BCL-2 is not useful in differentiating cortical tumors from those that are medullary. C-kit is not helpful in diagnosing adrenal tumors. Kit kinase inhibitor might have a limited role in treating adrenal tumors and paraganglioma due to the low incidence of c-kit expression in these tumors.

▶ Adrenal tumors are not a frequent occurrence in routine surgical pathology diagnostic reviews. The lack of experience is further compounded by histologic difficulty in distinguishing adrenal cortical from adrenal medullary tumors. This article provides some insight into immunohistochemical panels that can potentially improve diagnostic ability for separating adrenal cortical from adrenal medullary tumors. The results of this study indicate that calretinin could be useful since almost 100% of adrenal cortical lesions stained for this marker versus almost complete absence in pheochromocytomas. The authors have also investigated other immunohistochemical markers as part of this panel, with varying results. These markers would need further testing to validate their utility in clinical diagnostics.

R. Dhir, MD

Impaired ΔNp63 Expression Associated With Reduced β-Catenin and Aggresive Phenotypes of Urothelial Neoplasms
Koga F, Kawakami S, Kumagai J, et al (Tokyo Med and Dental Univ)
Br J Cancer 88:740-747, 2003   11–7

Background.—The normal development of stratified epithelia, including urothelium, relies on p63, a homologue of the *p53* gene. The possible roles of p63 in urothelial tumorigenesis were investigated.

Methods.—The expression of p63 was examined systematically in normal urothelium, low-grade papillary noninvasive urothelial tumors, and high-grade (invasive) carcinomas. An isoform-nonspecific or a ΔN–isoform-specific antibody was used. In addition, p63 expression profiles were examined in cultured cells.

Findings.—Immunoreactivity with the 2 antibodies in the tissue samples studied was virtually identical. This normal staining pattern was preserved in most low-grade papillary noninvasive tumors. In high-grade or muscle-invasive carcinomas, however, it was commonly impaired. Expression of ΔNp63 predominated over Tap63 at the mRNA level. Amounts of ΔNp63 mRNA were associated with p63 immunoreactivity. In cultured cells, ΔNp63 was expressed in both low-grade tumor and normal urothelial cells but was undetectable in high-grade cancer cells. Impaired ΔNp63 expression correlated significantly with decreased β-catenin expression possibly related to urothelial neoplasm progression.

Conclusion.—These data show that ΔNp63 accounts for p63 expressed in urothelial tissues. Impaired ΔNp63 expression is typical of aggressive urothelial neoplasm phenotypes.

▶ The tumor suppressor marker *p63* has been extensively studied over the last few years. Studies have shown 2 major isoforms of *p63*: one containing an acidic amino terminus (TAp63) and another with a truncated amino terminus (ΔNp63). This study evaluates the possible role of *p63* in urothelial carcinoma. The study assessed expression of the 2 variants of *p63* immunohistochemically using an isoform nonspecific antibody and a ΔN isoform specific antibody.

The study documents that p63 immunoreactivity in urothelium was predominately ΔNp63 in nature. The aggressive phenotypes of urothelial carcinoma showed decreased p63 expression. Studies using mRNA documented impaired ΔNp63 expression. This study provides an interesting insight into an abnormality involving an important tumor suppressor gene in urothelial carcinogenesis. This could provide a potential target for therapeutic intervention.

R. Dhir, MD

Metanephric Adenoma Lacks the Gains of Chromosomes 7 and 17 and Loss of Y That Are Typical of Papillary Renal Cell Carcinoma and Papillary Adenoma

Brunelli M, Eble JN, Zhang S, et al (Indiana Univ, Indianapolis; Università di Verona, Italy; Università di Sassari, Italy)
Mod Pathol 16:1060-1063, 2003   11–8

Background.—Morphologically, metanephric adenoma is similar to papillary renal cell neoplasms. In cytogenetic studies of papillary renal cell carcinoma and papillary adenoma, frequent gains of chromosomes 7 and 17 have been found, along with loss of the Y chromosome. Cytogenetic research investigating the hypothesis that metanephric adenoma is related to papillary renal cell neoplasia had yielded conflicting results. Seven metanephric adenomas were examined to further explore this issue.

Methods.—Fluorescence in situ hybridization in paraffin sections was applied with the use of centrometric probes for chromosomes 7, 17, and Y diluted 1:100 with tDenHyb1 buffer. In each tumor, signals in 100 to 200 nuclei were counted. A control group consisted of samples of histologically normal renal cortical tubule epithelium.

Findings.—Findings for chromosomes 7 and 17 were similar in all 7 metanephric adenomas. A high percentage of nuclei with 2 signals (median, 79%) were noted. Results were similar in normal kidney, with a median of 84%. All 3 tumors from male patients showed the Y chromosome, the median being 87%. This was similar to normal kidney. In addition, the presence of chromosomes 7, 17, and Y in metanephric adenomas was similar to that in normal kidney.

Conclusion.—This analysis showed that metanephric adenoma lacks the frequent gains of chromosome 7 and 17 and losses of the Y chromosome characteristic of papillary renal cell neoplasms. This supports the hypothesis that metanephric adenoma is unrelated to papillary renal cell carcinoma and papillary adenoma. In difficult cases, genetic analysis of chromosomes 7, 17, and Y may be useful for differentiating metanephric adenoma from papillary renal cell carcinoma.

▶ Metanephric adenoma is a benign lesion identified in the kidney that has morphological similarities to papillary neoplasms of the kidney. The primary differential consists of papillary renal carcinoma and papillary adenoma. Previous cytogenetic studies have documented frequent gains of chromosomes 7 and 17 and the loss of the Y chromosome in papillary renal tumors.

This study assessed the utilization of fluorescent in situ hybridization (FISH) performed on paraffin sections as a potential diagnostic tool for helping in distinguishing between metanephric adenomas and papillary neoplasm of the kidney. FISH centromeric probes were used for chromosomes 7, 17, and Y. The metanephric adenoma studied in this report demonstrated normal levels of 7, 17, and Y in a pattern similar to that identified in adjacent normal kidney. FISH evaluation of chromosome 7, 17, and Y may facilitate discrimination of metanephric adenoma from papillary renal carcinoma in difficult cases.

R. Dhir, MD

Molecular Serological Detection of DNA Alterations in Transitional Cell Carcinoma Is Highly Sensitive and Stage Independent
von Knobloch R, Brandt H, Schrader AJ, et al (Philipps-University, Marburg, Germany)
Clin Cancer Res 10:988-993, 2004   11–9

Background.—Approximately 3% of all newly diagnosed malignancies in Western countries are transitional cell carcinoma (TCC). The efficacy of fluorescent microsatellite analysis (MSA) in the serologic diagnosis of TCC of the urinary tract, analyzing free tumor DNA in serum from patients with cancer, was reported.

Methods.—Fluorescent MSA was applied to detect serum-DNA alterations in 61 patients with bladder and upper urinary tract TCC. Fresh tumor, peripheral blood, and serum were collected prospectively to determine corresponding DNA. Fluorescent MSA was done with a total 17 polymorphic markers from the chromosomal regions 5q, 8p, 9p, 9q, 13q, 14q, 17p, 17q, and 20q in the patients and in 20 healthy controls.

Findings.—Molecular serologic analysis resulted in tumor-specific diagnosis of TCC in 80.3% of the patients. Four persons in the control group were found to have serum-DNA artifacts, yielding a specificity of 80%. The highest frequency of serum-DNA alterations (36%) was identified for chromosomal region 8p. Eighteen percent to 21% of patients had serum-DNA changes in chromosomes 5q, 9p, and 20q. The finding of serum-DNA changes was unassociated with underlying local tumor stage but was more common in high-grade tumors.

Conclusion.—MSA is a very sensitive method for serologically diagnosing TCC. Simultaneous analysis of tumor DNA is recommended to exclude artifacts resembling allelic imbalance in MSA of serum DNA, thereby optimizing the specificity of MSA.

▶ The adoption of molecular technologies to diagnostic procedures related to diagnosis of cancers can have significant impact, especially in picking up neoplastic transformation at an earlier stage. This can be of special importance in neoplasia-like urothelial carcinomas, which cause significant morbidity and mortality, especially if they have progressed to a higher stage. This article describes utilization of MSA using serum as the biological material of interest. This technique is intriguing and interesting. It seems to be highly sensitive. However, specificity is an issue. Additional work needs to be done to decrease false-positive results before this methodology can be used clinically.

R. Dhir, MD

Transjugular Kidney Biopsy

Thompson BC, Kingdon E, Johnston M, et al (Royal Free Hosp, London)
Am J Kidney Dis 43:651-662, 2004   11–10

Background.—In most previous research showing the feasibility of transjugular kidney biopsy, a modified Colapinto aspiration biopsy needle was used. The outcomes of transjugular kidney biopsy using a transvenous side-cut needle was reported for a group of high-risk patients with contraindications to percutaneous renal biopsy.

Methods.—Twenty-five high-risk patients underwent the procedure. In selected patients, elective coil embolization was also used to reduce the risk of bleeding. Indications for obtaining renal histology and for transjugular biopsy were reviewed retrospectively.

Findings.—Renal tissue was obtained from 23 patients. Biopsy specimens were diagnostic in 91.3%. A mean of 3.5 cores were acquired with 9.9 glomeruli per procedure for light microscopy and 2.2 for electron microscopy. Adequate tissue for immunofluorescence was available from 11 of the 23 biopsy specimens. In all 23 biopsied patients, histologic findings affected patient management.

Capsular perforation was documented in 73.9% of the 23 biopsied patients. Six patients underwent elective coil embolization. There were 2 major complications. Both occurred in patients with multiple risk factors for bleeding, 1 of whom required coil embolization of an arteriocalyseal system fistula; in the other, renal vein thrombosis developed 6 days after a failed transjugular kidney biopsy.

Conclusion.—Transjugular kidney biopsy can provide a histologic diagnosis in high-risk patients with contraindications to percutaneous renal biopsy. This approach is a valuable addition to patient management.

▶ Performance of percutanoeus kidney biopsies has risks associated with it. These risks can sometimes be significant in the background of predisposing medical conditions. In certain instances, percutaneous kidney biopsies might not be feasible because of existence of risk factors. This article describes a new approach for performing kidney biopsies using a transjugular route. This technique does have associated complications, which are discussed in detail. However, it provides an alternative approach to performing kidney biopsies, especially in a high-risk medical setting. The use of this technique would need to be tempered by taking into account the existing medical condition of the patient.

R. Dhir, MD

12 Head and Neck

Do Frozen Sections Help Achieve Adequate Surgical Margins in the Resection of Oral Carcinoma?
Ribeiro NFF, Godden DRP, Wilson GE, et al (North Manchester Gen Hosp, England)
Int J Oral Maxillofac Surg 32:152-158, 2003   12–1

Background.—Up to 47% of patients with malignant oropharyngeal tumors have positive margins after resection. Thus, many centers perform frozen section analysis during the primary surgery to ensure free resection margins. Whether the routine use of frozen section is justified for patients with oropharyngeal carcinoma was investigated.

Methods.—The medical records of 82 patients (71% men, 36-89 years) who underwent attempted curative resection of oropharyngeal carcinoma between August 1994 and October 1998, and for whom frozen sections had been obtained, were examined. All patients were treated by the same surgeon. Frozen sections were taken from the mucosal and deep margins of the resection during the primary procedure. Resection margins with squamous epithelial dysplasia, carcinoma in situ, or infiltrating carcinoma, and margins within 5 mm of the tumor were considered positive for disease, and further resection was performed. The main specimen was also fixed in paraffin for analysis.

Results.—Most patients had stage III (19, or 23%) or stage IV (34, or 42%) tumors. Tumors were present in the tongue (30.5% of cases), floor of the mouth (28.0%), lower alveolus and mandible (9.8%), buccal mucosa (7.3%), palate (6.1%), retromolar area (6.1%), lips (3.7%), and other areas (8.5%). During this 4-year period, 350 mucosal, 179 deep tissue, and 22 nerve frozen sections were obtained from these 82 patients. Cryostat and paraffin preparations agreed in 548 of the 551 biopsies performed (concordance 99.5%), and frozen section did not produce any false-positive or false-negative findings for invasive tumor compared with paraffin sections. In 9 patients (11.0%) the frozen sections contained dysplastic squamous epithelium or invasive tumor, and these patients underwent further local resection (Table 4). Subsequent frozen sections ultimately indicated clear margins in 8 of these 9 patients. In 15 patients (18.3%) the frozen sections showed the margin of the main resected specimen was 5 mm or less from the tumor (Table 5). In addition, 5 patients (6.1%) had dysplasia or carcinoma in situ in the mucosal margins, and 12 patients (14.6%) had invasive tumor at a resec-

TABLE 4.—Patients Who Had Further Local Resection Dictated by Frozen Sections

Patient	pTNM	Frozen Section	Further Local Resection Tissue	Main Specimen Margins			Further Management	Local Recurrence/ Outcome
				Mucosal	Deep	Bone		
1	T4N1M0	2 Carcinoma in situ	Dysplasia	Dysplasia 4 mm	2 mm	Clear	Radiotherapy	NSR NCL
2	T4N1M0	2 Deep Frank tumour	Frank tumour		7 mm	—	Radiotherapy	NSR died of neck disease
3	T4N2M0	1 Frank tumour	Frank tumour	Frank tumour 10 mm	Frank tumour 10 mm	Frank tumour	Radiotheraphy	Yes died of disease
4	T1N0M0	2 FS Dysplasia PS inflammation only	Negative			—	—	NSR NCL
5	T2N2M0	FS reported positive found to be incidental neurofibroma on PS	Ca in tissue, dysplasia at the margin	8 mm	7 mm	—	Pt declined radiotherapy	NSR died of neck disease
6	T4N0M0	FS ?Reactive changes	Negative	6 mm	4 mm	Clear	Radiotherapy	NSR NCL
7	T2N0M0	3 Dysplasia	Negative	5 mm	7 mm	—	Radiotherapy	NSR died of neck disease
8	T4N2M0	1 Frank tumour	—	4 mm	Frank tumour 8 mm	Clear	Radiotherapy	NSR NCL
9	T1N0M0	1 FS Dysplasia 2PS Dysplasia	Negative	7 mm		—	—	NSR NCL Died of other disease

Abbreviations: NSR, No sign of local recurrence; *NCL,* no palpable cervical lymphadenopathy; *FS,* frozen section; *PS,* paraffin section.
(Courtesy of Ribeiro NFF, Godden DRP, Wilson GE, et al: Do frozen sections help achieve adequate surgical margins in the resection of oral carcinoma? *Int J Oral Maxillofac Surg* 32:152-158, 2003. Copyright 2003, with permission from the International Association of Oral and Maxillofacial Surgeons.)

TABLE 5.—Main Specimen Margins and Outcomes

Margins	No. of Patients	Frozen Sections			T Stage				Recurrence		Died of Disease
		Dysplastic	Ca *in situ*	Frank Tumour	T1	T2	T3	T4	Local	Neck	
Clear margins	50	6	—	—	11	22	5	12	2	14	13
Close margins (<5 mm)											
Mucosal	7	1	—	1	1	—	1	5	—	2	1
Deep	8	—	—	—	—	3	2	3	2	2	2
Dysplasia/Ca *in situ* in mucosal margins	5	2	1	—	1	2	1	1	2	1	1
Frank tumour at margin											
Mucosal	3	—	—	1	1	—	—	2	3	1	2
Deep	7	—	—	1	—	—	2	6	3	2	3
Bone	1	1	—	—	—	—	—	1	1	1	1
Mucosal deep and bone	1	—	—	1	—	—	—	1	1	1	1

(Courtesy of Ribeiro NFF, Godden DRP, Wilson GE, et al: Do frozen sections help achieve adequate surgical margins in the resection of oral carcinoma? *Int J Oral Maxillofac Surg* 32:152-158, 2003. Copyright 2003, with permission from the International Association of Oral and Maxillofacial Surgeons.)

tion margin. In 10 of these 12 patients with invasive tumor at a resection margin, intraoperative frozen section results were negative. During a mean follow-up of 55 months, 14 patients (17.1%) had a local recurrence. Recurrence was seen in only 1 of the 9 patients who had further local resection that was based on frozen section results.

Conclusion.—Intraoperative frozen section analysis can improve outcomes in patients with resection margins involved by oropharyngeal cancer. Care must be taken when obtaining the specimen, as sampling error is the largest shortfall with frozen section analysis.

▶ Few specimens present more anatomic complexity or greater intraoperative demands than those occasioned by complex resections of malignancies seated in the head and neck. These authors examine the relevance of frozen section margins in ultimately achieving adequate surgical resection. This study is remarkable in that more than 500 frozen sections were evaluated. These covered the entire spectrum of mucosal and deep soft tissue margins. Furthermore, frozen sections used to evaluate the possibility of identifying neural invasion at the limits of surgical resection are also described. A large number of patients are evaluated and their tumors involve an extensive range of head and neck sites. Of note, the authors have striven to identify not only invasive carcinoma but also squamous epithelial dysplasia and carcinoma in situ at the margins. Readers of these authors' results should note that invasive carcinoma within 5 mm was considered a positive margin. In this regard, it seems reasonable that when margins are close but free by frozen section, those of us in the surgical pathology suite may wish to comment on the distance between the carcinoma that is identified and the margin that is deemed free but close. No doubt, the response of different surgeons in varying clinical conditions to a range of tumor-margin measurements may vary widely. The very strong agreement between frozen section interpretation of margins and the ultimate determination by permanent section is heartening. The authors address in detail the difficulties of determining when a squamous epithelium shows dysplasia by frozen section. These authors justify routine performance of frozen sections during this type of surgical procedures because the patients with positive margins are more likely to show postoperative tumor recurrence. It seems very likely that those of us working in institutions that care for patients with advanced head and neck malignancy will continue to see requests for numerous frozen sections from large resection specimens. It is not clear from reading this article whether the authors limited their evaluations to patients with squamous cell carcinomas. The extensive discussion of dysplasias and carcinomas in situ suggest that this may be the case. However, the performance of 22 frozen sections from nerve margins suggest that other types of malignancies might have been involved. Those addressing this problem in the future may wish to consider the fact that not only are minimal squamous lesions difficult to evaluate by frozen section, but some salivary gland malignancies such as cribiform adenoid cystic carcinoma can be very difficult to identify confidently when minor salivary gland tissue is included in margins taken for frozen section.

M. W. Stanley, MD

Sentinel Lymph Node Biopsy for Head and Neck Melanomas

Chao C, for the Sunbelt Melanoma Trial Group (Univ of Louisville, Ky; et al)
Ann Surg Oncol 10:21-26, 2003   12–2

Introduction.—Melanomas of the head and neck (H&N) offer unique surgical challenges because of their complex lymphatic drainage patterns. These lesions are associated with an increased likelihood of recurrence and a reduced overall survival, compared with other sites. Lymphoscintigraphy has verified the fact that anatomical predictions of nodal drainage are not always reliable. The results of sentinel lymph node (SLN) biopsy were compared with those for H&N, truncal, and extremity melanomas.

Methods.—The Sunbelt Melanoma Trial was a multi-institutional, prospective, randomized trial performed between June 1997 and February 2002 and involved 79 centers in North America (Fig 1). Eligibility to participate included being 18 to 70 years old and having cutaneous melanomas of 1.0 mm or greater Breslow thickness, and being clinically negative (nonpalpable or N0) regional lymph nodes. Patients underwent wide local excision of the primary melanoma and SLN biopsy via intradermal injection of technetium sulfur colloid around the primary tumor site. The SLN was processed by hematoxylin and eosin (H&E) staining at multiple levels (minimum, 5 sections/block, along with 2 additional random sections for immunohistochemistry (IHC) of S100 protein). Completion lymph node

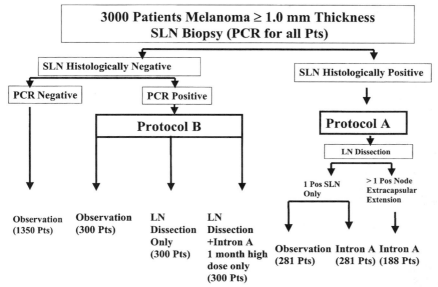

FIGURE 1.—The Sunbelt Melanoma Trial schema. *Abbreviations: SLN,* Sentinel lymph node; *PCR,* polymerase chain reaction; *LN,* lymph node; *Intron A,* interferon α-2b adjuvant therapy. (Courtesy of Chao C, for the Sunbelt Melanoma Trial Group: Sentinel lymph node biopsy for head and neck melanomas. *Ann Surg Oncol* 10(1):21-26, 2003.)

dissection of the involved node basin(s) was performed in patients with an SLN with metastatic disease by H&E or IHC.

Results.—A total of 2610 patients were assessed. The median follow-up was 18 months. The average number of SLN harvested per nodal basin for H&N, truncal, and extremity melanomas was 2.8, 2.7, and 2.1, respectively. No significant between-group differences were noted in median Clark level, Breslow thickness, and percentage of ulceration. Periparotid SLN were detected in 25% of patients. No facial nerve injuries were reported. The SLN biopsy for H&N melanoma had higher false-negative rates (1.5% vs 0.5% for trunk or extremity) but less histologically positive SLN (15% vs 23.4% for truncal and 19.5% for extremity melanoma; $P < .001$). Blue dye was visualized less frequently in the SLN of H&N melanoma patients compared with that of SLN of trunk or extremity melanomas.

Conclusion.—Preoperative lymphoscintigraphy, meticulous intraoperative inspection for blue or radioactive nodes, and a thorough anatomical knowledge of the region involved may improve results in H&N melanomas.

▶ Having written these commentaries for a number of years, I have had an opportunity to follow in detail the evolution of SLNs biopsies for various malignancies. As will be noted in this section and in the section on gynecologic pathology, application of what often seems to amount to microscopic staging of malignancy continues to expand. SLN biopsy for staging of malignant melanomas is not new. However, these authors offer a detailed look at problems unique to melanomas that occur in the head and neck.

This study is based on the fact that the lymphatic drainage of various H&N sites can be extremely complicated, thus introducing special problems into the efficacious identification and sampling of SLNs. This multicenter trial reports evaluation of a large number of patients with reasonable follow-up. Interesting findings include the fact that the incidence of positive SLNs appears to be lower in H&N melanomas than in lymph nodes draining similar malignancies occurring in other sites. Furthermore, the false-negative rate for these evaluations appears to be higher, albeit still low.

This work is especially interesting given what the authors describe as the "well known but not well understood phenomenon" of highly variable lymphatic drainage in this region of the body. Furthermore, the heightened lethality of melanomas in this area warrants our most careful study. Another strength of this study is central pathology review. Immunohistochemically, the workhorse marker in this study was S-100 protein. In a small number of centers, IHC for HMB-45 and MART-1 were also performed. This situation is appropriate, as S-100 protein is the most reliable marker of malignant melanomas occurring in H&N sites. One interesting result is that SLN biopsy in the area of the parotid never resulted in facial nerve damage.

One tantalizing aspect of this study which is not well described is the use of polymerase chain reaction for evaluation of minimal metastatic disease in protocol B (Fig 1). According to the authors' published algorithm, this assessment is essential for follow-up of patients with histologically negative SLNs. However, their discussion of this issue is relegated to generalities near the very end of the article. We should anticipate future articles in which this aspect of these authors' analysis is more fully described.

M. W. Stanley, MD

Sentinel Node Detection in N0 Cancer of the Pharynx and Larynx
Werner JA, Dünne A-A, Ramaswamy A, et al (Philipps-Univ of Marburg, Germany)
Br J Cancer 87:711-715, 2002   12–3

Background.—Sentinel lymph node (SLN) biopsy has been successfully used to limit the extent of lymph node dissection in patients with breast cancer or malignant melanoma. Whether SLN would be useful in patients with pharyngeal or laryngeal cancer with clinically negative nodes was investigated.

Methods.—The subjects were 50 patients (44 men and 6 women, 33-79 years) with squamous cell carcinoma of the oropharynx (n = 33), the larynx (n = 14), or the hypopharynx (n = 3). US showed no lymph node involvement in the neck (stage N0). At the start of surgery, technetium 99m was injected under microscopic control into multiple spots at the perimeter of the tumor. SLNs were identified intraoperatively via a collimated probe and a gamma probe. "Hot" nodes were dissected, followed by complete node dissection and excision of the primary tumor. All lymph nodes and the excised specimens were examined histologically.

Results.—A total of 90 SLNs was identified, and each patient had at least 1 SLN. On average, 36 lymph nodes were dissected per patient. Nine patients had nodal disease, and SLN identified 8 of them (sensitivity 89%) (Table 4). There was 1 false-negative finding, in which the SLN was histologically free of metastasis but a neighboring lymph node had a 0.65-cm metastasis.

Conclusion.—In these 50 patients with clinically N0 necks, 9 patients (18%) had occult disease. SLN biopsy correctly identified nodes in all but 1 of these patients. Still, skipping of nodal basins can occur, as shown by the 1 false-negative finding. These promising results support further research into

---

TABLE 4.—Predictiveness of Sentinel Lymphonodectomy in Pharyngeal and Laryngeal N0 Cancer

	No. of Cases and %	Post N-Status	Location
SN predictive	(49/50) 98%	41 × pN0	32/33 oropharynx
		7 × pN1	14/14 larynx
		1 × pN1 (mi)	3/3 hypopharynx
False-negative	(1/50) 2%	1 × pN1	1/33 oropharynx
Sensitivity	8/9 or 89% (95% confidence interval 63-100%)		

Abbreviation: SN, Sentinel lymph node.
(Courtesy of Werner JA, Düunne A-A, Ramaswamy A, et al: Sentinel node detection in N0 cancer of the pharynx and larynx. *Br J Cancer* 87:711-715, 2002. Used with permission. http://www.nature.com)

the use of SLN biopsy for limiting the extent of dissection in pharyngeal and laryngeal cancer patients.

▶ This article opens in what seems to this reviewer a somewhat self-congratulatory manner. Admittedly, the problem of what to do without lymph node dissections in clinically N0 patients with head and neck carcinoma is a reocurring problem. However, after reviewing the SLN literature in this series for the past several years, it seems to me that statements to the effect that a "potential excess of surgical therapy for the patient is currently achieved quite successfully in other tumor entities by applying the so-called SLN concept" is a bit premature. After all, it has not been that long since we were told that retrospective review of lymph nodes for missed micrometastases attach no great clinical significance to their detection. Furthermore, the natural history of diseases such as breast cancer are so long that frequent detection of micrometastases by immunohistochemical means continues to be of uncertain clinical significance. The bottom line in this study appears to be that, with proper clinical technique, SLNs can be identified in patients with squamous cell carcinomas of the pharynx and larnyx. However, it is still not clear whether identification of SLNs and a declaration that they are negative is sufficient to limit the extent of lymph node dissection in clinically N0 patients with these malignancies. The data in this article seemed to suggest that SLNs as assessed by these authors are predictive of the neck's true disease status. However, as noted in their discussion, the significance of micrometastases of uncertain prognostic significance remains unclear.

M. W. Stanley, MD

Sentinel Node Biopsy in Oral Cavity Cancer: Correlation With PET Scan and Immunohistochemistry
Civantos FJ, Gomez C, Duque C, et al (Univ of Miami, Fla)
Head Neck 25:1-9, 2003   12–4

Background.—The management of patients with mucosal squamous carcinoma of the head and heck with no clinical suspicion of lymph node involvement is controversial. Some researchers advocate a "watchful waiting" approach to avoid unnecessary morbidity, whereas others call for neck dissection or irradiation in patients at risk for cervical metastases. The possible use of lymphoscintigraphy and sentinel lymph node (SLN) biopsy in identifying patients with oral cavity cancer who would benefit from more extensive neck dissection was examined.

Methods.—The subject were 18 patients (16 men and 2 women, 34-79 years) with oral cavity cancers of the tongue (n = 11), buccal mucosa (n = 3), floor of the mouth (n = 2), alveolar ridge (n = 1), or oral vestibule (inner lip; n = 1). None of the patients had clinical evidence of lymph node involvement (stage N0). Preoperatively, patients underwent CT and [^{18}F] fluoro-D-glucose positron emission tomography (FDG PET). On the day of surgery, the tumor perimeter was injected with technetium 99m–sulfur colloid for

TABLE 1.—Results

Patient	Stage	CT	PET	Nuclear Imaging (# Hot Spots)	Histopathology of Sentinel Node: Frozen/Permanent		Neck Dissection
1	T_2	(−)	(−)	3	(−)	(−)	(−)
2	T_1	(−)	(−)	4 (2 supraclavicular)	(−)	(+)	(−)
3	T_2	(+/−) Some asymmetry	(−)	1	(−)*	(−) IHC only	(+) Matted
4	T_3	(−)	(−)	1	(+)	(+) (Omohyoid)	(+)
5	T_3	(+/−) More small nodes on side tumor	(−)	1	(+)	(+)	(+)
6	T_3	(+/−) Asymmetry present	(+) Unilateral	4	(+)	(+)	(+) 4
7	T_2	(−)	(−)	1	(−)	(+)	(−)
8	T_2	(+/−) Right glossotonsillar hypodensity	(−)	4	(−)	(−) IHC only	(−)
9	T_1	(−)	(−)	4	(−)	(−)	(−) 1 Papillary thyroid cancer
10	T_4	(+/−)	(+)	2	(−)	(+)	(−)
11	T_1	(−)	(−)	4	(+)	(+)	(−)
12	T_2	(−)	(+) Bilateral	3	(−)	(−)	(−)
13	T_2	(−)	(−)	2 Ipsilateral, 1 contralateral	(−)	(−)	(−)
14	T_1	(−)	(−)	2	(−)	(−)	(−)
15	T_1	(−)	(−)	2 Ipsilateral, 1 contralateral	(+)	(+)	(−)
16	T_2	(−)	(−)	2	(−)	(−)	(−)
17	T_2	(−)	(−)	1	(+)	(+)	(−)
18	T_2	(−)	(−)	2	(−)	(−)	(−)

*Patient had a histopathologically positive node without uptake noted during lymphoscintigraphy and sentinel lymph node biopsy.

Abbreviations: IHC, Immunohistochemistry.

(Courtesy of Civantos FJ, Gomez C, Duque C, et al: Sentinel node biopsy in oral cavity cancer: Correlation with PET scan and immunohistochemistry. *Head Neck* 25:1-9, 2003. Reprinted by permission of John Wiley & Sons, Inc.)

lymphatic mapping. At surgery, the primary tumor was excised first to re-duce background radioactivity; complete excision was confirmed by frozen section analysis. Next, SLNs were identified by the use of a gamma probe and "hot" nodes were excised. Subsequently, supraomohyoid neck dissec-tion was completed, and lymph nodes (including SLNs) were examined by histopathologic review and by immunoperoxidase staining to detect cyto-keratin.

Results.—At least 1 SLN was identified in all patients. Ten lesions (56%) were positive for disease (Table 1), 6 of which were identified on frozen sec-tions, 2 were identified on permanent sections, and 2 were identified only by IHC. Neither CT nor PET was predictive of histologic disease. SLN identi-fied all 10 true-positive lesions, and in 6 of these cases the SLN was the only node positive for disease. There was 1 false-negative finding on SLN biopsy, in which the SLN was negative but a neighboring node was "hot." In all, 2 patients (including the 1 with false-positive findings) had positive nodes that did not take up radioactivity; both of these nodes had been completely re-placed by tumor.

Conclusion.—Lymphoscintigraphy with SLN biopsy appears promising as a method for identifying which patients with oral cavity cancer will ben-efit from complete neck dissection. In 2 cases, involved nodes did not take up radioactivity; this suggests gross disease can replace the normal lymph node architecture, thus obstructing and redirecting lymphatic flow.

▶ Having just summarized an article describing SLN evaluation in head and neck squamous cell carcinomas, we turn now to oral cavity cancers for which evaluations of SLN study seems to be the most frequent of all head and neck sites. Albeit for a different primary tumor site, this article returns to the prob-lem of clinical management of the N0 neck in patients with squamous cell car-cinomas of the head and neck. The problem is that, because for many such patients the ultimate risk of neck disease is minimal, it is difficult to identify that minority who will have recurrences. This article attempts to focus on the relative minority of patients who will have occult metastases and for whom improved diagnostic techniques will allow increased survival while minimizing morbidity to the remaining majority of patients for whom increased treatment is not helpful. One of the most useful parts of this article is the detailed con-sideration of physiologic and anatomic considerations that may lead to aber-rant lymphatic drainage or to redirected lymphatic flow. The authors are to be commended for pointing out that, although their study is small, the false-negative rate for neck disease based on SLN evaluation was almost 10%. Al-though these results are encouraging, skepticism is clearly in order. (The com-ments regarding the complexity of head and neck lymphatic drainage noted in the second article in this series by Chao et al should be recalled at this point. [Abstract 12–2]) These authors go on to note that it is not rare to find metasta-ses in permanent section histology or based on postoperative immunohisto-chemistry that are not identified at the time of intraoperative frozen section. This article seems to emphasize a point we have made continually in these pages over the last several years. Interpretation of the SLN literature is ren-dered much more difficult by the fact that a wide range of intraoperative techniques for identification of these lymph nodes has been published. Furthermore, there is no consensus regarding optimum laboratory techniques either at the time of frozen section or subsequently for permanent sections and immunohistochemistry. Thus, this literature remains complex and difficult to interpret. Given the emergence of SLN information from a wide range of tumor types in various body sites, it seems essential that consensus panels be convened. Furthermore, in reading this year's selection of articles, I cannot escape the feeling that things are different in the head and neck. That is to say, a surface malignancy in 1 of these sites presents a much more complex physiologic and anatomic problem than might be experienced with malignancies of similar primary histology that arise in the trunk or extremities.

M. W. Stanley, MD

Expression of KIT (CD117) in Neoplasms of the Head and Neck: An Ancillary Marker for Adenoid Cystic Carcinoma
Mino M, Pilch BZ, Faquin WC (Harvard Med School, Boston)
Mod Pathol 12:1224-1231, 2003   12–5

Background.—Adenoid cystic carcinoma (ACC) of the head and neck is an indolent salivary gland malignancy with a poor long-term prognosis. Differentiating ACC from its many mimics is difficult, particularly in small biopsy samples. Recent studies suggest KIT (CD117) may be useful as a marker for ACC, yet it is unclear whether other tumors that mimic ACC also express CD117. Thus, KIT expression in ACC and a wide range of other head and neck malignancies were examined.

Methods.—Biopsy samples from 66 patients (35 males and 31 females, 13-81 years) with ACC of the head and neck (n = 53), trachea (n = 11), and breast (n = 2) were studied. Tumor sites included the minor salivary glands of the oral cavity (n = 12), parotid gland (n = 11), maxillary and ethmoid sinuses (n = 11), nasal cavity (n = 7), lacrimal gland/orbit (n = 6), submandibular gland (n = 4), ear canal (n = 2), tracheobronchial tree (n = 11), and breast (n = 2). In 40 cases the ACC was cribiform, in 9 it was tubular, in 8 it was solid, and in 9 it was of mixed morphology. ACC specimens were examined via immunohistochemistry with the use of 2 antibodies against KIT (H300 and A4502). These findings were compared with those from 98 patients with other neoplasms of the head and neck, including 16 cases of pleomorphic adenoma, 6 of basal cell adenoma, 5 of basal cell adenocarcinoma, 11 of basal cell carcinoma, 8 of polymorphous low-grade adenocarcinoma, 4 of adenosquamous carcinoma, 6 of basaloid squamous carcinoma, 6 of sebaceous carcinoma, 9 of mucoepidermoid carcinoma, 4 of salivary duct carcinoma, 8 of actinic cell carcinoma, 5 of oncocytoma, and 10 of Warthin's tumor.

Results.—The A4502 antibody detected KIT in 58 ACCs (82%), whereas the H300 antibody detected KIT in 54 ACCs (82%). Overall, 62 ACCs (94%) were positive for at least 1 antibody, and most (50, or 77%) were positive for both. KIT expression did not differ according to the site

TABLE 1.—KIT Expression in Head and Neck Neoplasms

Tumors (N)	Antibodies				
	H300		A4502		KIT
	Positive* % (N)	Strongly Positive† % (N)	Positive* % (N)	Strongly Positive† % (N)	Positive‡ % (N)
Adenoid cystic carcinoma (66)	30 (20)	52 (34)	18 (12)	71 (46)	94 (62)
Pleomorphic adenoma (16)	6 (1)	6 (1)	6 (1)	6 (1)	19 (3)
Basal cell adenoma (6)	0 (0)	17 (1)	17 (1)	0 (0)	17 (1)
Basal cell adenocarcinoma (5)	20 (1)	20 (1)	40 (2)	20 (1)	60 (3)
Basal cell carcinoma (11)	0 (0)	0 (0)	0 (0)	0 (0)	0 (0)
PLGC (8)	0 (0)	0 (0)	25 (2)	0 (0)	25 (2)
Adenosq. carcinoma (4)	0 (0)	0 (0)	0 (0)	0 (0)	0 (0)
Basaloid sq. carcinoma (6)	17 (1)	33 (2)	17 (1)	33 (2)	50 (3)
Sebaceous carcinoma (6)	17 (1)	0 (0)	17 (1)	0 (0)	17 (1)
Mucoepidermoid carcinoma (9)	11 (1)	0 (0)	0 (0)	0 (0)	11 (1)
Salivary duct carcinoma (4)	25 (1)	0 (0)	0 (0)	0 (0)	25 (1)
Acinic cell carcinoma (8)	0 (0)	13 (1)	0 (0)	0 (0)	13 (1)
Oncocytoma (5)	0 (0)	0 (0)	0 (0)	0 (0)	0 (0)
Warthin's tumor (10)	0 (0)	0 (0)	0 (0)	0 (0)	0 (0)
Total of other tumors (98)	6 (6)	6 (6)	8 (8)	4 (4)	16 (16)

*Cytoplasmic staining only.
†Cytoplasmic and membrane staining.
‡Positive staining with at least 1 of the 2 antibodies.
Abbreviations: PLGC, Polymorphous low-grade carcinoma; Adenosq, adenosquamous; sq, squamous.
(Courtesy of Mino M, Pilch BZ, Faquin WC: Expression of KIT (CD117) in neoplasms of the head and neck: An ancillary marker for adenoid cystic carcinoma. Mod Pathol 12:1224-1231, 2003.)

of the ACC, yet KIT expression did differ according to the histologic subtype: Staining with H300 and A4502 was positive in 37% and 61%, respectively, of the cribiform subtypes, 50% and 75% of the sold subtypes, 89% and 78% of the tubular subtypes, and 74% and 100% of the mixed subtypes. The sensitivity and specificity of the H300 antibody in detecting ACC were 82% and 88%, respectively, whereas corresponding values for the A4502 antibody were 89% and 87%. In contrast, only 8 of the non-ACC cases (8%) expressed both H300 and A4502. In particular, neoplasms that can mimic ACC (pleomorphic adenoma, basal cell adenoma, polymorphous low-grade adenocarcinoma, and basal cell carcinoma) had 25% or less staining with either antibody, and 5% or less staining with both antibodies (Table 1). However, 60% of basal cell adenocarcinomas and 50% of basaloid squamous carcinoma also had KIT expression.

Conclusion.—All but 4 cases of ACC expressed KIT, and KIT expression was significantly higher in ACC than in its mimics. These findings suggest KIT expression may be useful for distinguishing ACC from other neoplasms of the head and neck. Still, the high rates of KIT expression in basal cell adenocarcinoma and basaloid squamous carcinoma suggest KIT expression should not be the sole tool for distinguishing these 2 entities from ACC, especially in small samples.

▶ Identification of CD117 expression in chronic myelogenous leukemia and in gastrointestinal stromal tumors is 1 of the most exciting events in the recent history of pathology. Not only does this molecular marker suggest insights into tumor biology, it also provides significant heretofore unavailable therapeutic options. One of the most significant problems in head and neck disease is distinction of ACC from its many mimics. This problem is especially severe for those asked to approach these lesions by fine needle aspiration. Distinction of this often slowly progressive but ultimately lethal malignancy from less aggressive tumors such as polymorphous low-grade adenocarcinoma or from clearly benign entities including basal cell adenomas, is virtually impossible at the time of fine needle aspiration. Thus, a marker distinguishing these various entities has been sought. Among its other useful features, this article provides a concise but very informative review of CD117 expression in human neoplasia. Also, important warnings regarding the use of various immunoreagents is sounded clearly. Furthermore, the authors have evaluated the use of CD117 immunostaining in a very thorough manner by including a wide range of tumors that can be confused with ACC. Distinction of this entity from its mimics by CD117 studies is clearly far from perfect. However, it appears that support for this diagnosis can be obtained from such studies. The degree to which this study will translate into improved therapeutic options for patients who have ACC of the head and neck remains to be evaluated. Limitations of such evaluations become apparent when we consider the next article abstracted in this series (Abstract 12–6).

M. W. Stanley, MD

C-kit Expression in the Salivary Gland Neoplasms Adenoid Cystic Carcinoma, Polymorphous Low-Grade Adenocarcinoma, and Monomorphic Adenoma

Edwards PC, Bhuiya T, Kelsch RD (Long Island Jewish Med Ctr, New Hyde Park, NY)
Oral Surg Oral Med Oral Pathol Oral Radiol Endod 95:586-593, 2003   12–6

Background.—Differentiating between adenoid cystic carcinoma (ACC), polymorphous low-grade adenocarcinoma (PLGA), and the monomorphic adenomas (canalicular adenoma, trabecular adenoma, basal cell adenoma) can be difficult, particularly in small biopsy samples. Whether the expression of c-kit (CD117) could help differentiate between these salivary gland neoplasms was investigated.

Methods.—Formalin-fixed paraffin-embedded sections of ACC (n = 15), PLGA (n = 17), and monomorphic adenoma (n = 17) were stained with an antihuman c-kit polyclonal antibody, and the extent of immunoreactivity was examined. Staining was graded as weak (10%-25% of tumor cells stained positively), mild (26%-50%), moderate (51%-75%), and strong (76%-100%).

Results.—All 15 ACCs showed at least mild c-kit immunoreactivity, with most samples showing strong c-kit expression (Table 1). Interestingly, c-kit expression was stronger in ACCs of minor salivary glands than in ACCs of major salivary glands (Table 2). However, at least weak c-kit immunoreactivity was seen in all but 1 PLGA specimen (94%) and in all but 1 specimen of monomorphic adenoma (94%).

Conclusion.—All 3 tumor types expressed c-kit, yet immunoreactivity was stronger for ACCs than for PLGAs or monomorphic adenomas. Nonetheless, these findings suggest c-kit immunoreactivity is not useful for distinguishing between these 3 salivary gland neoplasms.

TABLE 1.—C-kit Immunoreactivity and Staining Intensity According to Tumor Type

	ACC	PLGA	Monomorphic Adenoma
Total number of cases	15	17	17
Negative staining	0	1	1
Weak staining (10% to 25% of cells)	0	4	1
Mild staining (26% to 50%)	1	4	1
Moderate staining (51% to 75%)	3	3	4
Strong staining (76% to 100%)	11	5	10
% Samples with positive staining	100%	94%	94%

(Courtesy of Edwards PC, Bhuiya T, Kelsch RD: C-kit expression in the salivary gland neoplasms adenoid cystic carcinoma, polymorphous low-grade adenocarcinoma, and monomorphic adenoma. *Oral Surg Oral Med Oral Pathol Oral Radiol Endod* 95:586-593, 2003.)

TABLE 2.—Summary of C-kit Immunoreactivity in ACC by Origin (Major Vs Minor Salivary Gland) and by Predominant Histologic Subtype (Tubular Vs Cribiform Vs Solid)

Predominant Histologic Subtype	Major Salivary Gland Origin ($n = 7$)			Minor Salivary Gland Origin ($n = 8$)		
	Tubular	Cribriform	Solid	Tubular	Cribriform	Solid
Negative staining	—	—	—	—	—	—
Weak staining (10% to 25% of cells)	—	—	—	—	—	—
Mild staining (26% to 50%)	1	—	—	—	—	—
Moderate staining (51% to 75%)	1	2	—	—	—	—
Strong staining (76% to 100%)	—	1	2	1	1	6
% Samples with >75% staining		43%			100%	

(Courtesy of Edwards PC, Bhuiya T, Kelsch RD: C-kit expression in the salivary gland neoplasms adenoid cystic carcinoma, polymorphous low-grade adenocarcinoma, and monomorphic adenoma. *Oral Surg Oral Med Oral Pathol Oral Radiol Endod* 95:586-593, 2003. Copyright 2003 by Elsevier.)

▶ If the last article abstracted (Abstract 12–5) in this series was cautiously optimistic about application of CD117 immunostaining to the differential diagnosis of ACC, the current article is frankly pessimistic regarding its clinical use. Some of this difference may be due to technical factors, including efficiency and specificity of the various immunoreagents used. An intriguing finding in the current study that is very difficult to understand at this time is the identification of more frequent CD117 staining in ACCs of minor salivary gland origin compared with those of major salivary gland origin. Although the numbers of cases in each category are small, this observation is intriguing. These authors provide a useful discussion of technical factors that might contribute to the different results in different studies. These will warrant careful consideration as future studies address the potential utility of CD117 immunostaining as a means of addressing what remains a very difficult differential diagnostic dilemma. Also, various mutations can be responsible for CD117 overexpression. Some of these result in a clinical response through recently developed pharmacologic agents, whereas others do not. Thus, the issue of patient treatment with these drugs is much more complex than immunostaining results alone would suggest. Given the dismal outlook of patients with ACC and the current level of noise regarding CD117 expression in these tumors, it is inevitable that some application of these agents to these patients will occur in the near future. Ultimately, immunostaining will take a backseat to clinical results.

M. W. Stanley, MD

Salivary Duct Carcinoma: Immunohistochemical Profile of an Aggressive Salivary Gland Tumour

Etges A, Pinto DS Jr, Kowalski LP, et al (Universidade de São Paulo, Brazil)
J Clin Pathol 56:914-918, 2003   12–7

Background.—Salivary duct carcinoma (SDC) is a rare, highly aggressive malignancy associated with a poor prognosis. Whether certain biomarkers might help identify patients with SDC at greater risk of death was investigated.

Methods.—Formalin-fixed, paraffin-embedded sections from 5 cases of SDC were examined immunohistochemically to determine the expression of cyclin D1, cyclin-dependent kinase 4, p16, retinoblastoma protein (pRb), E2F-1, p53, murine double minute 2, bcl-2, and c-erbB-2 oncoprotein. Patients were monitored to determine outcomes.

Results.—In all 5 cases, there was deregulation of the pRb and p53 pathways. Four cases had positive membranous staining for c-erbB-2 (Table 3), including 1 case with expression in more than 50% of the cells and 1 case with c-erbB-2 in 100% of cells. All 4 of these patients died of the disease within 1 year 4 months of diagnosis. In contrast, the 1 patient whose cells did not express c-erbB-2 was still alive at 10 years.

Conclusion.—The c-erbB-2 overexpression is associated with a poor prognosis in patients with SDC. The aggressive nature and potential for recurrence and metastasis of SDC are therefore more likely to be associated with the c-erbB-2 oncoprotein than with cell cycle deregulation (despite changes in the pRb and p53 pathways). The c-erbB-2 increases vessel permeability; endothelial cell growth, proliferation, migration, and differentiation; matrix degradation; and proteolytic activity. Its expression in SDC suggests aggressive behavior and a poor outcome.

TABLE 3.—Outcome and Immunohistochemical Protein Expression in 5 Cases of Salivary Duct Carcinoma

Case	Outcome	Cyclin D1	CDK4	p16	pRb	E2F-1	p53	mdm2	c-erbB-2	Bcl-2
1	DOD, 1 year	28.0	43.2	0.0	49.4	28.8	70.4	78.8	54.6	00
2	DOD, 7 months	0.0	0.0	23.2	49.4	23.4	0.0	0.0	5.0	0.0
3	DOD, 10 years	32.8	21.2	16.89	0.0	8.60	82.8	0.0	0.0	0.0
4	DOD, 1 year/4 months	29.8	20.2	0.0	51.0	15.6	0.0	0.0	12.4	0.0
5	DOD, 10 months	0.0	62.8	62.0	31.6	394	0.0	76.6	100.0	0.0

Abbreviations: CDK4, Cyclin-dependent kinase 4; *DOD,* died of disease; *mdm2,* murine double minute 2; *pRb,* retinoblastoma protein.

▶ SDC is primarily a tumor of elderly men and is most often seen in the parotid gland. Although its definition sounds fuzzy to nonpathologists, its identification as a tumor that histologically resembles breast cancer is a comfortable definition for those of us who do clinical microscopy on a daily basis. This article highlights 2 issues relevant to the clinical behavior of this tumor. First, this is a rare entity. This series of 5 cases is typical in size of many previously published studies. The second observation is that no matter what we do, this remains a very aggressive tumor regarding the biology of which we have very little understanding.

M. W. Stanley, MD

Oral Synovial Sarcoma: A Report of 2 Cases and a Review of the Literature

Meer S, Coleman H, Altini M (Univ of Witwatersrand, Johannesburg, South Africa)
Oral Surg Oral Med Oral Pathol Oral Radiol Endod 96:306-315, 2003   12–8

Background.—Synovial sarcomas usually occur in the para-articular regions of the extremities, but about 10% occur in the head and neck. Synovial sarcoma in the oral cavity, however, is rare, with only 29 cases reported in the literature. Two more cases of this malignancy are described, along with a literature review.

> *Case reports.*—The patients were 2 men, one man aged 43 years, with a 2 × 1.5 × 0.7-cm synovial sarcoma of the left mandibular and maxillary retromolar region, and the other man aged 49 years with a 4.5 × 3 × 1.5-cm synovial sarcoma of the floor of the mouth. On both clinical and pathologic examinations, these oral cavity tumors were similar to synovial sarcomas in other areas of the body. Outcome data are missing because both of these patients were lost to follow-up. Immunohistochemical analysis showed both tumors stained positively for epithelial membrane antigen, Bcl-2, CD99, vimentin, and calretinin.

Conclusion.—It is possible that synovial sarcoma of the oral cavity might be detected earlier and more easily accessed than sarcomas at other sites, and thus might be more amenable to surgery. Given the lack of follow-up, however, this remains to be proven. In general, synovial sarcomas in the oral cavity appear to be similar to sarcomas developing at other body sites, which have an aggressive nature and are associated with poor long-term outcomes. As shown by the literature review, about 20% of patients with synovial sarcoma have local recurrence develop, 30% have metastases develop, and almost 40% die of disease. To ensure accurate and early diagnosis, synovial sarcoma of the oral cavity should be included in the differential diagnosis of intraoral spindle cell malignancies.

▶ Typical examples of synovial sarcoma present little diagnostic difficulty. When this tumor occurs in young adults and is located near large joints, the diagnosis is usually obvious. Even the once controversial monophasic variant is usually readily recognized. One sometimes inadequately celebrated aspect of this tumor is its proclivity to occur in more central locations. Chief among these is the head and neck that hosts approximately 10% of synovial sarcomas. Although this report focuses on 2 examples of synovial sarcoma occurring in the oral cavity, the authors provide a useful review of its behavior in the head and neck. These authors do an excellent job of summarizing the immunohistochemical findings in synovial sarcoma of various sites. As is the case with many soft tissue tumors, as well as neoplasms of other sites, detailed cytogenetic analysis often provides considerable weight to a specific diagnosis. These authors highlight the ways in which molecular consequences of cytogenetic abnormalities will lead to improved methods of diagnosis in frozen or paraffin-embedded tissue. The importance of accurately diagnosing synovial sarcoma in head and neck sites is emphasized by these authors when they describe the frequent inadequacy of initial excisions and couple this to a 30% rate of metastases and a 20% rate of local recurrence. For those of us who do diagnostic pathology, the major problem with synovial sarcoma in the head and neck remains recognition of this uncommon entity.

M. W. Stanley, MD

Mucoepidermoid Carcinoma of the Larynx: Report of Three Cases
Prgomet D, Bilić M, Bumber Ž, et al (Zagreb Univ, Croatia)
J Laryngol Otol 117:998-1000, 2003   12–9

Background.—Mucoepidermoid carcinoma of the larynx is rare, and these tumors are often missed on histopathologic examination because of their close histologic similarity to squamous cell carcinoma. Three more cases of this malignancy are described, along with a literature review.

> *Case report.*—The subjects were 2 men and 1 woman, 48 to 66 years, with high-grade mucoepidermoid carcinoma of the larynx. The patients presented with dysphagia, hoarseness, and/or labored breathing. Supraglottic (2 cases) or total (1 case) laryngectomy was performed, with confirmation of complete tumor excision by frozen-section analysis. Postoperatively, all patients underwent radiation therapy and are free of disease at 39 months to 6 years of follow-up.

Conclusion.—According to the literature review, most patients with mucoepidermoid carcinoma of the larynx are treated by surgery only. However, given that up to 50% of these patients have recurrence, all 3 of these patients underwent both surgical excision and postoperative radiation therapy with good outcomes over more than 3 years of follow-up. Some evidence suggests distinguishing high- and low-grade mucoepidermoid carcinoma of the larynx may be important, because high-grade tumors behave aggressively, whereas low-grade tumors are often cured by local excision. Still, given the inconclusive evidence, the extent of excision depends on the size and localization of the tumor, and the need for postoperative radiation therapy depends on the pathohistologic findings and histologic grade of the tumor.

▶ It is easy to forget that virtually any type of carcinoma identified in the major salivary glands can occur in their minor counterparts elsewhere in the body. Thus, tumors such as mucoepidermoid carcinoma can be encountered in the larynx, trachea, bronchi, and even in the breast. These present differential diagnostic difficulties that can be severe, especially for those who study these tumors in fine needle aspiration samples. It has even been noted that salivary gland-type tumors occurring in the upper aerodigestive tract can present difficulties at the time of thyroid fine needle aspiration cytology. The authors of this article do an excellent job of highlighting not only the importance of these diagnoses, but also their rarity in clinical practice. Perhaps the major problem with diagnosis of this entity relates not only to the fact that it is extremely rare, but also to the finding that high-grade examples overlap histologically with the vastly more common squamous cell carcinomas. In this regard, the distinction of high-grade and low-grade mucoepidermoid carcinoma occurring in sites other than the major salivary glands is unclear. Experience with these more common locations for this tumor suggest that high-grade examples will behave aggressively, wheras low-grade tumors may be virtually cured by local excision. Literature reviewed by these authors appears to support this concept.

M. W. Stanley, MD

Sinonasal Adenocarcinoma: Evidence for Histogenetic Divergence of the Enteric and Nonenteric Phenotypes

Choi H-R, Sturgis EM, Rashid A, et al (Chonnam Natl Univ, Kwangju, Korea; Univ of Texas, Houston)
Hum Pathol 34:1101-1107, 2003   12–10

Background.—Adenocarcinomas of nonsalivary origin comprise 10% to 20% of all sinonasal malignancies. Varying histopathologic features and uncertain histogenesis characterize these adenocarcinomas. Sinonasal adenocarcinomas (SNACs) were investigated to better determine the histogenesis and phenotypic heterogeneity of these tumors.

Methods and Findings.—Immunohistochemical analyses for cytokeratin (CK) 7 and CK20 were performed on 12 primary SNACs representing the histopathologic spectrum of these lesions, adjacent normal mucosa, and 2 metastatic adenocarcinomas from colonic primary tumors. Histologically normal respiratory-type epithelium and submucosal seromucous glands demonstrated restricted reactivity to CK7. Epithelial metaplasia of surface

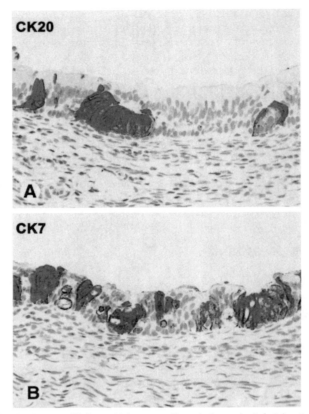

FIGURE 4.—Respiratory epithelium with interspersed intestinal metaplastic foci showing positive stain-ing for CK20 (**A**) and negative staining for CK7 (**B**). (Original magnification ×40.) (Courtesy of Choi H-R, Sturgis EM, Rashid A, et al: Sinonasal adenocarcinoma: Evidence for histogenetic divergence of the enteric and nonenteric phenotypes. *Hum Pathol* 34:1101-1107, 2003.)

epithelium related to enteric SNACs was associated with a conversion from CK7 positivity to CK20 positivity (Fig 4). All primary enteric-type carcino-mas and the 2 colonic metastases reacted to CK20. However, all nonenteric-type tumors were CK20 negative and CK7 positive. Coexpression of CK7 and CK20 were observed in some enteric types.

Conclusions.—Nonenteric-type adenocarcinoma may originate directly from surface respiratory-type epithelium or from seromucous glands. Meta-plastic transformation of surface respiratory to enteric-type epithelium pre-cedes enteric adenocarcinoma development. Coordinate analyses of CK7 and CK20 reactivity may be useful in the differential diagnosis of SNACs.

▶ The idea that enteric-type carcinomas occur in places as diverse as the sinonasal mucosa and the uterine cervix is fascinating. This work provides sup-port for the concept that an enteric type of metaplasia proceeds development of these carcinomas, as least in sinonasal sites. These authors also strengthen the concept that wherever enteric differentiation occurs, immunoreactivity for CK20 appears to be a useful surrogate biomarker that reflects an underlying shift in gene expression. It would be interesting to use this readily available tool to investigate the frequency of enteric metaplasia in this and other epithelia. The degree to which this change is an obligate precursor of malignancy is unclear.

M. W. Stanley, MD

Relative Paucity of Gross Genetic Alterations in Myoepitheliomas and Myoepithelial Carcinomas of Salivary Glands
Hungermann D, Roeser K, Buerger H, et al (Univ Hosp Muenster, Germany; Univ Hosp Eppendorf, Hamburg, Germany)
J Pathol 198:487-494, 2002   12–11

Background.—Salivary gland myoepithelioma has a heterogeneous cytomorphology and inconsistent immunophenotype. The diagnosis of this entity relies on conventional histology. However, cytomorphologic and immunophenotypic analysis cannot reliably predict the clinical course of this disease.

Methods and Findings.—The immunophenotype of 12 myoepitheliomas and 21 malignant myoepitheliomas was determined. Seven markers were tested. Antibodies against cytokeratins 5/6, S-100 protein, and vimentin yielded the most consistent reactivity profile. Comparative genomic hybridization (CGH) profiles revealed chromosomal losses in 3 of 12 myoepitheliomas. Of 19 myoepithelial carcinomas investigated by CGH, 10 lacked identifiable cytogenetic aberrations. In 5 cases, chromosome 8 showed aberrations, consistent with observations in salivary gland carcinomas of other differentiation. One case represented in 3 separately localized manifestations of disease yielded information on the relevance of gross aberration for tumor development because the tumor CGH profiles differed (Tables 1 and 2).

Conclusions.—In the work-up of myoepitheliomas, staining for cytokeratins 5/6 is useful because its expression is reliable in most cases and it may indicate the epithelial nature of the lesion. The value of CGH as a diagnostic adjunct appears to be limited. The presence of many gross cytogenetic aberrations should raise suspicion of malignancy. The low frequency of aberrations detected by CGH in overtly malignant myoepithelial neoplasms suggests that gross cytogenetic changes occurred during tumor progression. It also indicates the relevance of genetic changes not resolved by CGH.

▶ This article provides a useful review of concepts related to salivary gland tumors with myoepithelial differentiation. As outlined by these authors, these tumors can be difficult to diagnose with certainty. The morphologic findings depend heavily on adequate sampling to rule out other types of differentiation. Furthermore, while we expect positive immunostaining for S-100 protein and glial fibrillary acidic protein, even these most dependable markers of myoepi-

TABLE 1.—Myoepitheliomas: Summary of Clinical, Phenotypic, and CGH Data

Case No	Age (Years), Sex	Topography; Cytomorphology	Ck5/6	KL-1	SMA	Vim	ER	PR	S100	GFAP	Mitoses/10 HPF	Cytogenetic Alterations
1	59, m	Hard palate; epitheloid	+	(+)	–		–	–	(+)	(+)	<1	None
2	79, f	Palate; spindled	+	+	+		–	–	+	+	<1	None
3	26, m	Parotid gland; spindled	+	–	+	+	–	–	+	+	<1	None
4	35, m	Palate; plasmacytoid	+	–	+		–	–	+	+	<1	4p–
5	37, m	Parotid gland; epitheloid	+	+	(+)		–	–	+	+	<1	None
6	33, f	Parotid gland; epitheloid	–	–			–	–	+		2	None
7	60, f	Parapharyngeal; spindled	+	+	+		–	–	+	+	<1	8q–
8	57, m	Soft palate; plasmacytoid	+	–	–		–	–	+	+	<1	None
9	75, f	Parotid gland; spindled	+	+	(+)	+	–	–	+	+	<1	None
10	43, f	Parotid gland; spindled	+	–	+	+	–	–	+	+	<1	2p–, 2q–
11	57, f	Parotid gland; spindled	+	–	–		–	–		–	<1	None
12	53, ?	Parotid gland; spindled	+	–	(+)		–	–			<1	None

(Courtesy of Hungermann D, Roeser K, Buerger H, et al: Relative paucity of gross genetic alterations in myoepitheliomas and myoepithelial carcinomas of salivary glands. *J Pathol* 198:487-494, 2002. Reprinted by permission of John Wiley & Sons, Ltd.)

TABLE 2.—Myoepithelial Carcinomas: Summary of Clinical, Phenotypic, and CGH Data

Case No	Age (Years), Sex	Topography; Cytomorphology	Ck5/6	KL1	SMA	Vim	ER	PR	S100	GFAP	MIB-1	Mitoses	Cytogenetic Alterations
1	59, f	Lower lip; clear cell	(+)	+	+						np	<1	None
2	21, m	Parotid gland; epitheloid, ex PA	+	-	-						2%	<1	None
3	63, f	Paramandibular; epitheloid									<1%	<1	1q+, 5pq+, 8q+, 9q-11pq+, 17p+q+, 18p+q+, 22q+
4	56, f	Neck; spindled, ex PA	(+)	+	+						<1%	<1	8pq+
5	45, f	Palate; plasmacytoid	(+)	-	-		-		+	(+)	2%	<1	4q-
6	56, f	Palate; clear cell									<1%	<1	None
7	35, f	Parotid gland; spindled	+	+	-	+					<1%	<1	np
8	37, f	Parotid gland; spindled	+	+	-	+					15%	<1	5pq+
9	71, f	Parotid gland; plasmacytoid	+	+	+		-	-	+	+	2.5%	4	1p-q+, 4q-, 7p-+q+, 8pq+, 13q-, 16q-, 18pq+
10	63, f	Hard palate; spindled	+	+	+	+					3%	<1	np
11	60, f	Parotid gland; spindled	+	-	-	+	-	-	(+)	-	30%	8	np
12	62, m	Parotid gland; spindled	+	+	-	+	-	-	+	+	10%	2	np
13	28, m	Oropharynx; spindled				+					<1%	<1	None
14a	72, m	Pharynx; plasmacytoid, ex PA	+	+	(+)		-	-	+	+	np	<1	3p-, 4p-, 5pq+, 6q-
14b	72, m	Paravertebral; plasmacytoid, ex PA	+	+	+		-	-	+	+	np	2	None
14c	73, m	Orbit; plasmacytoid, ex PA	(+)	(+)	+	+			+	+	np	<1	1q+, 5pq+, 7p-, 8q+, 11pq+, 13q+, 17pq+, 18pq+, 22q+
15	72, f	Parotid gland; spindled	+	(+)	+	+					1%	<1	None
16	23, m	Parotid gland; spindled	+	+	-	+			+	+	5%	<1	None
17	49, m	Parotid gland; epitheloid	+	+	-	+					np	<1	None
18	62, m	Parotid gland; plasmacytoid	+	+	+	+					2%	<1	None
19	62, f	Tongue; plasmacytoid	+	+	+	-	-	-	-	-	np	<1	6q-
20	51, m	Parotid gland; plasmacytoid	+	+	+	-	-	-	+	+	np	<1	None
21	69, m	Parotid gland; plasmacytoid	-	-	-	-	-	-	+	-	8%	4	1p+q+, 2q-, 4q-, 5q-, 6p+q+, 8pq+, 9q-, 11p+q-, 12p+, 20q+

Abbreviations: PA, Pleomorphic adenoma; *np*, not performed.
(Courtesy of Hungermann D, Roeser K, Buerger H, et al: Relative paucity of gross genetic alterations in myoepitheliomas and myoepithelial carcinomas of salivary glands. *J Pathol* 198:487-494, 2002. Reprinted by permission of John Wiley & Sons, Ltd.)

thelial differentiation are not always helpful. In this study, immunostaining for cytokeratin 5/6 emerges as a very helpful diagnostic finding in both benign and malignant salivary gland tumors with myoepithelial differentiation. Our own experience with needle aspiration of salivary gland tumors indicates that most of the lesions in which we encounter myoepithelial differentiation are ultimately shown to be examples of mixed tumor. Thus, in those cases without clinical evidence of malignancy, confirmation of myoepithelial differentiation in a needle aspiration specimen would be very helpful and would most often point toward a benign ultimate diagnosis. In this regard, the potential utility of immunostaining for cytokeratin 5/6 opens up an intriguing possibility. These authors also do a good job of reviewing the literature and experience indicating that distinguishing between benign and malignant myoepithelial tumors can be very difficult, even in surgical resection specimens. At least for the methods used in this study, genetic analysis of myoepithelial tumors occurring in salivary gland sites appears to have little clinical utility. It would be interesting to apply the immunostaining information from this paper to a study of myoepithelial tumors of mammary origin.

M. W. Stanley, MD

The Relationship Between Tumor Thickness and Clinical and Histopathologic Parameters in Cancer of the Larynx
Yilmaz T, Gedikoğlu G, Gürsel B (Hacettepe Univ Faculty of Medicine, Ankara, Turkey)
Otolaryngol Head Neck Surg 129:192-198, 2003   12–12

Background.—The prognostic significance of tumor thickness has been shown in various carcinomas, including laryngeal cancer. However, the relation of tumor thickness to various clinical and histopathologic parameters in laryngeal cancer has not been elucidated. An attempt was made to link the thickness of a laryngeal tumor to clinical and histopathologic findings.

Methods.—The laryngectomy specimens of 111 surgically treated patients with T1 to T3 laryngeal cancer were retrospectively reviewed for tumor thickness, pathologic cervical lymph node metastasis, cartilage invasion, microscopic appearance, mode of invasion of the surrounding tissues, differentiation, lymphocyte infiltration, perineural and vascular invasion, and various histopathologic parameters. The 111 patients included 109 men and 2 women, all of whom smoked; their mean age was 51 years (range, 32-73 years).

Results.—Among the cases with cartilage invasion the mean tumor thickness was 9.7 mm; with no invasion, the mean was 5.4 mm, a statistically significant difference. Exophytic and endophytic tumors also showed a statistically significant difference in tumor thickness. No statistically significant differences were noted between well-differentiated, moderately differentiated, and poorly differentiated cases or between cases with and without vascular invasion. However, the difference in tumor thickness between cases with and without perineural involvement was statistically significant. Statistical analysis also found significant differences linked to mode of invasion of surrounding tissues; presence of mild, moderate, or marked lymphocytic infiltration; cases with and without cervical lymph node metastasis; clinical stages; and T stages. Factors found to independently determine tumor thickness were cartilage invasion and lymphocytic infiltration.

Conclusions.—With deeper invasion, the barriers of the larynx are breached by laryngeal cancers. Invasion of the cartilage and lymphocytic infiltration were found to independently determine tumor thickness, with good correlation also noted for most of the clinical and histopathologic parameters assessed. Therefore, measurement of tumor thickness offers reliable histopathologic indications for laryngeal cancer.

▶ These authors emphasize the potential utility of reporting depth of tumor invasion in laryngectomy specimens. In some instances, we tend to report this information in anatomic terms by describing such findings as perichondrium or cartilage invasion. However, these authors suggest that a numerical measurement of tumor depth might also be useful, as it seems to correlate with a number of other prognostic indicators.

M. W. Stanley, MD

13 Neuropathology

Aluminum-Induced Apoptosis in Cultured Cortical Neurons and Its Effect on SAPK/JNK Signal Transduction Pathway
Fu H-J, Hu Q-S, Lin Z-N, et al (Sun Yat-Sen Univ, Guangzhou, China)
Brain Res 980:11-23, 2003   13–1

Background.—Research on several neurodegenerative diseases has implicated aluminum exposure and apoptotic cell death. However, the mechanisms by which aluminum interacts with the nervous system are not well documented. The ability of aluminum to induce apoptosis of neurons was explored. The role of the SAPK/JNK (stress-activated protein kinase or c-jun N-terminal kinase) signal transduction pathway on the apoptosis induced by aluminum was also investigated.

Methods and Findings.—Cultured cortical neurons were examined. Aluminum-induced degeneration of cortical neurons involved the DNA fragmentation characteristic of apoptosis. Aluminum-treated neuron staining with the DNA-binding fluorochrome Hoechst 33258 showed the typical apoptotic condensation and fragmentation of chromatin. The apoptosis rate increased significantly, from 4.9% to 13.1%, 21.4%, and 59.8%, as assessed by TdT-mediated dUTP nick end labeling. Western blot analysis demonstrated that SAPK/JNK activities of cortical neurons varied with different $AlCl_3$ exposure times. Compared with control cultures, phosphorylation levels were 4.2 times greater at 6 hours, 3.3 times greater at 12 hours, 1.9 times greater at 24 hours, and 1.1 times greater at 48 hours. The JNK pathway inhibitor CEP-11004 inhibited SAPK/JNK activation to protect cortical neurons from apoptosis induced by aluminum chloride.

Conclusions.—Aluminum exposure can induce the apoptosis of cortical neurons. The current data also show that the SAPK/JNK signal transduction pathway may play an important role in the apoptosis.

▶ The neurotoxic effects of aluminum are controversial at best. Several studies have suggested a potential etiopathogenic role for aluminum in Alzheimer disease, amyotrophic lateral sclerosis, and dialysis-induced encephalopathy associated with extensive exposure to this element. These reports have raised considerable interest in the investigation of the potential deleterious effects of aluminum in the nervous system, with considerable effort being dedicated to identify possible mechanisms of action.

The current article investigated the effects of aluminum, in a dose-dependent manner, on primary cultures of rat cortical neurons. The results demonstrate that aluminum reduces neuronal viability, but the doses needed to induce apoptosis were very high, questioning the extrapolation of the results to an in vivo system. The authors show that the SAPK/JNK signaling pathway, which is a member of the mitogen-activated protein kinase, participates in the induction of neuronal apoptosis in their culture system. Given the reported data on the glial mediation in the neuronal cell death induced by aluminum, the possibility of an indirect effect of glial cells in this system could potentially be considered. The study brings significant contribution to the field by demonstrating the induction of apoptosis in neurons and showing a specific transduction pathway associated with this effect, which could potentially be the target of therapeutics. However, it is also clear from their studies that another signaling pathway, yet unidentified, is involved in the mechanisms of cell death. Future in vitro and in vivo studies will be needed to further characterize these findings.

M. E. Couce, MD, PhD

Correlation Between Genetic Alteration and Long-term Clinical Outcome of Patients With Oligodendroglial Tumors, With Identification of a Consistent Region of Deletion on Chromosome Arm 1p
Hashimoto N, Murakami M, Takahashi Y, et al (Kyoto Prefectural Univ, Japan; Saiseikai Shiga Hosp, Japan; Tokyo Med and Dental Univ)
Cancer 97:2254-2261, 2003   13–2

Introduction.—In oligodendroglial tumors, allelic losses on chromosome arms 1p and 19q are both diagnostic markers and statistically significant predictors of both chemosensitivity and longer recurrence-free survival. Twenty-one patients with diagnosed oligodendroglial tumors were genetically and clinically evaluated, with a focus on the associations between genetic alterations on arms 1p, 17p, and 19q and long-term therapeutic results.

Methods.—Of 21 patients who underwent surgery for oligodendroglial tumors, the surgical specimens revealed that 13 tumors were oligodendrogliomas, World Health Organization [WHO] grade II; 3 were anaplastic oligodendrogliomas, WHO grade III; 3 were oligoastrocytomas, WHO grade II; and 2 were anaplastic oligoastrocytomas, WHO grade III). Genetic testing for 1p deletions was conducted by using fluorescence in situ hybridization, and testing for 1p, 17p, and 19q deletions was performed via microsatellite analysis. Survival was calculated with the use of univariate and multivariate Cox regression models. In addition, a high-resolution map of 1p, which led to the discovery of a new deleted region on 1p, was acquired.

Results.—Both the loss of 1p and the loss of 19q independently and significantly predicted overall survival. A high-resolution deletion map, which demonstrated unusually narrow deletions, showed a new region of deletion between D1S513 and D1S458 (1p34.3-36.11).

Conclusion.—One of the putative tumor suppressor loci is situated more proximally than ever reported. Because of the finding that 1p and 19q deletions predicted survival, further use of diagnostic and prognostic genetic testing in the clinical setting is recommended.

▶ The determination of the status of chromosome arms 1p and 19q has become standard for the diagnosis of oligodendrogliomas. Numerous reports have shown that loss of 1p or combined 1p/19q loss is associated with better prognosis, and is present in 50% to 80% of these tumors, depending on the reports. However, the nature of the putative tumor suppressor gene is yet unknown.

The current study evaluates 21 patients undergoing partial or subtotal surgery for oligodendroglial tumors, including pure oligodendrogliomas and mixed oligoastrocytomas. The authors based their analysis on fluorescent in situ hybridization (FISH) for 1p, evaluation of 1p, 17p, and 19q deletion by microsatellite analysis, and a high-resolution deletion map of 1p. The goals of the study were to determine the long-term clinical outcome for these patients and to try to establish its association with the molecular genetic, pathologic findings. The authors demonstrated a loss of heterozygosity in a high percentage of the evaluated tumors, with both the loss of 1p and 19q being independent predictors of overall survival. Their results show that the 1p deletions seen in most samples were representative of a nearly complete arm deletion. The most important finding of the study was the identification of a common deleted region at 1p34.3-36.11 for the potential location of a putative tumor suppressor gene. This is the most precise and narrow approach reported yet, since previous studies have more broadly pointed at up to four 1p genomic regions as potential candidates for the location of tumor suppressor genes. Interestingly, chromosome arm 1p deletion determined by FISH was the most significant predictor among the variables studied. This is good news for the majority of the pathology labs that largely use FISH to determine the 1p/19q status of these tumors. The study additionally reemphasizes the importance of further use of diagnostic and prognostic genetic testing in the clinical setting.

M. E. Couce, MD, PhD

Ghrelin Main Action on the Regulation of Growth Hormone Release Is Exerted at Hypothalamic Level
Popovic V, Miljic D, Micic D, et al (Univ of Turin, Italy; Santiago de Compostela Univ, Spain)
J Clin Endocrinol Metab 88:3450-3453, 2003   13–3

Background.—Ghrelin has recently been identified as a hormone possibly involved in regulating growth hormone (GH) secretion and appetite. GH discharge has been stimulated by ghrelin administration in all species tested, including humans. The site of this action may be at the pituitary gland or the hypothalamus. The stimulatory effect of ghrelin on human GH secretion was assessed in patients with hypothalamopituitary disconnection. The goals included determining (1) whether ghrelin releases GH at the pituitary gland or hypothalamus, and (2) whether ghrelin offers promise as a treatment for GH-deficiency disorders.

Methods.—Nine patients with organic lesions located principally in the hypothalamic area and 9 age-matched and body mass index–matched controls were evaluated. After an insulin-induced hypoglycemia test (ITT) was performed, all patients had a severely GH-deficient response. In addition, patients' GH-releasing hormone (GHRH)-induced GH peaks were equal to or higher than those obtained with the ITT. Both patients and controls underwent 3 different tests administered on different days in random order and separated by at least 1 week. GHRH was given one day, ghrelin one day, and a combination of GHRH and ghrelin one day. Serum GH levels were determined and compared between the groups.

Results.—The mean GH peak in controls induced by GHRH was 21.2 µg/L; that in patients was 3.1 µg/L. The mean GH peak in controls after ghrelin was 75.1 µg/L; that in patients was 2.0 µg/L. The ghrelin-induced GH peak was lower than the GHRH peak in 7 of the 9 patients. In all patients, it was higher than that obtained after ITT. When the combination of GHRH and ghrelin was used, the mean GH peaks were 103.5 µg/L in controls and 9.6 µg/L in patients. Ghrelin was significantly more potent in the controls than in patients. The combination produced an additive effect. Among patients, the GHRH-mediated GH peak was higher than that after ITT, and the ghrelin-mediated GH secretion was lower than that elicited by GHRH. Patients exhibited potent blockage of the GH peak when GHRH and ghrelin were given together.

Conclusions.—The actions of ghrelin came mainly from suprapituitary structures, with the hypothalamic level being the most likely source. Thus, ghrelin will likely have no role in promoting GH secretion in patients with organic lesions of the hypothalamus, pituitary stalk, or pituitary itself. These patients failed to respond to ghrelin with increased GH release.

▶ Ghrelin is a new hormone mainly produced by the stomach and involved in the regulation of GH secretion and appetite. This study addresses the important question of whether ghrelin acts mainly at the hypothalamic level versus the pituitary. The data showed that individuals with an organic lesion in the hypothalamic area have an abnormal GH respond to ghrelin administration, either alone or in combination with GHRH, suggesting the hypothalamus as the main target for ghrelin action in humans.

This study helps us to better understand the mechanism of ghrelin action in humans, but also suggests that ghrelin, and probably its analogues, will have limited therapeutic efficacy in the treatment of GH deficiency in patients with abnormalities in the hypothalamic-pituitary area. An important question that remains to be answered is whether administration of exogenous ghrelin has any effect modulating appetite in individuals with hypothalamic-pituitary disconnection.

M. E. Couce, MD, PhD

Meningiomas: Loss of Heterozygosity on Chromosome 10 and Marker-Specific Correlations With Grade, Recurrence, and Survival

Mihaila D, for the NABTT CNS Consortium (Henry Ford Health Sciences Ctr, Detroit)

Clin Cancer Res 9:4443-4451, 2003

13–4

Background.—Loss of heterozygosity (LOH) on chromosome 10 has been linked to meningioma progression. A high incidence of LOH on chromosome 10 has been reported in benign meningiomas (73.4%), in atypical meningiomas (80%), and in malignant tumors (86.7%). Whether LOH at individual loci on chromosome 10 has any biologic or clinical predictive value for meningiomas was determined.

Methods.—In this study, with the use of laser capture microdissection and fluorescence-based detection of polymerase chain reaction products, LOH was evaluated at 11 microsatellite dinucleotide repeat loci in 208 sporadic and recurrent meningiomas from 173 patients. Correlations between LOH results and tumor location, histology, and grade; patient's race, age, and gender; and recurrence and survival data were noted.

Results.—Most (83.2%) of the 208 tumors were benign, with 9.6% atypical and 7.2% malignant. Significant differences were found between the histologic subtypes and LOH. In addition, tumors at certain locations showed relationships with LOH. Sphenoid tumors and LOH were linked, with a significant positive relationship noted between LOH at locus *D10S89* and these tumors. Parietal tumors showed a decreased likelihood of LOH, evidenced by a significant negative relationship with LOH at locus *D10S209* and these tumors. LOH was noted in all loci in benign tumors. The percentage of tumors with LOH increased with tumor grade at most loci. Patients having tumors with LOH at *D10S179*, *D10S89*, *D10S580*, or *D10S169* appeared to have an increased likelihood (10.94, 6.59, 4.99, and 6.61 times greater, respectively) of having a tumor that was atypical or malignant. No correlations were noted between LOH and race or between LOH and gender. Mean age and LOH status were significantly correlated for *D10S215*. Patients without LOH at this locus had a mean age of 52.6 years; patients with LOH at this locus had a mean age of 65.3 years. Thus, LOH at *D10S215* is more likely to occur in older patients. With respect to long-term survival, patients having LOH on locus *D10S209* had a 7.41 times greater risk of dying. Patients whose tumors had an LOH on this locus were more likely to have a shorter survival. Having LOH on *D10S169* was significantly predictive of recurrence, with patients having this situation 4.23 times more likely to experience tumor recurrence. A shorter time to recurrence also accompanied LOH at this locus.

Conclusions.—Significant correlations were noted between specific loci and tumor location, grade, recurrence, and patient age. Marginal correlations were found between specific loci and survival. Thus, genetic influences may underlie the development of tumors with respect to age at onset, histology, and location. Unfavorable prognostic signs were also found, with specific loci associated with higher tumor grade, shorter survival, and shorter time to recurrence. This information could be useful in choosing an appropriate clinical approach to the treatment of these patients.

▶ Over the years, we have learned much about meningiomas. We have been educated to recognize those aggressive variants, by means of recognizing histologic subtypes and World Health Organization grading. However, there are still a large number of those so-called typical meningiomas that do not follow the general rules and behave more aggressively, giving rise to multiple recurrences that increase significantly the morbidity and mortality for these patients.

Although several studies have addressed LOH of chromosome 10 in meningiomas, this study is particularly interesting, since it evaluates the association between LOH at specific loci and their correlation with clinical behavior in these tumors. The authors do so by examining a significant number of cases (173 patients and 208 specimens) with a long follow-up, and determined the status of 11 different loci on chromosome 10.

The study finds that for most of the evaluated loci, the percentage of tumors showing LOH was directly correlated with tumor grade, with 4 of the loci being strongly associated with atypical and anaplastic meningiomas. However, LOH of some of the markers determined were seen in benign tumors. Most importantly, LOH at the *D10S169* site was associated with recurrence in the studied meningiomas.

Although additional studies will be needed, this study significantly points to potential markers of clinical behavior in meningiomas, and is particularly helpful for those tumors classified as benign or typical, with the potential for progression and adverse clinical outcomes.

M. E. Couce, MD, PhD

EGF Amplifies the Replacement of Parvalbumin-Expressing Striatal Interneurons After Ischemia

Teramoto T, Qiu J, Plumier J-C, et al (Harvard Med School, Boston; Université de Liège, Sart-Tilman, Belgium)
J Clin Invest 111:1125-1132, 2003   13–5

Background.—Epidermal growth factor (EGF) and its various receptors take part in the proliferation of adult neural stem/progenitor cells. The intraventricular infusion of EGF increases the subventricular zone cell population, promoting the migration of cells into adjacent brain parenchyma. In an ischemic stroke, certain projection neurons and interneurons die, whereas others survive. Whether adult neurogenesis compensates for the dead neurons and promotes differentiation into specific neurons has not yet been determined. The ability of EGF to increase neurogenesis in an injured brain was evaluated, as well as whether EGF can promote the replacement of lost interneurons and projection neurons.

Methods.—The mouse model of injured adult striatum after cerebral ischemia was used in this study. EGF was administered in an albumin-containing vehicle for 1 week to an ischemic striatum. Neuronal replacement was assessed, looking for labeled subventricular zone cells to determine the number of neuronal precursor cells that eventually differentiate into neurons.

Results.—Neuronal replacement was enhanced 100-fold with the intraventricular administration of EGF and albumin. The newborn immature neurons migrated into the ischemic lesion, where 65% differentiated into mature parvalbumin-expressing neurons. More than 20% of the parvalbumin neurons lost after ischemia were replaced by the neurons induced by EGF infusion.

Conclusions.—The exogenous administration of factors such as EGF may be able to restore significant proportions of neuronal cells lost after ischemic injury. In the mouse model, EGF infusions for 1 week produced a 100-fold increase in the number of neuronal replacements made in comparison with those induced by vehicle alone. The newly created neurons traveled into the ischemic lesion and differentiated into needed neurons.

▶ Any well-conducted study addressing new avenues geared towards repair of injured adult brain draws considerable attention. Several studies have shown that regeneration of parvalbumin (PV)-containing neurons enhances the recovery after striatal injury. In addition, it is known that endogenous neural stem cells fail to produce enough functional replacement of neurons after brain injury. Given the known neuronal proliferation effects of EGF, the authors in this article propose the intraventricular administration of EGF in an ischemic striatal injury model, as a tool to induce proliferation of neuronal precursor cells that migrate into the neuronal deficient areas. Their findings are intriguing and indicate an exclusive PV⁺ neuronal proliferation after EGF treatment that could hypothetically be driven by ischemic cell injury. In addition, the results of this study indicate a concomitant proliferation of glial cells, induced by EGF, although the authors do not specifically address the role of these supporting glial cells in the neuronal repopulation of injured brain regions.

In summary, this article, although not the first addressing the potentially important role of EGF in neuronogenesis after brain injury, contributes significantly to the field, as it demonstrates significant restitution of a specific neuronal population in the affected area by the effective exogenous treatment of EGF.

M. E. Couce, MD, PhD

Phenotype *Versus* Genotype in Gliomas Displaying Inter- or Intratumoral Histological Heterogeneity

Walker C, du Plessis DG, Joyce KA, et al (Clatterbridge Hosp, Bebington, Wirral, England; Walton Centre for Neurology and Neurosurgery, Liverpool, England; Univ of Liverpool, England)
Clin Cancer Res 9:4841-4851, 2003   13–6

Conclusions.—The histopathologic diagnosis of gliomas is often challenging. Gliomas frequently have considerable histologic heterogeneity. The relationship between genotype and phenotype was examined for markers of potential clinical utility in histologically heterogeneous gliomas.

Methods.—The various histologic phenotypes in 42 tumors from 25 patients with gliomas, with either intertumoral or intratumoral histologic heterogeneity, were sampled by using laser capture microdissection. Multiple simultaneous polymerase chain reaction amplification of microsatellite markers and capillary electrophoresis were used to determine allelic imbalance in chromosome 1p, 19q, 17p, 10p, and 10q.

Findings.—Loss of 1p36 and 19q13 occurred only in oligodendroglial histology in 7 of 13 oligodendrogliomas. Loss of 17p13 was documented in 14 of 41 tumors in astrocytic, oligoastrocytic, oligodendroglial, and glioblastomatous histologies. All the high-grade histologies in all glioblastomas with an oligodendroglial component showed chromosome 10 loss. This loss was also seen in 1 of 5 low-grade oligodendroglial regions in high-grade tumors. No losses of any marker studied were detected in 7 tumors from 5 patients. Identical genetic losses were seen in all areas of histologic differentiation in 13 tumors with intratumoral heterogeneity. Additional losses were documented in some but not all histologies in 2 tumors. In 3 cases, these losses correlated with progression.

Conclusions.—The gliomas studied were more homogeneous in genotype than in histologic phenotype. Regions of differing histologic subtype were indistinguishable by the genetic markers used here, suggesting a monoclonal tumor origin.

▶ The authors of this article focus their study on a very interesting and debatable issue in tumoral neuropathology: Shall we follow strict histopathologic classification in gliomas, assisted by molecular testing; or shall we rather perform exclusive molecular testing in the ever-shrinking stereotactic CNS tumor biopsy? This question is driven by the common finding of histologic heterogeneity in gliomas, both in a single tumor specimen and in cases of subsequent recurrence of previously diagnosed homogeneous gliomas.

The study is carefully designed, and evaluates a significant number of cases with both astrocytic and oligodendroglial morphologic appearance, determining commonly affected molecular targets in gliomas (1p, 19q, 17p, 10p, and 10q) by microsatellite analysis. Although the authors found that the molecular classification of the gliomas studied did not show complete concordance with the histopathologic diagnosis, they also conclude that to arrive at an accurate genetic assessment, it is necessary to obtain proper samples from the most aggressive areas of the tumor. So, in spite of the finding of more homogeneity in these tumors from the genetic point of view, we will still need to rely on the finding of the most anaplastic areas from the histology to provide the most accurate genetic mapping in these tumors.

M. E. Couce, MD, PhD

The Pathological Basis of Temporal Lobe Epilepsy in Childhood
Bocti C, Robitaille Y, Diadori P, et al (Université de Montréal)
Neurology 60:191-195, 2003   13–7

Background.—Increasingly, temporal lobe epilepsy (TLE) in childhood is being defined as a different entity from adult TLE. The pathologic findings of TLE were described in children undergoing temporal lobectomy for refractory seizures, and these findings were correlated with clinical presentation.

Methods.—The charts of all 22 children undergoing anterior temporal lobectomy for refractory TLE between 1979 and 1999 at one center were reviewed. New neuropathologic analyses were performed without knowledge of the patients' clinical features and outcomes.

Findings.—The mean age at epilepsy onset was 3 years 7 months. The mean age at surgery was 10 years 11 months. All children had complex partial seizures with secondary generalization in 48%. In addition, most children had seizures daily. Forty-five percent had auras. The mean follow-up after resection was 5 years 2 months. Forty-one percent of the children were seizure free at follow-up. Another 14% had auras only. Cortical dysplasia of the temporal neocortex, and mesial temporal sclerosis were the most common neuropathologic abnormalities. Seven children had both. In 67%, mesial temporal sclerosis was associated with extrahippocampal pathology.

Conclusions.—In this population of children, mesial temporal sclerosis was commonly associated with cortical dysplasia. The high incidence of coexisting pathologies may explain the early seizure onset and high seizure frequency rate noted. Childhood TLE may be a different entity from TLE in adults, both clinically and neuropathologically.

▶ TLE appears as a clinically different entity in childhood. The pathologic basis of TLE in adults has been clearly defined, whereas this has not been so rigorously studied in the pediatric population. The findings of low-grade gliomas or gangliogliomas, and cortical dysplasia (CD) are more common in specimens from children with TLE, although one finds ample variability in the reported rates of these findings in the pediatric population. A high percentage of adult patients that come to surgery have mesial temporal sclerosis (MTS), defined first radiologically and then confirmed in the pathology specimen. Microscopically, this is defined as the finding of severe neuronal loss and gliosis in Sommer sector, end folium, and dentate granule layer. This finding of MTS is not commonly encountered in the pediatric specimens. There are, however, several well-documented studies that show a good correlation between the severity of MTS and a prolonged first convulsion in early childhood.

The authors of this article identify 80% prevalence of dual pathology (CD and MTS) in 22 children who underwent temporal lobectomy for refractory seizures. The authors conclude that this strong association suggests common causal factors and suggest the need for a better definition of TLE using better standarized criteria, particularly focusing on the pediatric population. The authors argue that the population studied had a very early onset of epilepsy, which differs with the usually later onset of seizures in the adult population with MTS. This is debatable, however, considering that others have reported a common early onset of seizures in the adult population. Nonetheless, rigorous prospective studies are needed to evaluate and compare children and adults with MTS undergoing temporal lobectomies, followed by thorough neuropathologic evaluations.

M. E. Couce, MD, PhD

Solitary Fibrous Tumors in the Central Nervous System: A Clinicopathologic Review of 18 Cases and Comparison to Meningeal Hemangiopericytomas
Tihan T, Viglione M, Rosenblum MK, et al (Johns Hopkins Univ, Baltimore, Md; Mem Sloan-Kettering Cancer Ctr, New York)
Arch Pathol Lab Med 127:432-439, 2003   13–8

Background.—Solitary fibrous tumors (SFTs) of the CNS are rare neoplasms that typically present as dura-based lesions. Most of these masses seem amenable to total resection, although their biologic behavior is not well understood. SFTs resemble meningiomas clinically, and histologically, they can appear similar to fibrous meningioma or hemangiopericytoma (HPC). Densely cellular regions observed in some SFTs may be indistinguishable from HPCs. The clinicopathologic spectrum of SFTs in the CNS was investigated.

Methods and Findings.—Eighteen patients with SFTs were studied, along with an age- and sex-matched cohort with HPCs. Eleven SFTs were supratentorial; 3, infratentorial; and 4, intraspinal. Four SFTs were intra-axial, including 2 in the lateral ventricles and 2 in the spinal cord. SFTs were histologically similar to HPCs. Six SFTs had densely cellular regions, and 1 had frankly anaplastic features. Fifteen patients had gross total resection, with no metastases or tumor-related mortality during a median follow-up of 40 months. In the HPC cohort, by contrast, 83% had local recurrences and 27%, extracranial metastases. Twenty-two percent of the patients with HPC died of tumor-related causes.

Conclusions.—SFTs are a distinct entity from meningiomas and HPCs. The biologic behavior of SFTs is more benign than that of HPCs, even when focal hypercellularity is present. The current data also demonstrate that SFTs can occur in the ventricular system and in the parenchyma of the spinal cord. Rarely do SFTs have anaplastic histologic features, the outcome of which is unclear.

▶ In this study, the authors report the largest and most comprehensive review of SFTs of the CNS, and compare them with the same number of the more aggressive HPCs in the same location. SFTs of the CNS are uncommon tumors, and their clinical behavior is not yet well understood. These tumors are commonly confused with meningiomas and represent a diagnostic challenge at the time of histologic examination. Classic examples are easy to recognize, whereas the distinction between less common examples and HPCs and meningiomas can be problematic.

The present review analyzed 18 examples of SFTs, perfectly matched with the same number of HPCs. The authors conclude that surgery alone is sufficient for successfully treating the majority of these tumors, although they remark that long-term prognosis is yet unknown. Examples of so-called malignant or anaplastic SFTs are scarce, and their prognosis is even more obscure. This study brings up the importance of the recognition of SFTs in the CNS and emphasizes the need for the definition of a histologic spectrum. In addition, the study prompts the crucial need of establishing clear histologic criteria to guide the pathologist to distinguish these tumors from HPCs and meningiomas.

M. E. Couce, MD, PhD

Molecular Analysis of Astrocytomas Presenting After Age 10 in Individuals With NF1
Gutmann DH, James CD, Poyhonen M, et al (Washington Univ, St Louis; Mayo Clinic Found, Rochester, Minn; Family Federation of Finland, Helsinki; et al)
Neurology 61:1397-1400, 2003   13–9

Background.—Low-grade astrocytomas develop in 15% to 20% of children with neurofibromatosis type 1 (NF1). Recent research has shown that older patients with NF1 are also at significantly greater risk of astrocytoma development. The genetic basis for astrocytoma development in patients with NF1 past the first decade of life was investigated.

Methods.—Genetic analyses were done on 10 NF-1–related astrocytomas representing all World Health Organization malignancy grades. Fluorescence in situ hybridization, loss of heterozygosity, immunohistochemistry, and direct sequencing were done.

Findings.—Unlike histologically identical sporadic astrocytomas, later-onset NF1-related astrocytomas showed *NF1* inactivation, indicating a direct correlation with NF1 instead of a chance occurrence. Some of the astrocytomas had homozygous *NF1* deletion. Genetic changes seen in high-grade sporadic astrocytomas were also observed in NF1-associated high-grade astrocytomas. These included *TP53* mutation and *CDKN2A/p16* deletion.

Conclusions.—In patients past the first decade of life, NF1-associated astrocytomas demonstrate genetic changes observed in sporadic high-grade astrocytomas. The risk of late-onset astrocytomas may be increased in patients with NF1 and germline *NF1* deletions.

▶ It is well known that a relatively high percentage of NF1 children develop low-grade astrocytomas, largely pilocytic astrocytomas, particularly involving the optic pathway. These tumors usually affect young children and are associated with *NF1* gene inactivation. The general management of these young patients is usually dictated by close follow-up with clinical and radiologic examination over the years, usually without surgical intervention, with chemotherapy or radiation therapy rarely being indicated. The clinical management of NF1-associated brain tumors in adults is not that well standardized. Recent reports also suggest that older NF1 patients have an increased risk of developing high-grade astrocytomas later in life.

This article reports the results of studying a fair number of older patients with NF1, diagnosed with astrocytomas of different grades. Half of the cases examined were characterized by large germline *NF1* deletions. Interestingly, those high-grade astrocytomas in the study also showed either *TP53* or *CDKN2A/p16* deletions, as in those sporadic gliomas of similar grade. The authors conclude that the finding of large *NF1* deletions might indicate an increased risk to develop malignant astrocytomas later in life for NF1 patients. The present study adds important information on the developing of brain tumors in older NF1 patients, particularly in those with large germline deletions.

Although the number of cases evaluated in this article is substantial, given the nature of the study, a significant number did not have sufficient material for complete genetic analysis. Additional studies, including a larger number of cases with sufficient material, will be needed to further confirm and possibly expand the shown genetic characteristics in this patient population.

M. E. Couce, MD, PhD

Neuronal Depletion of Calcium-Dependent Proteins in the Dentate Gyrus Is Tightly Linked to Alzheimer's Disease-Related Cognitive Deficits
Palop JJ, Jones B, Kekonius L, et al (Univ of California, San Francisco; Univ of California, San Diego)
Proc Natl Acad Sci U S A 100:9572-9577, 2003   13–10

Background.—The causes of Alzheimer disease (AD) are not yet clear, but investigations in related transgenic mouse models are revealing the pathogenic roles of some AD-associated molecules. The primary outcome measure in most of these studies is the development of amyloid plaques. Transgenic mice whose neuronal expression of human amyloid precursor proteins (hAPP) were directed by the platelet-derived growth factor β chain promoter were studied. These mice expressed familial AD-mutant hAPP (hAPP$_{FAD}$) and had high levels of human amyloid-β peptides (Aβ) in the hippocampus. The expression of calcium-dependent proteins in the hippocampus and their links to cognitive defects in hAPP$_{FAD}$ mice and AD were analyzed on the basis of the crucial role of neuronal calcium homeostasis and calcium signaling in learning, memory, and possibly in the pathogenesis of AD.

Methods.—Tissues from the brains of 15 humans with AD and 2 normal humans as well as transgenic mice were analyzed immunohistochemically. Immunoreactive structures were quantified by using digitized images. Sectioned hemibrains were analyzed for proteins with Western blot techniques. Quantitative fluorogenic reverse transcription–polymerase chain reaction analysis was also performed. Tasks involving learning and memory were used to test the mice.

Results.—Calbindin-D$_{28k}$ (CB) is usually abundant in hippocampal neurons, especially in granule cells of the dentate gyrus and pyramidal cells of the CA1 region, but both the dentate gyrus of the hAPP$_{FAD}$ mice and the humans with AD had significantly reduced levels of CB. Among the human samples, the greatest depletions of CB were noted in persons with the most severe dementia. These CB reductions were also age dependent in mice. The reductions in CB immunoreactivity correlated highly with CB protein and messenger RNA levels in the dentate gyrus of the opposite hemibrain in 6- to 7-month-old hAPP$_{FAD}$ mice. Even at the age of 4 to 5 months, hAPP$_{FAD}$ mice had a significant reduction in the c-Fos–immunoreactive neurons in the granular layer of the dentate gyrus. Further reductions were noted as the mice aged. The fact that these reductions were tightly correlated in the hAPP$_{FAD}$ mice implies that the underlying mechanism is not random and overlaps. These reductions in CB and c-Fos also correlated with the relative abundance of Aβ1-42. No correlation was found with either plaque load or gender. Deficits in learning and memory showed a clear relationship to the reductions of CB and c-Fos in neurons of the dentate gyrus. Nontransgenic controls showed the presence of spatial learning in hidden platform training, but hAPP$_{FAD}$ mice had spatial learning deficits in this area. Their CB levels correlated strongly with the presence of these deficits.

Conclusions.—A cause-effect relationship was present between the expression of hAPP$_{FAD}$/Aβ and age-dependent declines in CB and c-Fos among the neuronal population involved in learning and memory tasks. These calcium-dependent proteins were reduced in the granule cells of the dentate gyrus. Their levels were highly correlated with the presence of spatial learning deficits and depended on the relative abundance of Aβ1-42 but did not depend on the amount of Aβ deposited in plaques. Therefore, AD-related neuronal deficits result from small nonfibrous Aβ groupings instead of plaques. The reductions in CB and c-Fos in AD may contribute to cognitive deficits as well as reflect them.

▶ The pathogenesis of AD is largely unknown, and amyloid plaques are its most common pathologic finding. Numerous research groups try to uncover the significance of specific AD-associated molecules. One important line of research concentrates on hAPP.

This work from Palop et al focuses on neuronal calcium homeostasis and its role in learning and memory. The authors demonstrate that transgenic mice expressing hAPP, and humans with AD show reduced expression of the calcium-binding protein CB, which has been shown to be a protective factor for Aβ toxicity in neurons.

The authors establish a clear, direct relationship between CB reduction and the learning deficits shown in mice. In addition, they demonstrate that this finding is not associated with Aβ deposition of higher plaque load. The study suggests that the changes in CB are not only a reflection of the cognitive deficiency in AD patients, but also a contributing factor for its development. Therefore, they propose the detection of CB levels in patients with AD as a potential tool for their evaluation and assessment. Although we are still far from having a good measure of the correlation between severity of disease and CB reductions, the results of this study are exciting and could potentially be a significant contribution to the diagnosis and assessment of patients with AD.

M. E. Couce, MD, PhD

Survivin-Dependent Angiogenesis in Ischemic Brain: Molecular Mechanisms of Hypoxia-Induced Up-regulation
Conway EM, Zwerts F, Van Eygen V, et al (Univ of Leuven, Belgium)
Am J Pathol 163:935-946, 2003   13–11

Background.—Efforts are underway to determine the molecular events that regulate angiogenesis in stroke patients. If angiogenesis is regulated, the degree of parenchymal damage occurring after a stroke may be diminished. Survivin is an inhibitor of apoptosis protein. In vascular endothelial cells, it is upregulated in vitro by angiogenic factors, including vascular endothelial cell growth factor (VEGF). A mouse model of stroke was studied to determine the role of survivin in the brain exposed to hypoxia/ischemia.

Methods.—Normal adult BALB/c mice brains were assessed for survivin expression pattern. In addition, an infarct was surgically produced in mice brains, the mice were permitted to recover, then the brains were removed and prepared for histologic and vessel density analysis or immunofluorescent studies. Infarct volume measurements and messenger RNA levels were determined, and Western immunoblot analysis was done. Mice exposed to hypoxic conditions were killed, and cell culture tests were done.

Results.—In the normal mice brains, low survivin levels were detected in neurons in the CA-1, CA-2, and CA-3 regions of the hippocampus, dentate gyrus, and pyramidal cells of the cortex. For 6 hours to 7 days after infarct creation, survivin expression was maintained as in normal brain tissues. No survivin was detected in the infarct region itself. Six hours after infarction, the pia mater and pia vessels overlying the infarct region contained survivin, but the corresponding regions in the contralateral unaffected hemisphere did not. Survivin was detected 2 days after the infarct in microvessels in the peri-infarct and infarct regions, with a pattern suggesting endothelial cell staining. It remained in the pia and pia vessels but was absent from the unaffected hemisphere. Seven days after the insult, survivin levels and thrombomodulin expression in affected areas increased, and an irregular complex of vessels that extended from the penumbra and pia and leptomeninges and appeared to invade the infarct core was found. At baseline, VEGF was found in the hippocampus bilaterally. Six hours after the infarct, VEGF was noted in the leptomeninges and pia over the infarct region, and within the infarct in scattered glia-like cells. VEGF expression was most prominent over the peri-infarct and leptomeningeal regions 7 days after the infarct, with somewhat less intense expression in the infarct core, usually adjacent to microvessels. The spatial pattern of VEGF expression resembled that of survivin 3 to 7 days after the infarct. Vascularity and infarct size were partially affected by survivin expression. Its expression was augmented in the brains of mice exposed to hypoxia 1.8-fold more than in the brains of mice under normoxic conditions. VEGF levels were 8.6-fold higher in association with increased survivin expression, suggesting VEGF may serve a regulatory function. Survivin expression also responded to angiopoietin-1, basic fibroblast growth factor, and placental growth factor (Plgf) as well as VEGF. Enhanced survivin expression in the absence of hypoxia-inducible factor 1α (HIF1α) suggested that HIF1α may downregulate survivin. Plgf messenger RNA levels showed no change in response to hypoxia, so its effect may be limited.

Conclusions.—After cerebrovascular occlusion, survivin expression is increased by cerebral capillary endothelial cells of vessels in the peri-infarct and infarct regions as well as the overlying pia mater. Survivin helps to determine the extent of vascularization occurring in the first few days after occlusion. Survivin upregulation in response to hypoxia appears to depend on mechanisms that do not always require VEGF, HIF1α, or Plgf.

▶ Vascularization, or angiogenesis, is a key phenomenon responsible for diminishing cerebral tissue damage after a stroke. This study evaluated the role of an inhibitor of apoptosis known as survivin, in response to hypoxia/ischemia, in an animal model. Interestingly, the authors described that the expression of survivin is increased in endothelial cells of the cerebral capillary in the peri-infarct and infarct regions. They noticed that the extent of the vascularization in the first few days after cerebrovascular occlusions depended in part on survivin expression. They also reported that important growth factors such as VEGF and Plgf do not seem to mediate the upregulation of survivin in response to hypoxia.

Future studies determining the mechanisms involved in the regulation of the expression of survivin should be very useful in developing novel therapeutic approaches to treat and prevent stroke as well as other neurodegenerative disorders, where apoptosis may play an etiopathogenic role.

M. E. Couce, MD, PhD

14 Cytopathology

A Retrospective Review on Atypical Glandular Cells of Undetermined Significance (AGUS) Using the Bethesda 2001 Classification
Tam KF, Cheung ANY, Liu KL, et al (Univ of Hong Kong)
Gynecol Oncol 91:603-607, 2003   14–1

Introduction.—The Bethesda system for reporting cervicovaginal cytologic diagnoses was last revised in 2001. Pathologists are required to report whether a smear favors neoplastic changes, along with the origin of the abnormal cells. Before 2001, one of the diagnoses within the Bethesda system was "atypical glandular cells of undetermined significance." Archival smears and patient outcomes, including diagnoses and follow-up status, were reviewed to assess the usefulness of the new classification in atypical glandular cells (AGCs).

Methods.—Smears having AGCs that were obtained between January 1995 and December 1997 were investigated and subclassified by the revised Bethesda classification. Medical records were reviewed. Cases with discrepancies between the cytologic evaluation and the corresponding final histologic diagnoses were examined.

Results.—The mean patient age was 47 years (range, 18-78 years). Of 138 smears reviewed, 34 favored neoplasia and 104 were not otherwise specified. Sixty and 78 smears, respectively, favored endocervical and endometrial origin. Of 43 patients with significant pathology, 12 (8.7%) had high-grade cervical intraepithelial neoplasia, 2 (1.4%) had low-grade cervical intraepithelial neoplasia, 5 (3.6%) had human papilloma virus infection, 7 (5.1%) had carcinoma of the corpus, 1 (0.7%) had cervical adenocarcinoma in situ, 4 (2.9%) had adenocarcinoma of the cervix, 3 (2.2%) had endometrial hyperplasia, and 5 (3.6%) had carcinoma of the ovary. Two (1.4%) and 2 (1.4%) patients had double primary female genital malignancies and extragenital malignancies, respectively.

A significant association between smears favored neoplasia and a final diagnosis with significant pathology ($P < .05$). There was a significant link between AGC favored endocervical origin and a final diagnosis with cervical diseases ($P < .05$). Lesions were detected during subsequent visits in 4 of 43 patients with significant pathologies; all had cervical smears classified as AGC "favor neoplasia."

Conclusion.—An early and intensive investigation is recommended for patients in whom AGC is found on cervical smears.

▶ Articles now are being published based on the use of the newest Bethesda 2001 conference terminology. The article by Tam et al describes a retrospective study in which previously diagnosed atypical glandular cells of undetermined significance (AGUS) cases were reclassified using the newer AGCs terminology. Thus, a weakness in this manuscript is that the newer terminology is not tested on new cases but is tested on old AGUS cases. The results of this study are not surprising: A significant percentage of cases reclassified as AGC show clinically important abnormalities ranging from squamous dysplasia to adenocarcinoma.

To me, this shows a weakness of the Bethesda AGC reformulation. We still are not able to accurately predict which "atypical glandular" lesions will harbor clinically significant disease, and we still cannot remove the squamous abnormalities from the AGC mix. I should hope that, at some point in the future, the AGC category will not be just a hodgepodge of benign, neoplastic, and malignant glandular and squamous epithelial disease. That time is not now. The conclusion that AGC is a high-risk diagnosis should already be widely known.

S. S. Raab, MD

SUGGESTED READING

Solomon D, Davey D, Kurman R, et al: The 2001 Bethesda System—terminology for reporting results of cervical cytology. *JAMA* 287:2114-2119, 2002.

Geisinger KR, Stanley MW, Raab SS, et al: Atypical glandular cells of undetermined significance. *Modern Cytopathology*, Churchill Livingstone, 2004, pp 147-165.

Atypical Squamous Cells of Undetermined Significance in Liquid-Based Cytologic Specimens: Results of Reflex Human Papillomavirus Testing and Histologic Follow-Up in Routine Practice With Comparison of Interpretive and Probabilisitic Reporting Methods
Levi AW, Kelly DP, Rosenthal DL, et al (Johns Hopkins Med Institutions, Baltimore, Md)
Cancer 99:191-197, 2003   14–2

Introduction.—Human papillomavirus (HPV) DNA testing for high-risk types after Papanicolaou (Pap) smear interpretations of atypical squamous cells of undetermined significance (ASCUS) is a sensitive technique for identifying women harboring underlying high-grade squamous intraepithelial lesions. The application of HPV testing to ASCUS smears in routine practice with comparison of probabilistic and interpretive models of cytologic reporting has not been determined and was thus examined in Pap smears initially interpreted as ASCUS.

Methods.—The HPV DNA testing was performed reflexively on 216 liquid-based Pap smears initially interpreted as ASCUS. According to the interpretive model, ASCUS interpretations were altered and reported as either squamous intraepithelial lesions or low-grade squamous intraepithelial lesions when HPV-positive and as reactive when HPV-negative. With the use of the probabilistic model, ASCUS interpretations were maintained and reported with use of the HPV test result. Histologic follow-up data were analyzed.

Results.—Of 216 women with ASCUS cytology, 142 (65.7%) tested positive for high-risk HPV types. Of the 142 HPV-positive ASCUS smears, 101 (71.1%) were altered to an interpretation of low-grade squamous intraepithelial lesions (96 cases) or squamous intraepithelial lesions (5 cases) (Fig 3). Histologic follow-up of 55 of 101 HPV-positive smears in the interpretive group and 26 of the 41 HPV-positive smears in the probabilistic group produced similar percentages of lesions (18 lesions [32.7%] and 9 lesions [34.6%], respectively).

There was a preponderance of low-grade lesions in the interpretive group (89%). A nearly equal distribution of low-grade and high-grade lesions was observed in the probabilistic group (56% and 44%, respectively). Overall, 22% of lesions were classified as high-grade. Of 74 HPV-negative ASCUS smears, 71 (96%) were changed to reactive, and all 5 with histologic follow-up were classified as negative.

Conclusion.—Colposcopy with tissue studies was limited to HPV-positive cases, regardless of the reporting model used, indicating that clinicians are basing colposcopy triage on the HPV test result and not on the definitiveness of the cytologic interpretation. The similar yield of lesions in the

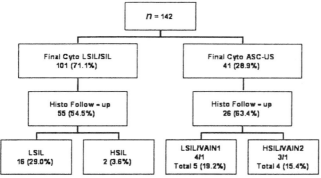

FIGURE 3.—Among the 142 specimens determined to be atypical squamous cells of undetermined significance (*ASC-US*) that were found to be positive for the human papillomavirus (HPV) by reflex HPV DNA testing. 71.1% (101 specimens) of the specimens were reclassified as low-grade squamous intraepithelial lesion (*LSIL*)/squamous intraepithelial lesion (*SIL*) and 28.9% (41 specimens) retained their ASCUS interpretations after final cytologic (*Cyto*) evaluation. The flow diagram compares the frequencies of low-grade and high-grade lesions on the tissue follow-up of cases from the interpretive and probabilistic groups. *Abbreviations: Histo*, Histologic; *VAIN 1*, vaginal intraepithelial neoplasia grade 1; *VAIN 2*, vaginal intraepithelial neoplasia grade 2. (Courtesy of Levi AW, Kelly DP, Rosenthal DL, et al: Atypical squamous cells of undetermined significance in liquid-based cytologic specimens: Results of reflex papillomavirus testing and histologic follow-up in routine practice with comparison of interpretive and probabilistic reporting methods. *Cancer* 99(4):191-197, 2003. ©2003 American Cancer Society. Reprinted by permission of Wiley-Liss, Inc., a subsidary of John Wiley & Sons, Inc.)

2 groups and the significant risk of high-grade lesions support the idea of not using the interpretive model to HPV-test ASCUS cases.

▶ This study evaluates the utility of 2 reporting systems for women with Pap tests diagnosed as ASC-US and followed by human papillomavirus HPV testing. At the Bethesda 2001 conference, interpretative (ie, changing the Pap test diagnosis from ASCUS to squamous intraepithelial lesions or low-grade squamous intraepithelial lesions or based on the HPV result) and probabilistic (ie, reporting the Pap test as ASCUS with the HPV result) reporting systems were debated. Most laboratories in the country report probabilistically.

A weakness in the study was that the pathologist could use either reporting mechanism, thus introducing individual preference and bias. Follow-up of these women showed that approximately one third had cervical intraepithelial neoplasia (CIN) and two thirds had no CIN. However, in the interpretative model, two thirds of the women were given a squamous intraepithelial lesion diagnosis (predominantly low-grade squamous intraepithelial lesion) and then had benign follow-up, which I imagine was frustrating for the clinicians. I believe that these data support the probabilistic reporting model. Data related to the HPV-negative cases in the interpretative model were scant, thus limiting conclusions. However, these data indicate that a number of women with ASCUS and a positive HPV test will have no CIN on follow-up. The importance of this finding is unclear.

S. S. Raab, MD

Suggested Reading

Solomon D, Schiffman M, Tarone R: Comparison of three management strategies for patients with atypical squamous cells of undetermined significance: Baseline results from a randomized trial. *J Natl Cancer Inst* 93:293-299, 2001.

Solomon D, Davey D, Kurman R, et al: The 2001 Bethesda System: Terminology for reporting results of cervical cytology. *JAMA* 287:2114-2119, 2002.

Wright TC Jr, Cox JT, Massad LS, et al: 2001 Consensus Guidelines for the management of women with cervical cytological abnormalities. *JAMA* 287:2120-2129, 2002.

Atypical Squamous Cells, Cannot Exclude High-Grade Squamous Intraepithelial Lesion: A Follow-up Study of Conventional and Liquid-Based Preparations in a High-Risk Population
Louro AP, Roberson J, Eltoum I, et al (Univ of Alabama at Birmingham)
Am J Clin Pathol 120:392-397, 2003   14–3

Introduction.—Since its introduction by the Bethesda System in 1988, the diagnostic category of atypical squamous cells has continued to evolve. The category of atypical squamous cells of undetermined significance was created to indicate squamous cellular changes that were more marked versus those attributable to reactive or inflammatory changes yet were not quantitatively or qualitatively diagnostic of a preneoplastic or neoplastic condition.

"Atypical squamous cell" (ASC) is a heterogeneous entity that can describe superficial or intermediate squamous cells or squamous metaplastic cells. The incidence of high-grade squamous intraepithelial lesions (ASC-Hs) in conventional and liquid-based preparations was evaluated in a high-risk population. The incidence of clinically significant cervical lesions after such an interpretation between conventional and liquid-based preparations and among different age groups was examined.

Findings.—The histologic follow-up of 368 smears or slides with an interpretation of ASC-H compared conventional and liquid-based preparations and age groups. The mean age of patients with an ASC-H interpretation was 36.8 years (17-87 years). There were 52 liquid-based specimens and 316 conventional smears. Follow-up was available in 218 cases (59.2%), including 28 liquid-based preparations (65%) and 190 conventional smears (58%).

In 20 liquid-based preparations (71%) and 152 conventional smears (80.0%), cervical intraepithelial neoplasia (CIN) or higher was observed on subsequent biopsy. Additional findings included liquid-based preparations, CIN1, 11 (55%); CIN2/3, 9 (45%); conventional smears, CIN1, 78 (51.3%); CIN2/3, 70 (46.1%); squamous cell carcinoma, 4 (2.6%). No statistically significant difference was observed in the incidence of CIN or higher on subsequent biopsy after an interpretation of ASC-H based on preparation types. The incidence of CIN in patients 40 years or older and patients younger than 40 years were 66% and 84%, respectively, a difference that was statistically significant.

Conclusion.—Due to the high rate of clinically significant lesions seen on subsequent follow-up, it is recommended that patients with an interpretation of ASC-H be closely observed and referred for colposcopic examination, regardless of age.

▶ The 2001 Bethesda Committee specifically recommended subclassifying ASC cases into the 2 categories of atypical squamous cells of undetermined significance (ASCUS) and ASC-H because of differences in the probability of a clinically significant lesion on follow-up. The ASC-H cases fall within a considerably higher risk category and warrant immediate colposcopy. The study by Louro et al justifies this separation with over 75% of women with ASC-H having a clinically significant lesion on follow-up. However, I was surprised that slightly more than 50% of women with CIN only had CIN1 on follow-up. This finding does not exactly go along with the cytologic appearance of atypical/dysplastic metaplastic cells.

Reasons for this finding may be lesion regression or biases in interpretation (eg, if a biopsy is obtained on a Pap test that is diagnosed as ASC-H, there could be a tendency to make an overcall on the histologic material). This study also illustrates another possible cause of failure in cervical cancer screening: 25% of women were lost to follow-up. Of the 89 patients lost to follow-up, the data of Louro et al would indicate that approximately 45 would have had CIN2 or CIN3 if colposcopy had been performed.

S. S. Raab, MD

SUGGESTED READING

Sherman ME, for the ALTS Group. Qualification of ASCUS: A comparison of equivocal LSIL and equivocal HSIL cervical cytology in the ASCUS LSIL Triage Study. *Am J Clin Pathol* 116:386-394, 2001.

Solomon D, Schiffman M, Tarone R: Comparison of three management strategies for patients with atypical squamous cells of undetermined significance: Baseline results from a randomized trial. *J Natl Cancer Inst* 93:293-299, 2001.

Virologic Versus Cytologic Triage of Women With Equivocal Pap Smears: A Meta-analysis of the Accuracy To Detect High-Grade Intraepthelial Neoplasia
Arbyn M, Buntinx F, Van Ranst M, et al (Scientific Inst of Public Health, Brussels, Belgium; Univ of Leuven, Belgium; Univ of Maastricht, The Netherlands; et al)
J Natl Cancer Inst 96:280-293, 2004   14–4

Introduction.—The appropriate management of women with minor cytologic lesions of the cervix is not clear. A meta-analysis was performed to evaluate the accuracy of human papillomavirus (HPV) DNA testing as an alternative to repeat cytology in women with equivocal results on a prior Pap smear.

Methods.—Data were extracted from previous reports published between 1992 and 2002 that contained results of virologic and cytologic testing followed by colposcopically directed biopsy in women with an index smear showing atypical squamous cells of undetermined significance (ASCUS). Fifteen trials were identified in which HPV triage and the histologic outcome (presence or absence of a cervical intraepithelial neoplasia of grade II or greater) was recorded.

Nine, 7, and 2 trials also documented the accuracy of repeat cytology when the cutoff for abnormal cytology was determined at a threshold of ASCUS or worse, low-grade squamous intraepithelial lesion, or high-grade squamous intraepithelial lesion or worse, respectively. Random-effects models were used to pool accuracy parameters in the event of interstudy heterogeneity. Differences in accuracy were examined by pooling the ratio of the sensitivity (or specificity) of HPV testing to that of repeat cytology.

Results.—The sensitivity and specificity were 84.4% (95% confidence interval [CI], 77.6%-91.1%) and 72.9% (95% CI, 62.5%-83.3%), respectively, for HPV testing overall and 94.8% (95% CI, 92.7%-96.9%) and 67.3% (95% CI, 58.2%-76.4%), respectively, for HPV testing in the 8 trials that used the Hybrid Capture II assay (Table 3). The sensitivity and specificity of repeat cytology at a threshold for abnormal cytology of ASCUS or

TABLE 3.—Triage of Atypical Squamous Cells of Undetermined Significance by Human Papillomavirus DNA Testing for the Detection of Histologically Confirmed Cervical Intraepithelial Neoplasia Grade II or Worse: Number of True and False Positives and True and False Negatives, Accuracy Parameters, Test Positivity Rate, and Prevalence of Disease Derived from Different Published Studies

Study	Type	True-positive	False-negative	False-positive	True-negative	Sensitivity	Specificity	Positive Predictive Value	Negative Predictive Value	Test Positivity Rate	Prevalence of Disease
Goff et al., 1993	VT	3	2	25	141	0.600	0.849	0.107	0.986	0.164	0.029
Slawson et al., 1994	VP	4	11	20	86	0.267	0.811	0.167	0.887	0.198	0.124
Cox et al., 1995	HC1	14	1	67	135	0.933	0.668	0.173	0.993	0.373	0.069
Wright et al., 1995	HC1	6	5	71	99	0.545	0.582	0.078	0.952	0.425	0.061
Fait et al., 1998	HC1	9	1	2	55	0.900	0.965	0.818	0.982	0.164	0.149
Ferris et al., 1998	HC1	5	5	53	106	0.500	0.667	0.086	0.955	0.343	0.059
Manos et al., 1999	HC2	58	7	326	582	0.892	0.641	0.151	0.988	0.395	0.067
Bergeron et al., 2000	HC2	10	2	38	61	0.833	0.616	0.208	0.968	0.432	0.108
Fait et al., 2000	HC1	48	8	5	165	0.857	0.971	0.906	0.954	0.235	0.248
Lin et al., 2000	HC2	27	0	12	35	1.000	0.745	0.692	1.000	0.527	0.365
Shlay et al., 2000	HC2	14	1	47	133	0.933	0.739	0.230	0.993	0.313	0.077
Morin et al., 2001	HC2	17	2	88	253	0.895	0.742	0.162	0.992	0.292	0.053
Rebello et al., 2001	HC2	18	3	13	41	0.857	0.759	0.581	0.932	0.413	0.280
Solomon et al., 2001	HC2	256	11	1050	984	0.959	0.484	0.196	0.989	0.568	0.116
Zielinski et al., 2001	HC2	11	1	63	138	0.917	0.687	0.149	0.993	0.347	0.056

Abbreviations: VT, ViraType; *VP,* ViraPap; *HC,* Hybrid Capture.
(Courtesy of Arbyn M, Buntinx F, Van Ranst M, et al: Virologic versus cytologic triage of women with equivocal pap smears: A meta-analysis of the accuracy to detect high-grade intraepithelial neoplasia. *J Natl Cancer Inst* 96:280-293, 2004. By permission of Oxford University Press.)

worse were 81.8% (95% CI, 73.5%-84.3%) and 57.6% (95% CI, 49.5%-65.7%), respectively.

Repeat cytology that used higher cytologic thresholds produced markedly lower sensitivity yet higher specificity than triage with the Hybrid Capture II assay. The ratio of sensitivity of the Hybrid Capture II assay to that of repeat cytology at a threshold of ASCUS or worse pooled from 4 trials that used both triage tests was 1.16 (95% CI, 1.04-1.29). The specificity ratio was not statistically significantly different from unity.

Conclusion.—The published literature suggests that the Hybrid Capture II assay has improved accuracy (higher sensitivity, similar specificity), compared with the repeat Pap smear using the threshold of ASCUS for an outcome of cervical intraepithelial neoplasia of grade 2 or greater among women with equivocal cytologic results. The sensitivity of triage at higher cytologic cutoffs is poor.

▶ Meta-analyses are helpful to assess the overall performance of tests when the individual reports may present conflicting data or head-to-head comparisons are not performed. A challenge in examining meta-analytic data is in explaining why individual studies present "outlying" data. Are outlining studies a reflection of the norm, differences in patient demographics, a difference in study design, or differences in a number of other variables?

Arbyn et al show that the Hybrid Capture II method has better performance than repeat Pap tests using the threshold of ASCUS for an outcome of cervical intraepithelial neoplasia 2 or greater. However, individual studies may show a spectrum of results, with some authors highlighting that repeat Pap testing possibly has a better specificity than overall meta-analytic data show. In addition, such studies do not show the optimum use of either test and include studies showing poor performance they may not equate with real laboratory settings.

S. S. Raab, MD

SUGGESTED READING

The Atypical Squamous Cells of Undetermined Significance/Low-Grade Squamous Intraepithelial Lesions Triage Study (ALTS) Group: Human papillomavirus testing for triage of women with cytologic evidence of low-grade squamous intraepithelial lesions: Baseline data from a randomized trial. *J Natl Cancer Inst* 92:397-402, 2000.

ASCUS-LSIL Triage Study (ALTS) Group: A randomized trial on the management of low-grade squamous intraepithelial lesion cytology interpretations. *Am J Obstet Gynecol* 188:1393-1400, 2003.

Location-Guided Screening of Liquid-Based Cervical Cytology Specimens: A Potential Improvement in Accuracy and Productivity Is Demonstrated in a Preclinical Feasibility Trial
Wilbur DC, Parker EM, Foti JA (ViaHealth, Rochester, NY)
Am J Clin Pathol 118:399-407, 2002   14–5

Background.—Improvements in specimen preparation and analysis have improved the accuracy of cervical cancer detection. The performance of a liquid-based slide preparation system (SurePath, TriPath Imaging, Burlington, NC) in concert with automated location-guided screening (FocalPoint System, TriPath Imaging) and review (SlideWizard 2, TriPath) was compared with that of routine manual screening.

Methods.—A total of 1275 slides prepared by the SurePath method were examined both by routine manual screening and by the FocalPoint System on a SlideWizard 2 automated review microscopy station. With the automated system, for slides flagged as abnormal the coordinates of the field of view (FOV) were downloaded directly from FocalPoint to the computer workstation and reviewed by a pathologist. The "true" diagnosis in each case was determined by pathologist adjudication.

Results.—The automated system accurately identified 218 slides (17.1%) as normal, and these required no further FOV or manual review. At all interpretation levels, the automated approach identified more abnormal cases and was more sensitive than routine manual screening. Of the 214 cases determined by adjudication to represent atypical squamous (or glandular) cells of undetermined significance and above (ASCUS+), the automated system identified 197 cases (sensitivity, 92.1%), whereas manual screening identified 183 cases (sensitivity, 85.5%). Of the 130 cases determined to be low-grade squamous intraepithelial lesion and above (LSIL+), the automated system identified 109 cases (sensitivity, 83.8%), whereas manual screening identified 100 cases (sensitivity, 76.9%). Of the 124 cases determined to be high-grade squamous intraepithelial lesion and above (HSIL+, including endocervical adenocarcinoma in situ), the automated system identified 103 cases (sensitivity, 83.1%), whereas manual screening identified only 73 cases (sensitivity, 58.9%). FOV review appropriately triaged 205 (95.8%) of 214 cases of ASCUS+, 128 (98.5%) of 130 cases of LSIL+, and all 124 cases (100%) of HSIL+ to full manual review. The automated method failed to identify 21 cases of HSIL+; 19 (90%) of these cases were captured as abnormal at the ASCUS+ level, and there were only 2 false-negative findings (10%). Manual screening failed to identify 51 cases of HSIL+; 38 (75%) cases were captured at the ASCUS+ level, 2 (4%) were deemed to be unsatisfactory samples, and 11 (22%) were false-negative results. Thus, the automated system identified (at any level) 122 of 124 cases of HSIL+ (sensitivity, 98.4%), whereas manual screening identified (at any level) 113 of 124 cases (sensitivity, 91.1%). Appropriate triage rates for identifying all abnormal cases were 92.1% for the automated system and 87.9% for manual screening.

Conclusion.—The automated method described was more accurate than routine manual screening in identifying cervical abnormalities, especially HSIL+. In almost 20% of cases, the automated system identified normal slides that did not require human review, thus improving the speed and efficacy of histopathologic reporting.

▶ During the past decade, of all areas of anatomic pathology, gynecologic cytology has had, by far, the greatest influx of new technologies. Wilbur et al report on TriPath's new automated screening with a location-guided screening system. Automated Pap test screening is the newest technology to change the cytology landscape. My impression is that these data show or will show an increased detection of squamous intraepithelial lesions (SILs) by using automated screening, and this probably will drive the market so that laboratories, particularly the larger ones, will adopt this technology. Unfortunately, true patient outcome data have always been lacking in the analysis of the newer Pap test technologies. Studies generally use the end point of SIL (which in and of itself does not cause mortality). Other studies then equate SIL to cancer progression, which is equated to mortality to determine if the technology is cost effective. It will be interesting to know if in 10 years the annual American cancer rate has decreased because of the use of all these new Pap test technologies.

S. S. Raab, MD

Suggested Reading

Lee KR, Ashfaq R, Birdsong GG, et al: Comparison of conventional Papanicolaou smears and a fluid-based, thin-layer system for cervical cancer screening. *Obstet Gynecol* 90:278-284, 1997.

Wilbur DC, Prey MU, Miller WM, et al: The AutoPap system for primary screening in cervical cytology: Comparing the results of a prospective, intended-use study with routine manual practice. *Acta Cytol* 42:214-220, 1998.

Education and Experience Improve the Performance of Transbronchial Needle Aspiration: A Learning Curve at a Cancer Center
Hsu L-H, Liu C-C, Ko J-S (Koo Found Sun Yat-Sen Cancer Ctr, Taipei, Taiwan)
Chest 125:532-540, 2004   14–6

Background.—Transbronchial fine needle aspiration (FNA) is a minimally invasive tool for diagnosing mediastinal lymphadenopathy and staging lung cancer. Despite its accuracy, it remains underused, in part perhaps because it is technically demanding. One center's experience with transbronchial FNA is described to characterize changes in the diagnostic yield and sensitivity of this method over time.

Methods.—The medical records of 549 patients who underwent diagnostic bronchoscopy from September 1999 to March 2003 were reviewed. All transbronchial FNAs were performed according to standard techniques with the use of 21-gauge cytology needles or 19-gauge histology needles.

The mediastinum and hilar lymph node mapping system was used in all cases. Specimens were examined in the operating room by a cytologist during FNA to determine specimen quality.

Results.—Transbronchial FNA was used in 90 patients (16.4%), including 66 patients with hilar-mediastinal lymphoadenopathies and 24 patients with submucosal and/or peribronchial lesions. Of these 90 patients, 78 (86.7%) were diagnosed with a malignancy. Transbronchial FNA results were positive in 45 of 66 patients (68.2%) with hilar-mediastinal lesions and in 17 of 24 patients (70.8%) with submucosal and/or peribronchial lesions. The sensitivity of transbronchial FNA diagnosis was 75% (45 of 60 patients) for hilar-mediastinal lesions and 80.9% (17 of 21 patients) for submucosal and/or peribronchial lesions.

Transbronchial FNA findings were diagnostic in 15 patients with mediastinal lesions whose airways appeared normal, and this was the only diagnostic tool used in 27 of these 90 cases (30%). Also, in 19 patients with non-small cell lung cancer, diagnostic and mediastinal staging were accomplished in 1 procedure. During the study period, the number of transbronchial FNAs performed per unit time increased steadily, and there were significant increases in both yield (inadequate specimens decreased from 21.1% to 6.9%) and sensitivity for detecting hilar-mediastinal lymphoadenopathies (from 33.0% to 80.5%). Also, as experience with the technique increased, there was a trend ($P = .06$) toward fewer inadequate specimens.

Conclusion.—The yield and sensitivity of transbronchial FNA improved as experience was gained. The ability to examine FNA specimens on-site during the procedure was crucial in improving diagnostic accuracy. Increased experience with this technique, combined with more focused education on its performance, will improve its use by bronchoscopists.

▶ This article by Hsu et al illustrates that it takes time for the clinicians to gain the skill at performing FNAs. The whole concept of false-negative results in FNA cytology is critically related to clinician or pathologist skill at performing the procedure. False-negative results in FNA cytology often lead to more invasive procedures associated with increased mortality, morbidity, and cost. Reducing morbidity, mortality, and cost are 3 of the reasons why we perform FNAs in the first place. Hsu et al also point out that the accuracy of FNA is increased with on-site rapid examination of transbronchial FNA specimens. Again, this illustrates the need for cytology services, particularly for those with FNA expertise in those centers that perform certain types of FNAs.

S. S. Raab, MD

SUGGESTED READING

Shure D, Fedullo PF: Transbronchial needle aspiration in the diagnosis of submucosal and peribronchial bronchogenic carcinoma. *Chest* 88:49-51, 1985.

Dasgupta A, Jain P, Minai OA, et al: Utility of transbronchial needle aspiration in the diagnosis of endobronchial lesions. *Chest* 15:1237-1241, 1999.

Mehta AC, Dasgupta A, Wang KP: Transbronchial needle aspiration, in Beamis JF, Mathur PN, (eds): *Interventional pulmonology.* New York, McGraw-Hill, 1999, pp 241-254.

Assessment of Utility of Ductal Lavage and Ductoscopy in Breast Cancer—A Retrospective Analysis of Mastectomy Specimens

Badve S, Wiley E, Rodriguez N, et al (Northwestern Univ, Chicago; Indiana Univ, Indianapolis)
Mod Pathol 16:206-209, 2003   14–7

Introduction.—Early detection of breast lesions remains an important goal in the management of breast cancer. Mammographic imaging, along with physical examination, is the primary screening method for detection of breast cancer. Fiberoptic ductoscopy and duct lavage have recently been used to assess patients at risk for breast cancer. Both methods examine the nipple and central duct area to identify intraductal lesions. The incidence of involvement of these structures in mastectomy specimens as a surrogate marker for estimating the utility of these methods was examined in patients with breast cancer.

Methods.—The presence and type of involvement of the nipple and central duct area were retrospectively examined in 801 mastectomy specimens obtained during a 4-year period. The specimens had been excised for infiltrating or in situ carcinoma. The presence of atypical proliferation or cells, when observed in the ducts of this region, were regarded as evidence of nipple involvement, even if definite evidence of malignancy was lacking.

Results.—Nipple and central duct involvement was observed in 179 cases (22%). Of 665 cases of infiltrating carcinoma, 17% did not involve an intraductal component.

Conclusion.—The relative rarity of nipple and central duct in mastectomy specimens and the lack of an in situ component in many cases brought into question the utility of fiberoptic ductoscopy and duct lavage as techniques for screening breast cancer. These techniques evaluate only 1 or 2 of the 15 to 20 ducts that open at the nipple and may therefore fail to identify focal abnormalities.

▶ Ductal lavage is one of the newest cytologic tests used to detect preneoplastic or neoplastic lesions in the breast. The data by Badve et al indicate that ductal lavage is not nearly as useful as some may believe because invasive and intraductal cancers often have neither a central component nor even an intraductal (for those tumors with an invasive carcinoma) component. A bias in this study is that Badve et al focused on mastectomies, which may not be representative specimens of all breast cancers (eg, mastectomies usually are not performed for localized in situ carcinomas). I think that ductal lavage is similar to other cytologic tests such as bronchial lavage or washing.

It may be unrealistic to expect that these tests detect the majority of neoplasms or preneoplastic lesions, but the unknown is the exact percentage of lesions these techniques may detect in experienced hands. Then, once these data are known, cost effectiveness studies need to be performed to determine the utility of such procedures and the tradeoff between cost and detection.

S. S. Raab, MD

SUGGESTED READING

Dooley WC, Veronesi U, Elledge R, et al: Detection of premalignant and malignant breast cells by ductal lavage. *Obstet Gynecol* 97(suppl 1):S2, 2001.

Dooley WC, Ljung BM, Veronesi U, et al: Ductal lavage for detection of cellular atypia in women at high risk for breast cancer. *J Natl Cancer Inst* 93:1624-1632, 2001.

Aspiration Biopsy of Mammary Lesions With Abundant Extracellular Mucinous Material: Review of 43 Cases With Surgical Follow-up
Ventura K, Cangiarella J, Lee I, et al (New York Univ)
Am J Clin Pathol 120:194-202, 2003   14–8

Introduction.—The diagnosis of malignancy on aspiration biopsy is straightforward when all of the characteristic features are present. Aspirates with abundant extracellular mucinous material originating from other mammary lesions, particularly those with increased cellularity, may be diagnostically challenging on fine-needle aspiration biopsy (FNAB). The FNAB smears and subsequent resected specimens from 43 mammary lesions containing abundant extracellular mucinous material on aspiration biopsy were examined to ascertain whether accurate classification of lesions yielding copious mucinous material can be achieved on FNAB.

Findings.—Of 43 FNAB smears, 26 were carcinoma. These included pure colloid carcinoma [CCA], 23 and mixed CCA/invasive ductal carcinoma, 3. Seventeen patients had benign lesions on follow-up. These included benign mucocele-like lesions (MLLs), 6; fibrocystic change [FCC], 6; and myxoid fibroadenoma [MFA], 5. All carcinomas were accurately identified as malignant on FNAB.

The initial cytologic diagnoses in benign cases were 8 benign, 8 atypical, and 1 suspicious for carcinoma. The CCAs were moderately to substantially cellular, with mild to moderate atypia. They lacked oval bare nuclei. Marked nuclear atypia was primarily confined to cases of mixed CCA/invasive ductal carcinoma. A distinct characteristic of CCA was thin-walled capillaries. Both FCCs and benign MLLs had overlapping cytologic characteristics and demonstrated variable or no or mild atypia.

The MFAs were strikingly cellular with dyscohesion and variable atypia. Stromal fragments and oval bare nuclei were observed in every case. Mucinous lesions may be divided into 2 categories by FNAB: adenocarcinomas and lesions that are not adenocarcinomas.

Conclusion.—The CCAs have unique characteristics that allow a definitive diagnosis on FNAB. Unnecessary surgery can be prevented in MFA by careful assessment of smear characteristics. Cytologic characteristics of FCC and MLL overlap. Due to the documented link of MLL with carcinoma, it is recommended that lesions that cannot be classified as adenocarcinoma or MFA be considered for conservative excision, even in the absence of atypia.

▶ In my opinion, the diagnosis of mucinous lesions of the breast on FNAB is highly dependent on clinical history. If the patient is older and the specimen is cellular, despite any blandness of the cytologic cellular features, a neoplastic lesion should be suspected. Younger patients pose more of a problem, but usually the mucin is attributable to a nonneoplastic condition. Thus, the key is the patient's age. Of course, any degree of cytologic atypia should result in an excision. In the end, this means that only lesions with bland cytology in a younger age group should not be biopsied. The amount of extracellular mucin is a much less important component than the cytologic atypia in determining if surgery should be performed.

S. S. Raab, MD

SUGGESTED READING

Dawson AE, Mulford DK: Fine needle aspiration of mucinous (colloid) breast carcinoma; nuclear grading and mammographic and cytologic findings. *Acta Cytol* 42:668-672, 1998.

Duane GB, Kanter MH, Branigan T, et al: A morphological study of cells from colloid carcinoma of the breast obtained by fine needle aspiration: Distinction from other breast lesions. *Acta Cytol* 31:742-750, 1987.

Fanning T, Sneige N, Staerkel G: Mucinous breast lesions: Fine needle aspiration findings (abstract). *Acta Cytol* 34:754-755, 1990.

Mammary Lesions Diagnosed as "Papillary" by Aspiration Biospy: 70 Cases With Follow-Up
Simsir A, Waisman J, Thorner K, et al (New York Univ)
Cancer 99:156-165, 2003   14–9

Introduction.—The accurate diagnosis of mammary papillary lesions by fine-needle aspiration biopsy (FNAB) is problematic due to overlapping cytologic characteristics of benign and malignant proliferations, along with true papillary neoplasms and their cytologic look-alikes. The accuracy of FNAB diagnosis of a papillary lesion in distinguishing true papillary from nonpapillary proliferations was examined. Cytologic criteria for the distinction of papillomas from true papillary malignancies and their cytologic look-alikes was assessed.

Methods.—A university medical center cytopathology database was searched for women who underwent surgical excision after a breast FNAB diagnosis of a papillary lesion. The FNAB smears and corresponding slides from excisional biopsy specimens were examined. Smears were assessed and graded for the following characteristics: cellularity, architecture, presence of fibrovascular cores, single cells, columnar cells, cellular atypia, myoepithe-lial cells, foamy histiocytes, and apocrine cells. The *F* test was used to ascertain the statistical significance of differences between true benign papillary lesions (papilloma) and adenocarcinomas (in situ and invasive).

Results.—Forty-six cases were benign (23 solitary intraductal papillomas, 6 intraductal papillomatosis, 11 examples of fibrocystic change, and 6 fibroadenomas); 24 (34%) were malignant (1 low-grade phyllodes tumor, 23 ductal in situ and invasive carcinomas). Of the 23 carcinomas, 3 (13%) were determined to be benign papillary lesions on FNAB and 19 were either atypical or suspicious. There was 1 case of low-grade phyllodes tumor that was originally classified as benign on FNAB.

Of the 4 false-negative diagnoses, 2 were due to sampling error and 2 to interpretive errors. A portion of lesions classified as papillary were fibroadenomas and were examples of fibrocystic change on excision; all were correctly classified as benign on FNAB. Of histologically proven papillomas, 62% were accurately classified as benign on FNAB; none were designated as being positive for malignancy.

Statistically significant characteristics of distinction between papillomas and carcinomas included cellularity ($P = .016$), cellular atypia ($P = .053$), and the presence of cytologically bland columnar cells ($P = .04$). Low-grade ductal carcinoma in situ (cribiform and micropapillary types) and tubular carcinoma represented the most challenging differential diagnostic problems.

Conclusion.—A significant number of lesions displaying a papillary pattern on FNAB are nonpapillary on follow-up. Among benign processes, fibrocystic change and fibroadenoma may closely simulate papilloma on cytology. Despite overlapping characteristics of true papillary lesions and their cytologic look-alikes, most can be reliably classified into benign or atypical (and above) categories by FNAB. Lesions that do not fit a definitive benign diagnosis should be placed in an indeterminate category and thus guide the surgeon to provide better patient management.

▶ FNAB of the breast has been shown to be accurate, in experienced hands, in classifying lesions along a categorical spectrum from benign to neoplastic. The challenge is in accurately placing lesions in the "in between" categories and in guiding the clinician in the most appropriate clinical management strategies. I think the cytologic category of "papillary lesion" has value only if we consider this category in the context of the categorical scale and how we want clinicians to behave. My impression is that the category of "papillary lesion" usually implies that a lesion is atypical and should be excised.

Simsir et al implied that the authors classify lesions as benign papillary lesions (and presumably do not excise these lesions), although given a 13% false-negative frequency. I do not think that most clinicians would find this acceptable. I think the take-home message from this article is that a high percentage of lesions classified as papillary by FNAB are not papillary at all. Thus, I wonder why we should use this category, unless we qualify it by saying "atypical" and suggest excision.

S. S. Raab, MD

SUGGESTED READING

Jeffrey PB, Ljung B-M: Benign and malignant papillary neoplasms of the breast: A cytomorphologic study. *Am J Clin Pathol* 101:500-507, 1994.

Michael CW, Buschmann B: Can true papillary neoplasms of breast and their mimickers be accurately classified by cytology? Cancer (Cancer Cytopathol) 96:92-100, 2002.

Yield of Endoscopic Ultrasound–Guided Fine-Needle Aspiration Biopsy in Patients With Suspected Pancreatic Carcinoma: Emphasis on Atypical, Suspicious, and False-Negative Aspirates
Eloubeidi MA, Jhala D, Chhieng DC, et al (Univ of Alabama, Birmingham)
Cancer 99:285-292, 2003   14–10

Introduction.—Atypical or suspicious cytology may support a clinical diagnosis of malignancy, yet it is frequently not adequate for the implementation of therapy in patients with pancreatic carcinoma. Endoscopic US-guided fine-needle aspiration biopsy (EUS-FNAB) is a somewhat new technique for obtaining cytology samples. It may reduce the number of atypical/suspicious diagnoses. The yield of EUS-FNAB in the diagnosis of patients seen with solid pancreatic lesions was assessed, along with the significance of atypical, suspicious, and false-negative aspirates.

Methods.—All patients with a solid pancreatic lesion who underwent EUS-FNAB during a 13-month period were evaluated. On-site examination of specimen adequacy by a cytopathologist was available for all patients. Follow-up included histologic correlation in 21 patients and clinical or imaging follow-up in 80 patients, including 38 patients who died of the disease.

Results.—A total of 101 patients underwent EUS-FNAB. The mean patient age was 62 years (range, 34-89 years); the male-to-female ratio was 2:1. Locations of the lesions were 65%, head of the pancreas; 12%, uncinate; 17%, body; and 6%, tail. The mean tumor size was 3.3 cm (range, 1.3-7 cm). Patients underwent a median of 4 needle passes (range, 1-11 passes). Biopsy interpretations were as follows: 62 (61.4%), malignant on cytologic evaluation; 5 (5%) suspicious for a malignancy; 6 (5.9%), atypical/indeterminant; and 26 (25.7%), benign processes.

Of 76 malignant lesions, 71 were adenocarcinoma, 3 were neuroendocrine tumors, 1 was lymphoma, and 1 was metastatic renal cell carcinoma. All except 1 of the suspicious/atypical aspirates were subsequently verified as malignant. The agreement was complete for all atypical cases. Of these, 2 of the 5 were identified as carcinoma by 1 cytopathologist and as suspicious lesions by the other (40% disagreement between the 2 cytopathologists). For the 10 atypical or suspicious cases that later were verified as malignant, the final diagnosis of malignant disease was not made due to scant cellularity that was attributed to sampling error in 8 cases and to interpretive disagreement in 2 cases (20%).

All 4 false-negative diagnoses were attributed to sampling error. Two percent of biopsy specimens were insufficient for interpretation. Of 99 adequate specimens, 72, 23, and 4, respectively, yielded true-positive results, true-negative results, and false-negative results. There were no false-positive results. The sensitivity, specificity, positive predictive vale, and negative predictive value of EUS-FNAB for solid pancreatic masses were, respectively, 94.7%, 100%, 100%, and 85.2%.

Conclusion.—The EUS-FNAB is both safe and highly accurate in tissue diagnosis of patients with solid pancreatic lesions. Patients with suspicious and atypical EUS-FNABs deserves further clinical examination.

Intraductal Papillary-Mucinous Neoplasm of the Pancreas: The Findings and Limitations of Cytologic Samples Obtained by Endoscopic Ultrasound–Guided Fine-Needle Aspiration
Stelow EB, Stanley MW, Bardales RH, et al (Hennepin County Med Ctr, Minneapolis; Univ of Minnesota, Minneapolis)
Am J Clin Pathol 120:398-404, 2003   14–11

Introduction.—Several recent trials have examined the value of cytologic evaluation of intraductal papillary-mucinous neoplasms (IPMNs), based on material obtained via endoscopic retrograde cholangiopancreatography or fine needle aspiration (FNA). The reported sensitivities are highly variable and may depend on sampling technique, cytopathologist experience, and the thoroughness with which clinicopathologic correlation is achieved. Described was an experience using endoscopic US (EUS) with FNA, a specific and sensitive diagnostic modality that allows visualization, sampling, and diagnosis of pancreatic and other gastrointestinal lesions. Eighteen lesions clinically, sonographically, and cytologically consistent with IPMNs were evaluated.

Methods.—All clinically and ultrasonographically suspected examples of IPMN aspirated between January 2000 and September 2002 were reviewed and analyzed for follow-up. The age range of the 18 patients in whom IPMNs were suspected was 52 to 87 years. All of the FNA slides were reviewed for the following cytologic features: presence and characteristics of extracellular mucin, presence and cellularity of neoplastic cells, cytomorphologic features of neoplastic cells, presence of goblet cells, presence of intracellular mucin, and mucicarmine positivity.

Results.—All 18 patients had dilated pancreatic ducts; 3 had intraductal papillary lesions. Five patients had adjacent cystic or solid pancreatic masses. Cytologic preparations revealed thick, glistening, viscid, abnormal mucus in all patients. Aspirates from 13 lesions (72%) were acellular or sparsely cellular.

Entrapped single or loosely cohesive molecules were seen in 16 patients (89%) Goblet cell morphological characteristics were frequently observed (6/18 or 33%). Papillary clusters and dysplastic changes were uncommon (3 or 17%, each) (Table 1). Confirmatory histologic follow-up was available

TABLE 1.—Clinical, Endoscopic, US, and Cytologic Findings in 18 Cases of Suspected Intraductal Pancreatic Mucinous Neoplasm

| Case No./ Sex/Age (y) | Adjacent Mass | | Endoscopic Ultrasound Findings | | | | | Fine-Needle Aspiration Findings | | | |
| | | | Duct Dilatation | | | Architectural | | | Cytologic | | |
	Cystic (cm)	Solid	Main Duct Only	Side Branches	Both	Thick Mucus	Papillae*	Smear Cellularity†	Goblet Cells	Cytoplasmic Mucin	Atypia‡
1/M/55	+ (2.8)	–	+	–	–	+	–	1+	+	–	–
2/F/52	–	–	–	–	+	+	–	2+	–	–	–
3/M/70	+ (2.8)	–	+§	–	–	+	–	1+	–	–	–
4/F/69	–	–	–	–	+	+	–	1+	–	–	–
5/F/78	–	Ill-defined	–	–	+	+	–	3+	–	–	–
6/F/78	–	–	–	–	–	+	+	4+	+	–	+
7/F/57	–	–	+§	–	+§	+	+	3+	+	–	+
8/F/79	–	–	–	–	–	+	–	2+	+	–	–
9/M/71	+	–	–	–	+	+	–	2+	–	+	–
10/M/78	–	–	–	+	–	+	–	1+	–	+	–
11/F/62	–	–	–	–	+	+	–	1+	–	–	–
12/F/68	–	–	–	+	–	+	+	0	–	–	–
13/F/74	+	–	–	–	+	+	+	4+	+	+	+
14/M/65	–	–	–	–	+	+	–	1+	+	+	–
15/M/87	–	–	–	+	+	+	–	4+	+	+	–
16/F/75	–	–	–	+	–	+	–	1+	–	+	–
17/M/82	–	–	–	+	–	+	–	2+	–	+	–
18/F/83	–	–	–	+	–	+	–	0	–	–	–

* A papilla was defined as a fibrovascular core covered by an epithelium. It may or may not show branching.
† Cellularity was graded semiquantitatively as follows: 0, acellular; 1+, very low; 2+, low; 3+, moderate; and 4+, high.
‡ Atypia was defined by comparing neoplastic cells with normal biliary ductal or duodenal mucosal cells and featured variable degrees of increased nucleolar prominence.
§ Endoscopic US showed intraluminal papillary projections.

Abbreviations: +, Present; –, absent; —, not applicable or stain not performed owing to insufficient material.
(Courtesy of Stelow EB, Stanley MW, Bardales RH, et al: Intraductal papillary-mucinous neoplasm of the pancreas: The findings and limitations of cytologic samples obtained by endoscopic ultrasound-guided fine-needle aspiration. *Am J Clin Pathol* 120:398-404, 2003. Copyright 2003 by the American Society of Clinical Pathologists. Reprinted with permission.)

for only 4 patients (22%), since most individuals with lesions clinically, sonographically, and cytologically consistent with IPMNs are elderly and frequently have co-morbid conditions.

Conclusion.—The EUS FNAs have important limitations. Gross and cytologic findings can be helpful in verifying the suspected diagnosis. Integration of complete clinical, sonographic, and cytologic information may be the best approach for achieving the most accurate diagnosis possible.

▶ US-guided FNA biopsy of the pancreas is becoming increasingly popular and the articles by Eloubeidi et al (Abstract 14–10) and Stelow et al (Abstract 14–11) attempt to address 2 important current issues: (1) diagnostic accuracy and (2) IPMNs. Eloubeidi et al report that the sensitivity and specificity of EUS-FNA of solid pancreatic lesions is high, although several points should be made. First, in this study, pathologists made immediate interpretations and thus, presumably, good material was obtained in each case. The accuracy is lower if pathologists do not perform an immediate interpretive service. Second, accuracy is highly dependent on the skill of the radiologist. The Alabama radiologists seem to perform this procedure with frequency that has probably increased their skill. Not all institutions will have these highly skilled radiologists. Third, some IPMNs present as solid masses, and it is uncertain how these lesions were addressed in this study since these lesional types are not described. This biases the study and makes accuracy data less valid.

The study by Stelow et al addresses the issue of IPMNs, tumors that generally were not aspirated by the previously used transabdominal approach. These tumors are a challenge, partly because they have a very bland appearance (Table 1). I think the US findings need to be known before this tumor may be suggested by cytologic findings that are not obviously malignant.

S. S. Raab, MD

SUGGESTED READING

Adsay NV, Longnecker DS, Klimstra DS: Pancreatic tumors with cystic dilatation of the ducts: Intraductal papillary mucinous neoplasms and intraductal oncocytic papillary neoplasms. *Semin Diagn Pathol* 17:16-30, 2000.

Fukushima N, Mukai K, Kanai Y, et al: Intraductal papillary tumors and mucinous cystic tumors of the pancreas: Clinicopathologic study of 38 cases. *Hum Pathol* 28:1010-1017, 1997.

Cytologic Findings of Marginal Zone Lymphoma: A Study of 14 Specimens
Crapanzano JP, Lin O (Mem Sloan-Kettering Cancer Ctr, New York)
Cancer 99:301-309, 2003   14–12

Introduction.—Low-grade lymphomas can be challenging to diagnose in cytology specimens, particularly marginal zone B-cell lymphomas (MZLs). These low-grade lymphomas are characterized by a heterogeneous lymphoid population which may be difficult to distinguish from reactive processes in cytology specimens.

Methods.—Fourteen cytology specimens of MZL from 11 patients (10 with histologically verified MZL and 1 with flow cytometry (FC)-verified MZL) were examined. The 14 specimens included 12 fine-needle aspiration biopsy specimens (salivary gland, lung, lymph node, and breast, in 6, 3, 2, and 1, respectively, and 1 each soft tissue and pleural effusion). Cytologic preparations involved air-dried and alcohol-fixed direct smears, ThinPrep slides, and cell blocks. Six specimens had FC studies available.

Results.—All 13 fine-needle aspiration biopsy specimens were composed predominantly of intermediate-sized lymphoid cells, which were interspersed with small, round lymphocytes and transformed cells. The intermediate-sized cells exhibited a moderate amount of cytoplasm, slight nuclear membrane irregularities, and inconspicuous to absent nucleoli. The pleural fluid contained primarily small to intermediate-sized, round lymphocytes. The intermediate-sized cells in 10 specimens frequently demonstrated plasmacytoid morphology, which was best visualized in Diff-Quik–stained slides.

Monocytoid cells, plasma cells, lymphohistiocytic aggregates, and tingible body macrophages were variably identified in 6, 7, 11, and 5 specimens, respectively. Lymphoepithelial lesions were not seen. Three specimens with FC studies revealed a phenotype compatible with MZL and 3 were nondiagnostic.

Conclusion.—Cytologic features suggestive of MZL included abundant intermediate-sized lymphoid cells with mild atypia in a background of small lymphocytes and transformed cells, frequently with plasmacytoid morphology. FC was useful only in selected MZL cytology specimens. Surgical correlation may be needed to verify the diagnosis.

▶ Articles outlining the features of low-grade malignant lymphomas are useful when they provide clues to prevent us from making a false-negative diagnosis. Many argue that FC is necessary, even in those cases that may appear benign, regardless of the patient age. For some malignant lymphomas, such as MZL, the lymphoid population is mixed and few clues are available. The diagnosis depends on clinical history and the ancillary studies.

S. S. Raab, MD

SUGGESTED READING

Wakely PE Jr: Fine-needle aspiration cytopathology in diagnosis and classification of malignant lymphoma: Accurate and reliable? *Diagn Cytopathol* 22:120-125, 2000.

Meda BA, Buss DH, Woodruff RD, et al: Diagnosis and subclassification of primary and recurrent lymphoma: The usefulness and limitations of combined fine-needle aspiration cytomorphology and flow cytometry. *Am J Clin Pathol* 113:688-699, 2000.

15 Hematolymphoid

Subcutaneous, Blastic Natural Killer (NK), NK/T-Cell, and Other Cytotoxic Lymphomas of the Skin: A Morphologic, Immunophenotypic, and Molecular Study of 50 Patients
Massone C, Chott A, Metze D, et al (Univ of Graz, Austria; Univ of Genoa, Italy; Univ of Vienna, Austria; et al)
Am J Surg Pathol 28:719-735, 2004   15–1

Background.—A new group of subcutaneous, natural killer (NK) cell, NK/T cell, and other cytotoxic T-cell lymphomas of the skin was recently described. Some of these lymphomas have been included as distinct clinicopathologic entities in the classification of hematologic malignancies. They would be classified as CD30− large T-cell lymphoma, small/medium pleomorphic T-cell lymphoma, or subcutaneous T-cell lymphoma in the European Organization for Research and Treatment of Cancer system. Precise clinicopathologic and prognostic features of all of these new entities have not yet been delineated.

Methods and Findings.—Eighty-one biopsy specimens from 50 patients with subcutaneous, blastic NK cell, NK/T cell, or other nonmycosis fungoides cytotoxic T-cell lymphomas of the skin were examined retrospectively. Clinical, morphological, phenotypic, and genetic data—as well as data on Epstein-Barr virus association—were used to classify these cases. There were 7 categories: subcutaneous "panniculitis-like" T-cell lymphoma, which included 10 patients; blastic NK-cell lymphoma, consisting of 12 patients; nasal-type extranodal NK/T-cell lymphoma, including 5 patients; epidermotropic CD8+ T-cell lymphoma, including 5 patients; cutaneous γ/δ T-cell lymphoma, consisting of 8 patients; cutaneous α/β pleomorphic T-cell lymphoma, including 8 patients; and cutaneous medium/large pleomorphic T-cell lymphoma, not otherwise specified, including 2 patients. The estimated 5-year surviva rate was 80% for patients in the first group, compared with 0 in the other groups.

Conclusion.—Cutaneous lymphomas can be classified precisely into diagnostic categories. Except for subcutaneous panniculitis-like T-cell lymphoma, these groups of lymphomas have an aggressive course, irrespective of diagnostic category.

▶ This article summarized the diagnostic features of NK, NK/T-cell, and other cytotoxic lymphomas involving the skin. Although there have been several articles this year related to the diagnosis of NK and related neoplasms, this area still remains confusing. There appear to be 2 broad categories of NK-related neoplasms; those composed of mature cells and those composed of blasts.

Probably the best-defined blastic tumor is the "blastic NK-cell lymphoma" also known as "agranular CD4+ CD56+ haematodermic neoplasm." Knowledge about this entity is still growing, and there is recent evidence that this tumor represents a proliferation of plasmacytoid type-2 dendritic cells rather than true NK cells. Although the morphological and phenotypic features of blastic NK-cell lymphoma are somewhat variable, recognition of this entity is usually assisted by the presence of prominent involvement of the skin.

Distinction of other leukemia blastic NK-cell neoplasms from acute myeloid leukemia and precursor T-cell acute lymphoblastic leukemia remains problematic. One possible source of confusion is the overlap in phenotypes since T-cell and NK-cell associated antigens can be expressed in acute myeloid leukemia and myeloid antigens can be expressed in acute lymphoblastic leukemia and possibly on immature NK cells. There is also confusion over the classification of mature NK-cell neoplasms, with authors emphasizing different aspects including the presence of NK-associated antigens, cytotoxic granule-associated proteins, or the structure of the T-cell receptor (α/β versus γ/δ).

However, as this article outlines, there has been some progress in the recognition of distinct disease entities and the criteria for their diagnosis. The consensus seems to be that the diagnosis of T/NK-cell neoplasms requires a multiparametric approach. Clinical information is of paramount importance, with particular attention to whether the disease is primarily leukemic, nodal, or extranodal. Recognition of 1 of the defined entities within each of these groups usually requires evaluation for NK-associated antigens such as CD56 and CD57, cytotoxic molecular such as TIA-1 and granzyme-B or perforin, the presence of Epstein-Barr virus, and possibly the components of T-cell receptor. I can only hope that as distinct entities emerge, recognition of the most important defining features will make their diagnosis less complicated.

F. Craig, MD

SUGGESTED READING

Jaffe ES, Krenacs L, Raffeld M: Classification of cytotoxic T-cell and natural killer cell lymphomas. *Semin Hematol* 40:175-184, 2003.

Cheung MMC, Chan JKC, Wong K-F: Natural killer cell neoplasms: A distinctive group of highly aggressive lymphomas/leukemias. *Semin Hematol* 40:221-23, 2003.

Expression and Function of KIR and Natural Cytotoxicity Receptors in NK-Type Lymphoproliferative Diseases of Granular Lymphocytes

Zambello R, Falco M, Chiesa MD, et al (Università di Padua, Italy; Istituto Giannina Gaslini, Genova, Italy; Università di Genova, Genoa, Italy; et al)
Blood 102:1797-1805, 2003   15–2

Background.—In natural killer (NK) cell type lymphoproliferative disease of granular lymphocytes (LDGL), proliferation of large granular lymphocytes (LGLs) displaying a typical NK phenotype is abnormal. The different forms of LDGL range from mild, asymptomatic conditions to aggressive, usually fatal diseases. Monoclonal antibodies (mAbs) specific for different NK receptors were used to study the lymphocyte population from a group of patients with NK-type LDGL.

Methods and Findings.—Eighteen patients were included in the study. Analysis of resting and cultured NK cell populations showed NK cells exhibiting a homogeneous staining with given anti-killer immunoglobulin-like receptor mAbs in 11 patients. In most patients, NK cells were characterized by the CD94/NKG2A+ phenotype. A small proportion of the cases expressed CD94/NKG2C. The function of the various NK receptors was also assessed in 7 patients.

The killer immunoglobulin-like receptor (KIR) molecules that homogeneously marked the NK cell expansion in each patient displayed an activating function as determined by cross-linking with specific anti-KIR mAbs. The KIR genotype analysis done in 13 cases showed that certain activating KIRs and infrequent KIR genotypes occurred at higher frequencies than in healthy persons. Most KIR genotypes in patients with LDGL included multiple genes coding for activating KIRs.

In an analysis of non–HLA-specific triggering receptors, the natural cytotoxicity receptors were expressed at significantly low levels in NK cells freshly drawn from most patients. However, in most cases, the expression of NKp46 and NKp30 could be upregulated on culture in interleukin 2.

Conclusion.—In NK-LDGL, the expanded subset is characterized by the expression of a given activating KIR. This suggests that these molecules play a direct role in the pathogenesis of NK-LDGL.

► LGL leukemia is a disorder characterized by a persistent increase in the number of LGLs, without a clearly identified cause. Unfortunately, there are many causes of a reactive increase in LGLs. Therefore, it would be useful to have a test to separate reactive LGL proliferations from LGL leukemia. Sometimes flow cytometry immunophenotyping can assist in the diagnosis by identifying an abnormal phenotype such as loss of a pan–T-cell antigen. Immunophenotypic studies can also be used to distinguish 2 types of LGL leukemia: T-cell LGL leukemia and NK-cell LGL leukemia. Molecular diagnostic studies for clonal T-cell receptor rearrangement can be used to further evaluate T-cell LGL leukemia, but an equivalent test is not available for NK-cell LGL leukemia.

This article describes evaluation of additional antigens expressed on NK cells and identification of abnormal patterns of expression in NK-cell LGL leukemia. NK cells express a variety of cell surface receptors that either trigger or inhibit NK-mediated cytolytic activity. The inhibitory NK receptors include the KIRs. There are many different KIRs that are specific for different groups of HLA class I alleles. Reactive populations of NK cells appear to express a heterogeneous mixture of receptors that are mainly inhibitory rather than activating.

Using multiple KIR-specific mAbs, the authors studied 18 cases of NK-cell LGL leukemia and identified a relatively homogeneous staining pattern or an abnormal lack of all tested KIRs. These results support the clonal nature of NK-cell LGL leukemia and suggest that evaluation of KIR expression might be a useful clinical test.

F. Craig, MD

SUGGESTED READING

Morice WG, Kurtin PJ, Leibson PJ, et al: Demonstration of aberrant T-cell and natural killer-cell antigen expression in all cases of granular lymphocytic leukemia. *Br J Haematol* 120:1026-1036, 2003.

CD10 Expression in Extranodal Dissemination of Angioimmunoblastic T-Cell Lymphoma
Attygalle AD, Diss TC, Munson P, et al (Univ College, London)
Am J Surg Pathol 28:54-61, 2004   15–3

Background.—Patients with angioimmunoblastic T-cell lymphoma (AITL), a systemic disease, are commonly found to have extranodal involvement at presentation. In recent research, these authors demonstrated that neoplastic T cells in most cases of AITL can be identified by an aberrant expression of CD10. The aim of this study was to investigate whether CD10 expression by the neoplastic T cells is maintained in extranodal sites.

Methods.—Ten patients with AITL and histologic and immunophenotypic evidence of extranodal dissemination were included in the study. A control group consisted of 7 patients with peripheral T-cell lymphoma unspecific, who had biopsies of involved extranodal sites; 2 patients with enteropathy type T-cell lymphoma; and 1 patient with extranodal NK/T lymphoma, nasal type. Findings on diagnostic lymph node biopsies and biopsies of extranodal sites were re-examined. In addition, polymerase chain reaction was done for T-cell clonality and single-layer immunostaining for CD3, CD20, CD10, and CD21 and double-layer immunostaining for DC20/CD10.

Findings.—All 10 patients with AITL had characteristic histologic features. Molecular evidence of the disease in lymph node biopsy specimens was also noted in all cases. Aberrant CD10 expression was maintained in the lung, cecum, tonsil, and nasopharynx as well as in 1 of 6 involved bone marrow trephines. The CD10-positive tumor cell distribution in these extranodal biopsy specimens correlated with the distribution of the follicular dendritic cell meshwork (FDC). The 5 bone marrow trephines without aberrant CD10 expression showed no morphological or immunohistochemical evidence of FDC. These 5 cases showed evidence of aberrant CD10 expression in other involved sites with FDC. In patients with peripheral T-cell lymphoma unspecific; enteropathy type T-cell lymphoma; and extranodal NK/T lymphoma, nasal type, the neoplastic cells were CD10 negative.

Conclusion.—Aberrant CD10 expression appears to be a useful phenotypic marker for diagnosing AITL in most involved extranodal sites, except for bone marrow. This suggests a possible role for FDC in the pathogenesis of AITL.

▶ AITL is considered a type of nodal peripheral T-cell lymphoma that has frequent evidence of extranodal disease at the time of diagnosis. Attygalle and colleagues previously described the identification of CD10-positive T cells in AITL, used molecular diagnostic studies performed on microdissected samples to suggest that these cells were neoplastic, and proposed that the identification of these cells could assist in the distinction of AITL from other types of peripheral T-cell lymphoma.[1]

In the more recent article from this group, they report the presence of CD10-positive T cells at several extranodal sites involved by AITL, including the lung, cecum, tonsil, and nasopharynx. However, CD10-positive T cells were only identified in 1 of 6 bone marrow specimens involved by AITL. The authors also noted that the presence of CD10-positive T cells appeared to correlate with the presence of an FDC. Although the authors suggest that the presence of CD10-positive T cells could be used to diagnose AITL at extranodal sites, I think the results should be interpreted with caution.

The study by Cook and colleagues identified benign CD10-positive T cells in reactive lymphoid proliferations and accompanying B-cell lymphoma.[2] Interestingly, the benign CD10-positive T cells were located in follicular germinal centers. Therefore, the presence of CD10-positive T cells should not be used by itself to diagnose lymphoma. However, if an extranodal site is involved by T-cell lymphoma, the presence of CD10-positive T cells or the presence of an FDC might be used to favor the AITL subtype.

F. Craig, MD

References

1. Attygalle A, Al-Jehani R, Disse TC, et al: Neoplastic T cells in angioimmunoblastic T-cell lymphomas express CD10. *Blood* 99:627-633, 2002.
2. Cook JR, Craig FE, Swerdlow SH: Benign CD10-positive T cells in reactive lymphoid proliferations and B-cell lymphomas. *Mod Pathol* 16:879-885, 2003.

Flow Cytometry in the Differential Diagnosis of Lymphcyte-Rich Thymoma From Precursor T-Cell Acute Lymphoblastic Leukemia/Lymphoblastic Lymphoma

Li S, Juco J, Mann KP, et al (Emory Univ, Atlanta, Ga)
Am J Clin Pathol 121:268-274, 2004   15–4

Background.—Thymocytes, immature T lymphocytes with varying degrees of maturation, are common in anterior mediastinal masses. Often they are a significant component of hyperplastic thymus or lymphocyte-rich thymoma. Precursor T-cell acute lymphoblastic leukemia/lymphoblastic lymphoma (ALL/LBL) also occurs frequently in the anterior mediastinum. A comprehensive analysis of antigen-expression profiles of thymocytes in lymphocyte-rich thymomas and T-cell ALL/LBL lymphoblasts was conducted to determine whether the expression pattern of certain antigens can differentiate these entities by using 4-color flow cytometry.

Methods and Findings.—Fifteen thymomas were studied. In all cases, thymocytes showed 3 distinct subpopulations. The least mature cells expressed low-density CD2 and CD5, high-density CD7, CD10, CD34, and heterogeneous CD4 and CD8. These entities had the lowest density CD45 expression and were negative for surface CD3. Immature cells were CD10− and CD34− and expressed CD2, CD5, CD7, CD4, CD8, heterogeneous surface CD3, and intermediate-density CD45. Mature cells expressed CD2 and surface CD3, CD5, and CD7. They also expressed CD4 or CD8.

A characteristic smearing pattern for these antigens resulted from the heterogeneous expression of surface CD3, CD4, and CD8. Lymphoblasts in all 15 T-cell ALL/LBL cases formed a tight cluster with no discrete subpopulations or smearing pattern. Four of 5 double-negative cases showed a loss of CD2, CD10, or CD34 expression. Five of 7 double-positive cases had complete loss of surface CD3, CD2, or CD5. Four of these were CD10+ and 2 were CD34+. Two of the 3 single-positive cases demonstrated a loss of CD2 or aberrant CD34 expression.

Conclusion.—Analysis of the antigen expression pattern can help clinicians differentiate thymoma from T-cell ALL/LBL. The presence or absence of T cell-associated antigen deletion and the expression of CD10 and CD34 by 4-color flow cytometry are useful for this differentiation.

▶ Flow cytometry has a well-established role in the diagnosis of mature B-cell neoplasms. More recent studies have confirmed the utility of this technique in the diagnosis of mature T-cell malignancies and in the distinction between precursor B ALL/ABL (B-ALL/LBL) and hematogones. This article describes immunophenotypic differences that could assist in the distinction between precursor T ALL/LBL (T-ALL/LBL) and thymoma. T-ALL/LBL often presents as a large mediastinal mass and may be difficult to distinguish from normal thymic tissue or the reactive thymocytes present in a thymoma.

In this article, all 15 cases of thymoma studied demonstrated a maturation sequence that was represented by 3 subpopulations of thymocytes each with a characteristic phenotype (CD4 and CD8 double-negative, CD4 and CD8 double-positive, and CD4 or CD8 single-positive). For example, the double-negative population expressed low-density CD45, CD2, and CD5; high density CD7, CD10, and CD34; and lacked surface CD3. Knowledge of these distinct sub-populations assisted in identification of abnormalities in the phenotype of most cases of T-ALL/LBL.

Cases of T-ALL/LBL displayed a more uniform phenotype and frequently demonstrated loss of the antigens characteristic of that stage of maturation. For example, double-negative cases of T-ALL/LBL demonstrated loss of CD2, CD10, or CD34. Therefore, flow cytometric immunophenotypic studies may assist in the evaluation of samples from the mediastinum, especially when material is limited, such as is obtained by fine-needle aspiration.

F. Craig, MD

SUGGESTED READING

Jamal S, Picker LJ, Aquino DB, et al: Immunophenotypic analysis of peripheral T-cell neoplasms: A multiparametric approach. *Am J Clin Pathol* 116:512-526, 2001.

McKenna RW, Washington LT, Aquino DB, et al: Immunophenotypic analysis of hematogones (B-lymphocyte precursors) in 662 consecutive bone marrow specimens by 4-color flow cytometry. *Blood* 98:2498-2507, 2001.

ALK-Positive Diffuse Large B-Cell Lymphoma Is Associated With *Clathrin-ALK* Rearrangements: Report of 6 Cases

Gascoyne RD, Lamant L, Martin-Subero JI, et al (Centre de Physiopathologie de Toulouse-Purpan, Toulouse, France; British Columbia Cancer Agency, Vancouver, Canada; Univ Hosp Schleswig-Holstein Campus, Kiel, Germany; et al)
Blood 102:2568-2573, 2003   15–5

Background.—T-cell and null anaplastic large-cell lymphoma (ALCL) result from a novel fusion created by the anaplastic lymphoma kinase (*ALK*) gene on chromosome 2p23 and the nucleophosmin (*NPM*) on 5q35 or other variant translocation partners. A rare variant of diffuse large B-cell lymphoma (DLBCL) has been described. This variant was believed to overexpress full-length ALK, in contrast to a chimeric protein characteristic of ALCL. However, full-length ALK protein lacks tyrosine kinase activity. Thus, the mechanism of oncogenesis continues to be unclear.

Methods and Findings.—Six cases of ALK-DLBCL were examined. They were characterized by a simple or complex t(2;17)(p23;q23) involving the clathrin gene (*CLTC*) at chromosome band 17q23 and the *ALK* gene at chromosome band 2p23. Fluorescence in situ hybridization was used in all cases, complemented in 1 by standard cytogenetic analysis, multicolor karyotyping (M–fluorescence in situ hybridization), and reverse transcriptase-polymerase chain reaction. Analysis clearly showed that most cases of ALK+ DLBCL share the same mechanism of deregulated ALK expression. The presence of *CLTC-ALK* fusions was demonstrated.

Conclusion.—Most cases of ALK + DLBCL share the same mechanism of deregulated ALK expression. The presence of *CLTC-ALK* fusions in these tumors extended the list of diseases associated with this genetic abnormality to include classic T-cell or null ALCL, ALK + DLBCL, and inflammatory myofibroblastic tumors.

▶ Immunohistochemical staining for ALK protein is most often performed in the evaluation of ALCL of a T or null phenotype. Many cases of ALCL harbor the translocation t(2;5) that leads to fusion of the *ALK* and *NPM* genes. The fusion transcript can be detected by immunohistochemical staining for ALK protein and is usually located in both the nucleus and cytoplasm. In addition to the translocation t(2;5), several other variant translocations, fusing *ALK* with other partner genes, have been associated with ALK protein staining in ALCL.

This article describes cases of ALK protein–positive B-cell lymphoma and demonstrates an association with the translocation t(2;17) involving the clathrin gene and the *ALK* gene. These cases of ALK-positive DLBCL have distinct morphological and immunophenotypic features, including a sinusoidal growth pattern, immunoblastic and/or plasmablastic appearance, and the following phenotype: CD20 negative, CD79a negative, CD30 negative, and CD138 positive. Some cases stained for cytoplasmic immunoglobulin demonstrated an apparent preference for lambda immunoglobulin light chain. Two cases demonstrated weak focal staining for CD4 and 1 case was CD57-positive.

These B-cell lymphomas demonstrated a staining pattern for ALK protein (fine granular cytoplasmic staining) similar to that described for ALCL with the variant clathrin-*ALK* translocation. There is also a recent report of an ALK-positive DLBCL with similar morphological and immunophenotypic findings to those described by Gascoyne and colleagues but harboring the t(2;5) NPM-ALK translocation and demonstrating nuclear and cytoplasmic ALK staining. Therefore, ALK-positive DLBCL seems to be a distinct entity that can be recognized by a combination of characteristic morphological and immunophenotypic features. The clinical significance of recognizing this subtype of DLBCL remains uncertain.

F. Craig, MD

SUGGESTED READING

Adam P, Katzenberger T, Seeberger H, et al: A case of diffuse large B-cell lymphoma of plasmablastic type associated with the t(2;5)(p23;q35) chromosome translocation. *Am J Surg Pathol* 27:1473-1476, 2003.

Diffuse Large B-Cell Lymphomas With Plasmablastic Differentiation Respresent a Heterogeneous Group of Disease Entities

Colomo L, Loong F, Rives S, et al (Univ of Barcelona; Natl Cancer Inst, Bethesda, Md; Hosp Galdakao, Vizcaya, Spain)
Am J Surg Pathol 28:736-747, 2004   15–6

Background.—Initially, plasmablastic lymphoma was reported as a variant of diffuse large B-cell lymphoma (DLBCL) of the oral cavity in patients positive for HIV. It is characterized by immunoblastic morphology and a plasma cell phenotype. However, similar morphological and immunophenotypic features may be found in other lymphomas. The significance of plasmablastic differentiation in DLBCL and the heterogeneity of lymphomas with these characteristics were investigated.

Methods and Findings.—Fifty DLBCLs with low or absent CD20/CD79a and an immunophenotype indicating terminal B-cell differentiation were examined. Several distinct subgroups were identified. Twenty-three tumors showing a monomorphic population of immunoblasts with little or no plasmacytic differentiation were classified as plasmablastic lymphoma of the oral mucosa type. Most patients in this group were HIV-positive, and three fourths were positive for the Epstein-Barr virus. Forty-eight percent of the lesions in this group first appeared in the oral mucosa, but 39% first occurred in extranodal sites and 13% in nodal sites.

Another 16 cases were designated plasmablastic lymphoma with plasmacytic differentiation. These were composed mainly of immunoblasts and plasmablasts. In addition, however, they showed more differentiation to mature plasma cells. Only 33% of the patients in this group were HIV-positive, with 62% having Epstein-Barr virus. Forty-four percent of these lesions had a nodal presentation. In 9 cases, the lesions were indistinguishable morphologically from the previous group but were secondary extramedullary plasmablastic tumors. These lesions occurred in patients with previous or synchronous plasma cell neoplasms. In 7 of 9 cases, they were classified as multiple myeloma.

Another 2 neoplasms were HHV-8+ extracavitary variants of primary effusion lymphoma and an ALK+ DLBCL. In an additional 39 cases, HHV-8 was examined and proved to be negative in all all them.

Conclusion.—These findings show that DLBCLs with plasmablastic differentiation are a heterogeneous group of neoplasm. The clinicopathologic characteristics of these tumors are different and may correspond to different entities.

▶ The category of DLBCL, as defined in the World Health Organization classification, contains a heterogeneous group of lymphomas with unpredictable outcome. In this study, the authors identified cases of DLBCL with plasmablastic features and documented that many of these patients had aggressive disease. They also used morphological and immunophenotypic findings to separate out groups of plasmablastic lymphoma that appeared to represent distinct disease entities. Therefore, recognition of plasmablastic differentiation may be of diagnostic value.

Plasmablasts are large cells that usually resemble immunoblasts rather than lymphoblasts and have abundant basophilic cytoplasm and occasionally a perinuclear hof. They usually lack staining for CD20, are negative or only weakly positive for CD45, and stain for plasma cell associated antigens such as CD138 and CD38. The identification of plasmablastic differentiation in DLBCL should raise the possibility of several entities: plasmablastic lymphoma of the oral cavity; extramedullary plasmablastic tumors associated with plasma cell neoplasms such as multiple myeloma; primary effusion lymphoma and its solid extracavitary variant, plasmablastic lymphoma associated with multicentric Castleman disease; and ALK-positive DLBCL.

This and other recent articles have recognized cases of plasmablastic lymphoma of oral mucosa type in other extranodal locations. However, this group of lymphomas appears to be united by lack of differentiation to more typical plasma cells, frequent presence of Epstein-Barr virus, and association with HIV infection. Cases of plasmablastic lymphoma that demonstrated some differentiation to plasma cells included those occurring in patients with a prior or synchronous plasma cell neoplasm. Staining for CD56 and cyclin-D1 assisted in identification of some of these secondary tumors.

This article also confirmed the presence of plasmablastic differentiation in primary effusion lymphoma and ALK-positive DLBCL. Therefore, in cases of DLBCL demonstrating plasmablastic features or lacking staining for CD20, it might be worth considering several of these entities and possibly pursuing stains for plasma cell–associated antigens, Epstein-Barr virus, HHV-8, and ALK1.

F. Craig, MD

SUGGESTED READING

Simonitsch-Klupp I, Hauser I, Ott G, et al: Diffuse large B-cell lymphomas with plasmablastic/plasmacytoid features are associated with TP53 deletions and poor clinical outcome. *Leukemia* 18:146-155, 2004.

Chetty R, Hlatswayo N, Muc R, et al: Plasmablastic lymphoma in HIV+ patients: An expanding spectrum. *Histopathology* 42:605-609, 2003.

The B-Cell Transcription Factors BSAP, Oct-2, and BOB.1 and the Pan–B-Cell Markers CD20, CD22, and CD79a Are Useful in the Differential Diagnosis of Classic Hodgkin Lymphoma
Browne P, Petrosyan K, Hernandez A, et al (IMPATH, Los Angeles; Kaiser Found Hosp, Los Angeles)
Am J Clin Pathol 120:767-777, 2003   15–7

Background.—Most Hodgkin lymphomas, both classic Hodgkin lymphoma (CHL) and nodular lymphocyte predominant Hodgkin lymphoma (NLPHL), are of B-cell origin. However, the differentiation of CHL from diffuse large B-cell lymphoma (DLBCL) or anaplastic large cell lymphoma can be difficult. The reasons for incomplete development of the B-cell phenotype and the lack of immunoglobulin expression in CHL have not been fully explained. Crippling immunoglobulin gene mutations have been proposed as the cause of absent immunoglobulin expression in CHL. However, recent studies have focused on impaired activation of the immunoglobulin promoter secondary to defective interaction with, or lack of expression of, transcription factors as the dominant mechanisms. It has been proposed that the transcription factors B cell–specific activator protein (BSAP), octamer-binding transcription factor 2 (Oct-2), and B-cell Oct-binding protein 1 (BOB.1) and the pan–B-cell markers CD20, CD22, and CD79a may aid in the clarification of the diagnosis. It was determined whether decreased expression of these transcription factors is correlated with the varied expression of the pan–B-cell markers in both types of Hodgkin lymphoma.

Methods.—Routinely processed formalin-fixed, paraffin-embedded tumor specimens were obtained for 57 cases of CHL, 5 cases of NLPHL, and 33 cases of non-Hodgkin lymphoma. Diagnoses were confirmed and classified according to the World Health Organization Classification of Tumors. Diagnoses were established according to standard procedures, including morphologic examination, immunohistochemical analysis, flow cytometric analysis, gene rearrangement studies by polymerase chain reaction, and chromosomal abnormalities by cytogenetic and fluorescent in situ hybridization techniques, when necessary.

Results.—The transcription factor phenotype BSAP+ and either Oct-2− or BOB.1− were predictive of CHL. BSAP+/Oct-2+/BOB.1+ was predictive of NLPHL or DLBCL, whereas BSAP− was predictive of anaplastic large cell lymphoma. The expression of all 3 pan–B-cell markers was observed only in NLPHL and DLBCL. Positivity for a single B-cell marker was present only in CHL.

Conclusions.—The transcription factors and pan–B-cell markers may be useful in the differential diagnosis of CHL.

▶ Which immunohistochemical stains are appropriate in the diagnosis of Hodgkin lymphoma? Although the following stains usually suffice—leukocyte common antigen, CD30, CD15, and CD20—recent articles have documented cases of "grey-zone" lymphoma where the distinction between subtypes of Hodgkin lymphoma and non-Hodgkin lymphoma is more problematic. The article by Browne and colleagues reports on the performance of several additional stains that may assist in the diagnosis of Hodgkin lymphoma. The authors also propose a diagnostic algorithm for their use. BSAP, encoded by the *PAX*-5 gene, is a marker of B cells and is found in most cases of DLBCL, NLPHL, and CHL. However, staining for BSAP would be unusual in anaplastic large cell lymphoma. Lymphoma positive for BSAP but lacking staining for both Oct-2 and BOB.1 would be most characteristic of CHL. The presence of staining for both Oct-2 and BOB.1 in addition to several pan–B-cell antigens would strongly favor DLBCL or NLPHL over CHL. In my experience, the BSAP stain works well, and the nuclear staining pattern is easy to interpret. The authors also mention that the Oct-2 and BOB.1 stains were reproducible and easy to interpret. Therefore, these stains might make a useful addition to the diagnostic armamentarium for CHL.

F. Craig, MD

SUGGESTED READING

Rudiger T, Jaffe ES, Delsol G, et al: Workshop report on Hodgkin's disease and related diseases ('grey zone' lymphoma). *Ann Oncol* 9:S31-S38, 1998.

The Molecular Signature of Mediastinal Large B-Cell Lymphoma Differs From That of Other Diffuse Large B-Cell Lymphomas and Shares Features With Classical Hodgkin Lymphoma

Savage KJ, Monti S, Kutok JL, et al (Dana-Farber Cancer Inst, Boston; Whitehead Inst, Cambridge, Mass; Brigham and Women's Hosp, Boston; et al)
Blood 102:3871-3879, 2003   15–8

Background.—Mediastinal large B-cell lymphoma (MLBCL) is a recently identified subtype of diffuse large B-cell lymphoma (DLBCL). The characteristic presentation of MLBCL is as localized tumors, usually in young female patients. The pathologic features of MLBCL are distinctive, but its clinical manifestations are similar to those of the nodular sclerosis subtype of classical Hodgkin lymphoma (cHL). Combined modality therapy is only partially effective in treating these tumors because more than 40% of MLBCL patients die of their disease. In addition, involved-field radiation therapy has been associated with long-term side effects, including secondary malignancies and cardiac dysfunction. Additional insights are therefore needed into the molecular signature of MLBCL to identify potential rational treatment targets. The molecular features of MLBCL were determined.

Methods.—The gene expression profiles of newly diagnosed MLBCL and DLBCL were compared, and a classification system for these diseases was developed.

Results.—MLBCLs were found to have low levels of expression of multiple components of the B-cell receptor signaling cascade, a profile similar to that of Reed-Sternberg cells in cHL. MLBCLs, like cHLs, were found to have high levels of expression of the interleukin-13 receptor and downstream effectors of interleukin-13 signaling (Janus kinase-2 and signal transducer and activator of transcription-1 [STAT1]), tumor necrosis factor (TNF) family members, and TNF receptor–associated factor-1 (TRAF1). The increased expression of STAT1 and TRAF1 in MLBCL was confirmed by immunohistochemistry. The findings of TRAF1 expression and the known link to nuclear factor-κB (NF-κB) prompted evaluation of MLBCLs for nuclear translocation of c-REL protein. In almost all cases, c-REL was localized to the nucleus, consistent with activation of the NF-κB pathway.

Conclusions.—A molecular link, as well as a shared survival pathway, was found between MLBCL and cHL.

Molecular Diagnosis of Primary Mediastinal B Cell Lymphoma Identifies a Clinically Favorable Subgroup of Diffuse Large B Cell Lymphoma Related to Hodgkin Lymphoma

Rosenwald A, Wright G, Leroy K, et al (NIH, Bethesda, Md; Hôpital Henri Mondor, Créteil, France; Univ of Nebraska, Omaha; et al)
J Exp Med 198:851-862, 2003   15–9

Background.—Under current criteria, primary mediastinal B-cell lymphoma (PMBL) cannot be reliably distinguished from other types of diffuse large B-cell lymphoma (DLBCL). The imprecision in the diagnosis of PMBL may account for some of the heterogeneity in clinical responses. At present, there are no molecular tests routinely available for the diagnosis of PMBL. Gene expression profiling was used to develop a more precise molecular diagnosis of PMBL.

Methods.—Quantitative polymerase chain reaction assays were used to assess the genomic copy number of the *PDL2* gene relative to the control *PRKCQ* gene. Control samples of genomic DNA from peripheral blood mononuclear cells of normal volunteers yielded a *PDL2* to *PRKCQ* ratio of 0.99, with a standard deviation of 0.08. A threshold *PDL2* to *PRKCQ* ratio for gain/amplification was set at 1.31, which is 4 standard deviations above the mean. A biopsy specimen composed of 100% malignant cells would be expected to yield a *PDL2* to *PRKCQ* ratio of 1.5 if the malignant cells had a gain of a single chromosome copy.

Results.—The patients with PMBL were significantly younger than other DLBCL patients, and their lymphomas often involved other thoracic structures but not extrathoracic sites that are typically involved in other DLBCLs. Patients with PMBL had a relatively favorable clinical outcome, with a 5-year survival rate of 64% compared with 46% for other DLBCL patients. Results of gene expression profiling were strongly supportive of a relationship between PMBL and Hodgkin lymphoma. More than one third of the genes that were more highly expressed in PMBL than in other DLBCLs were also characteristically expressed in Hodgkin lymphoma cells. *PDL2*, which encodes a regulator of T-cell activation, was the gene that best discriminated PMBL from other DLBCLs, and was also highly expressed in Hodgkin lymphoma cells. Amplification of the genomic loci for *PDL2* and several neighboring genes was observed in more than half of the PMBLs and in Hodgkin lymphoma cell lines.

Conclusions.—The heterogeneity of DLBCL is emphasized in these results. Clinical trials in DLBCL will have to include gene expression profiling so that the 3 distinct disease entities that characterize DLBCL can be differentiated. The molecular diagnosis of these subgroups is the initial step in understanding the oncogenic mechanisms involved.

▶ These 2 articles (Abstracts 15–8 and 15–9) renewed my excitement over gene expression profiling. Two independent groups, using different techniques (Affymetrix and Lymphochip DNA microarray systems), identified similar findings in their analyses of large B-cell lymphoma primary to the mediastinum. In addition, the information obtained from these studies not only improves our understanding of the pathobiology, but may also be useful in diagnosis. Primary mediastinal large B-cell lymphoma appears to be a distinct entity with a characteristic profile of expressed genes. Some of the expression results confirm previous findings—for example, the characteristic expression of MAL and FIG1, and increased expression of genes located at the site of the frequent chromosome aberrations on the short arm of chromosome 9. The studies identified low levels of expression of several components of the B-cell receptor signaling cascade that probably lead to the characteristic lack of surface immunoglobulin. Both studies also identified similarities between the gene expression profiles of classical Hodgkin lymphoma and primary mediastinal large B-cell lymphoma, as well as confirming differences such as the expression of CD19, CD20, CD79a, and Oct-2 by primary mediastinal large B-cell lymphoma. The study by Savage and colleagues (Abstract 15–8) identified 2 pathways that might be important in the pathogenesis of primary mediastinal large B-cell lymphoma: a cytokine pathway involving the interleukin-13 receptor and a pathway leading to NF-κB activation. Rosenwald and colleagues (Abstract 15–9) identified a group of genes that could be used to distinguish primary mediastinal large B-cell lymphoma from diffuse large B-cell lymphoma, and suggest that molecular diagnostic techniques could be used as a diagnostic tool. I don't think I'm ready to put aside my microscope, but feel that information such as this will assist in the definition of these disease entities and possibly in the identification of diagnostic tools.

F. Craig, MD

Diffuse Large B-Cell Lymphoma of Bone: An Analysis of Differentiation-Associated Antigens With Clinical Correlation
de Leval L, Braaten KM, Ancukiewicz M, et al (Massachusetts Gen Hosp, Boston; Univ of Liège, Belgium)
Am J Surg Pathol 27:1269-1277, 2003   15–10

Background.—The bone marrow is frequently involved in lymphoma, but localized bone lesions are less often produced. Morphologically, most primary bone lymphomas are composed of large centroblastic cells, frequently with multilobated nuclei and abundant sclerosis, and are classified as diffuse large B-cell lymphomas (DLBCLs) according to the World Health Organization criteria for classification of hematologic malignancies. Molecular genetic studies have shown that most DLBCLs arising in lymph nodes or in various extranodal locations harbor somatic mutations in the variable regions of their immunoglobulin genes, which is a hallmark of the germinal center (GC) reaction. It has been hypothesized that DLBCLs involving bone are also likely to derive from B cells at a post-GC stage of differentiation. Patients with DLBCLs that presented with bone involvement were studied. Patients with primary osseous tumors were compared with patients with extraosseous disease at diagnosis to determine the relationship of primary DLBCL of bone to DLBCL in other locations.

Methods.—The study included 29 patients with DLBCLs presenting with bone involvement, including 18 localized primary bone lymphomas, 2 multifocal primary bone lymphomas, and 9 patients with extraskeletal disease at diagnosis. The tumors were classified according to the World Health Organization classification criteria and evaluated by immunohistochemistry for expression of antigens associated with GC and non-GC stages of B-cell differentiation. The presence of a BCL-2/IgH gene rearrangement was investigated by polymerase chain reaction.

Results.—All the cases were characterized by similar clinicopathologic and morphologic features and had similarly good overall outcome. Distribution of the tumors was in the long bones in 14 patients, axial skeleton in 8 patients, limb girdles in 3 patients, and multiple sites in 4 patients. Most of the tumors (n = 24) were centroblastic, with multilobated cells in 12 cases. Nearly half of the tumors (48%) were bcl-6+CD10+ (GC-like), 31% were bcl-6+CD10− (indeterminate phenotype), and 21% were CD10−bcl-6− (post–GC-like). The indeterminate phenotype was observed only in primary bone lymphoma. MUM-1 was frequently expressed in GC-like and non–GC-like categories. No evidence was found of plasmacytic differentiation by CD138, and VS38c immunoreactivity was rare, occurring in only 2 of 29 patients. CD44 was detected in 6 tumors, all of which were CD10−. Bcl-2 was expressed by 70% of the tumors, but only 1 of 23 cases tested showed a Bcl-2/JH rearrangement by polymerase chain reaction. Survival analysis showed that GC-like tumors had a longer overall survival than non–GC-like tumors.

Conclusions.—A GC-like immunophenotype is found in approximately half of large B-cell lymphomas of bone and is associated with an improved survival.

▶ Some patients with DLBCL present with primary involvement of bone. Although several characteristic features have been described, including the presence of multilobated nuclei and sclerosis, the relationship of primary DLBCL of bone to DLBCL in other locations is uncertain. This study evaluated 29 patients with DLBCL who presented with symptoms related to one or multiple bone lesions. Although there were 2 groups of patients (those with lymphoma confined to bone and those with extraosseous disease at the time of diagnosis), both groups had similar morphologic and immunophenotypic features. In addition, many of the cases had features considered typical for DLBCL of bone. The authors used immunohistochemical stains to further evaluate the lymphoma cells for stage of B-cell differentiation. They concluded that there was no evidence of plasmacytic differentiation, approximately one half of the case had a GC-like phenotype, and expression of CD10 was associated with a better survival. These results would suggest that primary DLBCL of bone has similar phenotypic features to DLBCL in other locations, and confirm that identification of a GC-like phenotype might be of prognostic value.

F. Craig, MD

Primary Cutaneous Diffuse Large B-Cell Lymphoma: Prognostic Significance of Clinicopathological Subtypes

Goodlad JR, for the Scotland and Newcastle Lymphoma Group (Raigmore Hosp, Inverness, Scotland; et al)
Am J Surg Pathol 27:1538-1545, 2003   15–11

Background.—The classification and subdivision of primary cutaneous diffuse large B-cell lymphoma (PCDLBCL) are subjects of continuing debate. Criteria advanced by the World Health Organization would result in categorization of these lesions as diffuse large B-cell lymphoma (DLBCL), a heterogeneous disorder that encompasses several disease entities. The EORTC classification of cutaneous lymphomas would also assign large B-cell lymphomas with a diffuse growth pattern to 1 of 2 categories, mainly on the basis of anatomic location. The morphologic, immunophenotypic, and clinical features of PCDLBCL were assessed.

Methods.—From a review of all primary cutaneous B-cell lymphomas in the Scotland and Newcastle Lymphoma Group database, 30 cases of PCDLBCL were selected for review of the morphologic, immunophenotypic, and clinical features. In addition, the number of cases harboring t(14;18) was determined by using a polymerase chain reaction and primers to the major breakpoint cluster region. The effect on prognosis of a variety of clinical and pathologic factors was assessed for the group of 30 PCDLBCLs, and the 5-year disease-specific survival of this group was compared with that of 195 cases of stage I DLBC arising primarily in lymph nodes identified from the same database.

Results.—A location on the leg was the only independent prognostic factor for determining the outcome in PCDLBCL. The presence of multiple lesions, involvement of more than one body site, and expression or not of CD10, bcl-2, bcl-6, and CD10 and bcl-6 had no effect on survival. When compared with cases arising above the waist, cases on the leg occurred more often in females, and the patients were older and had a significantly higher incidence of bcl-2 expression as well as a poorer prognosis. These patients also showed more frequent coexpression of CD10 and bcl-6, supporting a follicle center cell origin for some, but the difference was not statistically significant. There was no significant difference in the 5-year disease-free survival between the cases of PCDLBCL and those of stage I nodal DLBCL, but the latter cases were generally treated with more aggressive therapy. A significant difference in 5-year disease-free survival was observed when the nodal DLBCLs were compared with PCDLBCLs arising above the waist (78% vs 100%, respectively).

Conclusions.—The results were supportive of the current EORTC approach of subdividing PCLBCL on the basis of site to produce prognostically relevant groupings.

▶ B-cell non-Hodgkin lymphoma may arise in the skin or may spread to the skin as a result of systemic involvement. Several recent articles have addressed differences in behavior between primary cutaneous and systemic lymphoma. For example, primary cutaneous follicular lymphoma is more often bcl-2 negative, t(14;18) negative, and more often responds to localized therapy than systemic follicular lymphoma. Differences such as these have been used to justify a separate classification scheme for primary non-Hodgkin lymphoma of the skin. What about PCDLBCL? For the most part, DLBCL that is primary to the skin also appears to have a better prognosis than systemic DLBCL. However, this study investigating 30 PCDLBCLs confirms previous reports that location on the leg is an important adverse prognostic factor. Although the survival results for DLBCL of the leg are similar to those for nodal DLBCL, the authors comment that the patients with nodal lymphoma had received more aggressive therapy. Another large study of PCDLBCL reported that although location on the leg was associated with a worse prognosis, bcl-2 expression was the strongest independent predictor of death from lymphoma. Therefore, it remains uncertain whether DLBCL of the leg represents a distinct biologic entity. The study by Goodlad and colleagues also performed immunohistochemical stains and identified that a subset of PCDLBCL appeared to be of follicle center cell origin, as demonstrated by staining for CD10 and bcl-6. However, there was a low incidence of the t(14;18) translocation using PCR studies. Therefore, the relationship between primary cutaneous follicular lymphoma and DLBCL also needs further investigation. However, it can be concluded that when diagnosing B-cell lymphoma involving the skin, one should consider the possibility of primary cutaneous lymphoma because this disease may not require intensive systemic therapy. In addition, it may be important to identify primary DLBCL of the leg.

F. Craig, MD

SUGGESTED READING

Kim BK, Surti U, Pandya AG, et al: Primary and secondary cutaneous diffuse large B-cell lymphomas: A multiparametric analysis of 25 cases including fluorescence in situ hybridization for t(14;18) translocation. *Am J Surg Pathol* 27:356-364, 2003.

Grange F, Petrella T, Beylot-Barry M, et al: Bcl-2 protein expression is the strongest independent prognostic factor of survival in primary cutaneous large B-cell lymphomas. *Blood* 103:3662-3668, 2004.

Confirmation of the Molecular Classification of Diffuse Large B-Cell Lymphoma by Immunohistochemistry Using a Tissue Microarray
Hans CP, Weisenburger DD, Greiner TC, et al (Univ of Nebraska, Omaha; British Columbia Cancer Agency, Vancouver, Canada; Norwegian Radium Hosp, Oslo, Norway; et al)
Blood 103:275-282, 2004   15–12

Background.—Diffuse large B-cell lymphoma (DLBCL) is the most common type of non-Hodgkin lymphoma, accounting for 30% to 40% of new diagnoses. However, DLBCL is both clinically and morphologically heterogeneous. Persistent remission is achieved in only 40% to 50% of patients despite the use of anthracycline-based chemotherapy; thus, it is important to identify at diagnosis patients who might benefit from more aggressive or experimental therapies. DLBCL can be divided by means of complementary DNA (cDNA) microarray into prognostically significant subgroups with germinal center B-cell–like (GCB), activated B-cell–like (ABC), or type 3 gene expression profiles. The GCB group has significantly better survival than the ABC group. Another study in which an oligonucleotide array was used demonstrated that DLBCL can be divided into 2 molecularly distinct populations. However, this technology is expensive and not generally available, so there is a need for a simpler, more widely available method for classification of DLBCL with immunohistochemistry. The use of immunoperoxidase staining for predictive markers to accurately subdivide DLBCL into prognostically relevant subgroups was evaluated, using the cDNA microarray results as a gold standard.

Methods.—Tissue microarray blocks were created from 152 cases of DLBCL, of which 142 had been successfully evaluated by cDNA microarray. Sections were stained with antibodies to CD10, bcl-6, MUM1, FOXP1, cyclin D2, and bcl-2.

Results.—Expression of bcl-6 or CD10 was associated with better overall survival, whereas expression of MUM1 or cyclin D2 was associated with worse overall survival. Cases were subclassified by using CD10, bcl-6, and MUM1 expression, and 64 cases (42%) were considered GCB, and 88 cases (58%) were considered non-GCB. The 5-year overall survival for the GCB group was 76%, compared with only 34% for the non-GCB group. These survival findings were similar to those reported with the cDNA microarray. Bcl-2 and cyclin D2 were found to be adverse predictors in the non-GCB group. Multivariate analysis showed that a high International Prognostic Index score (3-5) and the non-GCB phenotype were independent adverse predictors of survival.

Conclusions.—Immunostains are useful in determining the GCB and non-GCB subtypes of DLBCL and predicting survival similar to the cDNA microarray.

▶ Gene expression profiling has been used to identify prognostically significant groups of DLBCL. However, these techniques are not widely available, have a significant failure rate, and require collection of fresh or frozen tissue that is representative of the lymphoma. Therefore, several investigators have attempted to identify the same prognostic groups using paraffin section immunohistochemistry. The study by Hans and colleagues used gene expression profiling results as the gold standard for comparison with immunohistochemical stains performed on tissue microarrays. The authors developed an algorithm for using the immunohistochemical stain results to separate GCB from non-GCB lymphoma. Cases with the following phenotypes were designated as GCB: CD10+ or CD10− plus bcl6+ and MUM1 −. All other combinations of stain results were designated as non-GCB. For the most part, the results of these 3 stains could accurately predict the gene expression profiling results. Although there were 22 discrepant cases out of 142 comparisons, the immunohistochemical stain results in these cases appeared to more accurately predict prognosis. Therefore, it was suggested that the material studied by gene expression profiling might not have been representative. Although there is still controversy over the role of individual immunohistochemical stains as predictors of prognosis in DLBCL, this study suggests that a combination of stains might be of value in separating the GCB and non-GCB groups. Other studies have failed to identify a combination of stains that predicts outcome; therefore, the algorithm proposed by Hans and colleagues warrants further investigation.

F. Craig, MD

SUGGESTED READING

Alizadeh AA, Eisen MB, Davis RE, et al: Distinct types of diffuse large B-cell lymphoma identified by gene expression profiling. *Nature* 402:503-511, 2000.

Colomo L, Lopez-Guillermo A, Perales M, et al: Clinical impact of the differentiation profile assessed by immunophenotyping in patients with diffuse large B-cell lymphoma. *Blood* 101:78-84, 2003.

Chang C-C, McClintock S, Cleveland RP, et al: Immunohistochemical expression patterns of germinal center and activation B-cell markers correlated with prognosis in diffuse large B-cell lymphoma. *Am J Surg Pathol* 28:464-470, 2004.

A Subset of t(11;14) Lymphoma With Mantle Cell Features Displays Mutated *IgV$_H$* Genes and Includes Patients With Good Prognosis, Nonnodal Disease

Orchard J, Garand R, Davis Z, et al (Royal Bournemouth Hosp, England; Univ Hosp, Nantes, France; Univ Hosp, Southampton, England; et al)

Blood 101:4975-4981, 2003   15–13

Background.—The t(11;14)(q13;q32) translocation is important in B-cell malignancy because it results in the juxtaposition of the *BCL1* gene and the immunoglobulin heavy chain locus, with consequent overexpression of cyclin D1. The t(11;14) is the hallmark of mantle cell lymphoma (MCL), but this translocation is not exclusive to MCL. However, the incidence of t(11;14) in diseases other than MCL or myeloma is difficult to define. The question as to whether all cases of lymphoma with t(11;14) circulating lymphocytes are MCL variants or whether they encompass other diseases has not been answered definitively. Sequencing the variable region of the immunoglobulin heavy chain (*IgV$_H$*) genes has provided new insights into the clonal origin of the chronic B-cell malignancies. Some studies in patients with MCL have found mutations in the *IgV$_H$* gene sequences in a minority of cases. It was determined whether cases of MCL with a more favorable course can be identified at presentation, and whether a knowledge of the *IgV$_H$* gene status can facilitate resolution of the diagnostic uncertainty surrounding patients who do not have palpable lymphadenopathy.

Methods.—Lymphocyte morphology, histology, immunophenotype, IgV_H gene mutations, and clinical course were analyzed in 80 unselected patients with circulating t(11;14) lymphocytes.

Results.—Of the 80 patients, 43 had peripheral lymphadenopathy (nodal group), and histologic evaluation confirmed MCL in all of these patients. There were 37 patients with no lymphadenopathy (the nonnodal group), of whom 13 had histologic findings, all showing MCL. IgV_H genes were unmutated in 90% of nodal and 44% of nonnodal cases; CD38 was positive in 94% of nodal and 48% of nonnodal cases. Immediate treatment was required in 95% of nodal patients compared with 49% of nonnodal patients who had indolent disease. Median survival was 30 months in the nodal group and 79 months in the nonnodal group. Mutation status had no statistical effect on survival, but of the 6 long-term survivors, all were nonnodal and 5 of 5 had mutated IgV_H genes.

Conclusions.—There was no evidence against a diagnosis of MCL in the nonnodal patients. Mutated IgV_H genes may aid in the identification of patients with indolent disease.

▶ Recent classification schemes for non-Hodgkin lymphoma emphasize the importance of distinguishing MCL from the other small lymphoid B-cell malignancies because of its more aggressive course. The World Health Organization classification recommends a multiparametric approach with identification of the characteristic morphologic features in conjunction with the typical phenotype and presence of the characteristic translocation t(11;14). However, there has been a trend towards considering the presence of t(11;14), after exclusion of multiple myeloma and hairy cell leukemia, as synonymous with MCL. Indeed, as discussed in the 2003 Year Book, some authors have used the presence of the translocation t(11;14) in cases of B-cell prolymphocytic leukemia to reclassify these cases as MCL. The article by Orchard and colleagues identifies patients with t(11;14)-positive lymphoma involving the peripheral blood that appears to meet the criteria for MCL but is associated with a good prognosis. This observation confirms the need to either refine the criteria for the diagnosis of MCL or to identify biologic differences that can be used as prognostic markers within the disease entity. In this study, patients who had a good prognosis lacked lymphadenopathy, more frequently had the mutated form of the IgV_H gene, and were more often CD38 positive. It is interesting that some of the prognostic markers recently identified in B-cell chronic lymphocytic leukemia also seem to play a role in MCL. Therefore, it appears that the MCL story is still evolving.

F. Craig, MD

SUGGESTED READING

Wong K-F, So C-C, Chan JKC: Nucleolated variant of mantle cell lymphoma with leukemic manifestations mimicking prolymphocytic leukemia. *Am J Clin Pathol* 117:246-251, 2002.

Nodit L, Bahler DW, Jacobs SA, et al: Indolent mantle cell lymphoma with nodal involvement and mutated immunoglobulin heavy chain genes. *Hum Pathol* 34:1030-1034, 2003.

Patterns of Bone Marrow Involvement in 58 Patients Presenting Primary Splenic Marginal Zone Lymphoma With or Without Circulating Villous Lymphocytes

Audouin J, Le Tourneau A, Molina T, et al (Hôtel Dieu, Paris; Hôpital Gilles de Corbeil, Corbeil-Essonnes, France)
Br J Haematol 122:404-412, 2003   15–14

Background.—A group of patients with primary splenic marginal zone lymphoma (PSMZL) has been observed for more than 2 decades by a hospital pathology department in Paris. Before the description of PSMZL in the 1990s, most of these patients received a diagnosis of lymphoplasmacytic immunocytoma, according to the updated Kiel classification. Recently, 31 patients with PSMZL were described, including some who were previously reported as having lymphoplasmacytic lymphoma. The patterns of bone marrow involvement in 58 of the 70 patients identified at the Paris hospital were described. The remaining 12 patients were excluded because of the absence of bone marrow biopsy for these patients.

Methods.—A total of 86 bone marrow biopsy specimens from 58 patients with PSMZL were studied. A splenectomy was performed in 42 patients, which enabled a histopathologic diagnosis. In these patients, 44 biopsies were performed before splenectomy, and 25 were performed after splenectomy. In 16 recently observed patients, the results of 17 bone marrow biopsies led to a diagnosis of PSMZL, and these patients were treated without splenectomy.

Results.—Seven different infiltrate patterns were recognized, including intravascular, interstitial, nodular (2 types), massive, plasmacytic mimicking myeloma, and transformation into large B-cell lymphoma. The association of an intravascular infiltrate and nodules with a germinal center or a marginal zone favored a diagnosis of marginal zone lymphoma. Immunohistochemical findings demonstrated the expression of B cell–associated antigens and, in 40% of patients, a monotypic lymphoplasmacytic cell component. These patients often had a serum M component and autoimmune disorders. Bone marrow involvement was found in all the patients. Successive biopsies showed progression and, after chemotherapy, a slight decrease in infiltrates. Transformation into large B-cell lymphoma occurred in 11 of 34 patients.

Conclusions.—The infiltrate patterns of bone marrow involvement described in these patients with PSMZL are not specific to this disease but occur also in primary nodal marginal zone lymphoma and, more rarely, in mucosa-associated lymphoid tissue (MALT)-type lymphoma.

▶ If you're faced with making the initial diagnosis of lymphoma from a bone marrow sample, how certain can you be of the subtype? Although the availability of immunophenotyping and genotyping studies has made this task less formidable, the pattern of bone marrow infiltration can still provide useful diagnostic clues. This article describes the pattern of infiltration associated with splenic marginal zone lymphoma (SMZL). Although several patterns were identified, features favoring SMZL included intravascular infiltration; the presence of nodules with a recognizable germinal center or marginal zone, or both; and a monotypic lymphoplasmacytic component. The infiltrates of SMZL seemed to progress over time from predominantly intravascular and intersitial to become more nodular. The intravascular infiltrates described in this study appear to correspond to the intrasinusoidal pattern reported in other publications. The authors comment that these patterns may also be seen in nodal and MALT-type marginal zone lymphoma, and to a lesser extent in other subtypes of lymphoma. Although other authors have challenged the specificity of this finding, the presence of prominent intrasinusoidal infiltration in an initial diagnostic specimen, with supporting phenotypic data, should at least raise the possibility of marginal zone lymphoma. The authors also mention that intravascular infiltrates may be difficult to identify on hematoxylin and eosin–stained sections, but are highlighted with immunohistochemical staining for CD20.

F. Craig, MD

SUGGESTED READING

Kent SA, Variakojis D, Peterson L: Comparative study of marginal zone lymphoma involving the bone marrow. *Am J Clin Pathol* 117:698-708, 2002.

Schenka AA, Gascoyne RD, Duchayne E, et al: Prominent intrasinusoidal infiltration of the bone marrow by mantle cell lymphoma. *Hum Pathol* 34:789-791, 2003.

Histopathologic Features of Splenic Small B-Cell Lymphomas: A Study of 42 Cases With a Definitive Diagnosis by the World Health Organization Classification
Kansal R, Ross CW, Singleton TP, et al (Univ of Michigan, Ann Arbor)
Am J Clin Pathol 120:335-347, 2003   15–15

Background.—In patients with malignant lymphomas, the spleen is frequently involved secondarily as part of generalized disease. Lymphomas will occasionally manifest with prominent splenomegaly, with or without overt evidence of lymphadenopathy, and in these cases a splenectomy is performed for diagnostic purposes. The differential diagnosis of small B-cell lymphomas (SBLs) involving the spleen can be difficult, particularly in patients with prominent splenomegaly only, in which no additional diagnostic interpretation can be made from a lymph node specimen. However, precise diagnostic subclassification is required because of the significant differences in therapy and prognosis within various subclasses of SBLs. The morphologic features of SBL involving the spleen was defined by studying the cases of SBL in which a definitive diagnosis and subclassification was established according to the recent World Health Organization (WHO) classification after integration of all available clinical and pathologic information.

Methods.—A total of 42 cases of splenic SBL with a definitive diagnosis by the WHO classification was studied. The patients included 21 men and 21 women ages 32 to 82 years, with a median of 65 years. The diagnoses were chronic lymphocytic leukemia in 8 patients, mantle cell lymphoma in 9 patients, follicular lymphoma in 12 patients, and marginal zone lymphoma in 13 patients.

Results.—Splenectomy was performed for diagnosis or therapy, and splenic weights ranged from 0.2 to 3.8 kg, with a median of 1.4 kg. Splenic SBLs generally showed white pulp expansion, and the morphologic features of the nodules recapitulated the corresponding lymph node histopathologic features. Marginal zones were a common finding in splenic marginal zone lymphomas and follicular lymphomas. These marginal zones may be present in mantle cell lymphoma involving the spleen and may present in hilar lymph nodes in SBLs other than splenic marginal zone lymphomas. Follicular lymphomas may simulate splenic marginal zone lymphomas and can be differentiated by the presence of neoplastic follicles and hilar lymph node morphologic features.

Conclusions.—It would appear from this study that well-characterized cases of small B-cell lymphomas involving the spleen often have typical morphologic features of the splenic white pulp and red pulp nodules reminiscent of the histopathologic features of lymph nodes involved by the corresponding lymphoma. The overall assessment and correlation of the histologic features with peripheral blood and bone marrow morphologic, immunophenotypic, and clinical features usually results in precise subclassification of small B-cell lymphomas involving the spleen.

▶ This article describes the features of 42 cases of small B-cell lymphoma involving the spleen. All cases involved the splenic white pulp and the morphologic and immunophenotypic features in that compartment resembled those described in lymph nodes. This finding should be reassuring for those of us less familiar with evaluation of splenectomy specimens. Most types of lymphoma also involved the red pulp in either a diffuse or a nodular pattern. Interestingly, the 2 cases of mantle cell lymphoma that demonstrated diffuse infiltration of the red pulp were also leukemic. The most frequent diagnosis in this study was splenic marginal zone lymphoma (SMZL). Most of these cases had a recognizable marginal zone and most demonstrated foci with a typical "biphasic pattern" composed of a central zone of small lymphocytes surrounded by a paler marginal zone. However, the authors also mentioned that marginal zones were frequently identified in follicular lymphoma, and were occasionally seen in mantle cell lymphoma. Indeed, because of the similar growth patterns, the authors sometimes encountered difficulty in distinguishing SMZL from follicular lymphoma. Often lymphoma present in splenic hilar lymph nodes had a more typical appearance. Therefore, the authors recommend routine sampling of hilar nodes in splenectomy specimens. They also recommend bcl-2 staining in these difficult cases to distinguish the bcl-2 positive neoplastic follicles of follicular lymphoma from the reactive follicles that were seen in most of their cases of SMZL. However, the authors did caution that rarely residual reactive germinal center could be seen in follicular lymphoma involving the spleen. Therefore, this article provides a good summary of the morphologic and immunophenotypic findings in small B-cell lymphoma involving the spleen, warns of potential pitfalls, and suggests some practical ways to avoid them.

F. Craig, MD

Using 4-Color Flow Cytometry to Identify Abnormal Myeloid Populations
Kussick SJ, Wood BL (Univ of Washington, Seattle)
Arch Pathol Lab Med 127:1140-1147, 2003   15–16

Background.—Diagnosis of myeloproliferative disorders (MPDs) and myelodysplastic syndromes (MDSs) has relied on the combination of clinical information with the morphologic features of the peripheral blood and bone marrow to determine a final diagnosis. However, objective evidence of a myeloid stem cell neoplasm in the form of a clonal cytogenetic abnormality is obtained in only 30% to 40% of nonchronic myeloid leukemia (CML) chronic MPDs (non-CML MPDs) and in a similar percentage of MDSs. Normal patterns of antigen expression during myeloid maturation were identified and whether flow cytometric evaluation of myeloid maturation is representative of an additional objective method for assessment of the likelihood of a stem cell neoplasm was determined.

Methods.—Retrospective evaluations were performed of 4-color flow cytometry data from more than 400 bone marrow aspirates obtained since 1998 from patients with suspected non-CML MPD or an MDS.

Results.—Reproducible patterns of antigen expression were present in normal myeloid maturation as in benign reactive settings such as marrow degeneration. In addition to these findings, data from another retrospective comparison of the sensitivity of flow cytometry with conventional cytogenetics in a large number of bone marrow aspirates on which both types of studies were performed showed that more than 90% of non-CML MPD and MDS cases with a clonal cytogenetic abnormality will be identified as abnormal with 4-color flow cytometry. These findings will provide validation of the use of flow cytometry in the diagnosis of MPDs and MDSs.

Conclusions.—These findings are supportive of the value of 4-color flow cytometry in experienced laboratories for the workup of patients with non-CML MPD and MDSs.

▶ This article summarizes the results of 4-color flow cytometric analysis performed on 76 specimens being evaluated for non-CML MPD and 333 specimens being evaluated for a MDS. The analysis performed was a little different from that used in most clinical flow cytometry laboratories; more cells were acquired (100,000-150,000 viable cells per tube in most cases and 400,000 cells in a minority of cases), the analysis was performed with software created inhouse, and analysis included evaluation of monocytes and maturing granulocytes in addition to blasts. However, the procedure described could be reproduced by most laboratories. The authors identified the normal patterns of antigen expression seen during myeloid maturation and then used deviations from these patterns to identify abnormal myeloid populations. They commented that the use of 4-color analysis allowed identification of more complex relationships among antigens than fewer colors. Abnormal myeloid populations were identified in many cases and were found more frequently in cases with abnormal cytogenetics. The abnormalities identified included alterations in antigen intensity, abnormally homogeneous expression of 2 or more myeloid antigens, dyssynchronous expression of 2 myeloid antigens, and aberrant expression of nonmyeloid antigens. As reported in previous studies, abnormal patterns of expression of CD11b versus CD16, and CD13 versus CD16 were among the most frequent abnormalities identified. Aberrant expression of nonmyeloid antigens and loss of expression of CD10 on neutrophils were less frequent findings. Therefore, it was suggested that the identification of abnormal populations of myeloid cells by flow cytometry might assist in the diagnosis of a few cases MPD or MDS where morphologic and cytogenetic findings are not diagnostic. However, the authors do describe several "abnormalities" in myeloid phenotype seen in bone marrow regeneration with and without growth factor therapy. These benign abnormalities included low to absent expression of CD16, low-level expression of CD11b, and low-level expression of CD56 on maturing granulocytes and monocytes. Therefore, it is important that flow cytometry laboratories become familiar with these reactive changes before interpreting case of potential MDS and MPD.

F. Craig, MD

SUGGESTED READING

Stetler-Stevenson M, Arthur DC, Jabbour N, et al: Diagnostic utility of flow cytometric immunophenotyping in myelodysplastic syndrome. *Blood* 98:979-987, 2001.

Wells DA, Benesch M, Loken MR, et al: Myeloid and monocytic dyspoiesis as determined by flow cytometric scoring in myelodysplastic syndrome correlates with the IPSS and with outcome after hematopoietic stem cell transplantation. *Blood* 102:394-403, 2003.

Chronic Myeloid Leukemia Following Therapy With Imatinib Mesylate (Gleevec): Bone Marrow Histopathology and Correlation With Genetic Status
Frater JL, Tallman MS, Variakojis D, et al (Northwestern Univ, Chicago; Oregon Health and Science Univ, Portland; Novartis, Basel, Switzerland)
Am J Clin Pathol 119:833-841, 2003   15–17

Background.—The Philadelphia (Ph) chromosome is the hallmark of chronic myeloid leukemia (CML). This chromosome arises from a reciprocal translocation between 9 and 22, the molecular consequence of which is a bcr-abl chimeric gene whose protein product (bcr-abl) shows enhanced tyrosine kinase activity. This enzyme activity is essential to the transforming function of bcr-abl and is a major factor in the pathophysiology of CML. The presence of bcr-abl in all patients with CML and the requirement of kinase activity for bcr-abl function have made this an attractive target for a selective kinase inhibitor. Imatinib mesylate has been shown to inhibit bcr-abl activity. In 1 study, treatment with imatinib mesylate reduced the leukocyte count to less than 10,000/µL within weeks in patients with chronic-phase CML. The bone marrow biopsy characteristics of patients with CML who were treated with imatinib mesylate are reported. Bone marrow findings in these patients were correlated with the genetic status of the patients at the time of the biopsies.

Methods.—Bone marrow pathologic features and cytogenetic and molecular genetic status were evaluated in 13 patients with interferon-resistant, chronic-phase CML, treated with imatinib mesylate. All the patients had morphologic evidence of CML in the blood and bone marrow and were positive for bcr-abl by reverse transcription polymerase chain reaction, fluorescence in situ hybridization (FISH), or both. Follow-up marrow biopsies, interphase FISH for bcr-abl, and conventional cytogenetics were performed at 3-month intervals for up to 24 months after the initiation of therapy.

Results.—Reduced bone marrow cellularity and decreased myeloid/erythroid ratios were observed in all patients at 3 to 6 months after therapy. The percentage of bcr-abl–positive cells by FISH was decreased in all patients, from a median of 73% before therapy to a median of 47% at 3 months. Data from cytogenetic and FISH analysis defined 2 groups after 6 months of follow-up, with 5 patients becoming negative for bcr-abl by FISH and 8 patients remaining positive, of whom 4 had signs of clonal cytogenetic evolution develop. The patients who became negative for bcr-abl had no morphologic evidence of CML at 15 to 24 months of follow-up, whereas patients who remained positive had morphologic features of CML redevelop as cellularity increased. There were signs of progression in some bcr-abl–positive patients, including 2 patients who had myeloid blast phase develop.

Conclusions.—All the patients in this study showed an initial decrease in bone marrow cellularity after imatinib mesylate therapy, yet continued follow-up showed that histopathologic findings correlated with genetic response.

▶ Many patients with CML receive treatment with imatinib mesylate (Gleevec; formerly known as STI571). This article describes some of the changes that may be seen on routine bone marrow evaluation. During the first 3 to 6 months of therapy, all 13 patients demonstrated a response as evidenced by a decrease in bone marrow cellularity, a decrease in the myeloid/erythroid ratio, and a decrease in the percentage of bcr-abl positive cells detected by FISH. After 6 months, some patients became negative for the bcr-abl translocation with FISH and, although some bone marrows were hypercellular, there was no definitive morphologic evidence of residual disease at 15 to 24 months. Patients who remained positive for bcr-abl by FISH regained the morphologic features of CML. Sea-blue histiocytes were a prominent feature in some patients who retained bcr-abl probably because of increased cell turnover. The authors also reported decreased fibrosis in a few patients even with persistent disease. Therefore, this article describes some of the changes that may be seen with imatinib mesylate therapy for CML, indicates that an initial morphologic response does not predict a maintained response, and that reappearance of the features of CML may predict persistence of a positive FISH result. This article also demonstrates the value of conventional cytogenetics in documenting clonal evolution that may precede blast crisis. Other recent articles in this area have evaluated the use of peripheral blood quantitative real-time polymerase chain reaction (RT-PCR) for bcr-abl messenger RNA. The level of bcr-abl detected in the peripheral blood with the use of this technique appears to correlate with the bone marrow cytogenetic findings and the levels at 2 months may predict the cytogenetic response at 6 months. In addition, serial quantitative studies may be used to detect the development of resistance to imatinib mesylate therapy. However, it is important to realize that a negative quantitative RT-PCR assay for bcr-abl in most laboratories should not be used as evidence of molecular remission, because the conventional manual PCR methods, especially those using nested primers, are often more sensitive.

F. Craig, MD

SUGGESTED READING

Ross DM, Hughes TP: Cancer treatment with kinase inhibitors: What have we learnt from imatinib? *Br J Cancer* 90:12-19, 2004.

Wang L, Pearson K, Pillitteri L, et al: Serial monitoring of bcr-abl by peripheral blood real-time polymerase chain reaction predicts the marrow cytogenetic response to imatinib mesylate in chronic myeloid leukemia. *Br J Haematol* 118:771-777, 2002.

16 Pediatrics

A Report of Dizygous Monochorionic Twins
Souter VL, Kapur RP, Nyholt DR, et al (Univ of Washington, Seattle; Regional Med Ctr, Seattle; Queensland Inst of Med Research, Brisbane, Australia; et al)
N Engl J Med 349:154-158, 2003   16–1

Introduction.—It is accepted as medical doctrine that monochorionic twins are expressly monozygous. Reported is a case of sex-discordant monochorionic twins conceived by in vitro fertilization.

Case Report.—Woman, 48, conceived twins by in vitro fertilization using donor oocytes without intracytoplasmic sperm injection. Three oocytes were successfully fertilized, cultured to the blastocyte stage of development, and placed in the patient's uterus. A US scan at 6 weeks of gestation revealed a viable twin pregnancy, with findings suggestive of monochorionic diamniotic twinning, including a thin intertwin membrane, a T-shaped insertion of the membrane, and absence of the lambda sign (a triangular projection of placental tissue extending into the base of the intertwin membrane, which is identifiable at this stage of development in dichorionic twins). At 20 weeks of gestation, a US scan was consistent with earlier evidence of monochorionicity; yet the twins appeared to be discordant for sex. The pregnancy was otherwise uncomplicated. At 37 weeks of gestation, a healthy boy (weighing 2114 g) and a healthy girl (weighing 2183 g) were delivered. There was no evidence of sexual ambiguity. Both infants had O Rh-positive blood and a negative Coombs' test. Pathologic evaluation revealed a monochorionic, diamniotic placenta. Blood samples were obtained from each infant at 1 week of age for zygosity determination. At 3 months, blood was obtained for cytogenetic examination. Assessment of the twins at 5 months of age revealed unremarkable physical examination findings and normal, sex-appropriate external genitalia. Abdominal US scan of the female twin verified the presence of a uterus and ovaries. Both peripheral-blood samples and skin-biopsy specimens were obtained at 5 months of age for additional cytogenetic and zygosity evaluations. There were no tissue samples available from either of the biological parents.

Conclusion.—The embryologic events that resulted in monochorionic placentation for these dizygous twins can only be speculated. The influence of in vitro fertilization on early embryonic development warrants further investigation.

▶ For those who question the value of case reports on the basis that they provide only anecdotal information, here is one that challenges that contention. A detailed examination of the placenta confirmed by histology and fluorescent in-sito hybridization for X-Y chromosomes was complemented by cytogenetics and a detailed polymerase chain reaction-based DNA zygosity study.

This revealed that sex-mismatched, genetically different infants were monochorionic, a finding that flies in the face of conventional wisdom that decrees that monochorionic = monozygotic. The finding has implications for genetic mechanisms, epidemiology, and tissue transplantation. The authors can only speculate on how this might have happened, but since the twins were the product of an in vitro fertilization, there is clear indication that there is more to be learned yet about the biohazards of this type of intervention.

R. Jaffe, MB, BCh

Maternal Diabetes: Effects on Embryonic Vascular Development: A Vascular Endothelial Growth Factor-A-Mediated Process
Madri JA, Enciso J, Pinter E (Yale Univ, New Haven, Conn)
Pediatr Dev Pathol 6:334-341, 2003   16–2

Background.—Vasculogenesis, angiogenesis, and the formation of cardiac structures are complex processes that give rise to highly orchestrated, temporospatially regulated signaling pathways. The vascular endothelial growth factor (VEGF) family is prominent among the many soluble factors involved in signaling during the development of the cardiovascular system. Major congenital malformations, many of which are the result of abnormal cardiovascular patterning, are the leading cause of infant mortality and morbidity. The targeted mutation of several genes, including VEGF and VEGF receptors, and certain teratogenic agents, including excess α-D-glucose, gives rise to embryonic lethal phenotypes that are associated with failure in the formation of a functional vitelline circulation and aberrant organogenesis. Congenital abnormalities are responsible for a significant amount of infant mortality and morbidity, affecting 2% to 3% of the more than 4 million births in the United States and having a 21% mortality. Maternal diabetes is known to be associated with a decreased rate of pregnancy and an increased rate of postimplantation loss. The authors summarized their work to date examining the effects of hyperglycemic insults on yolk sac vascular development in vivo in streptozotocin-treated mice and in whole conceptus cultures, and on the formation of endocardial cushions in streptozotocin-treated mice, in whole conceptus cultures, and in atrioventricular canal explant cultures.

Overview.—Yolk sac vasculopathy and the failure of endocardial cushion epithelial-mesenchymal transformation occur in hyperglycemic conditions in whole conceptus cultures from mice and in embryos from streptozotocin-induced diabetic mice. These cardiovascular abnormalities are associated with changes in the expression and the phosphorylation state of adhesion molecules such as platelet endothelial growth factor-1 and the expression of growth factors such as VEGF-A.

Conclusions.—A more thorough understanding of the effects of maternal diabetes on yolk sac and embryonic vasculogenesis/angiogenesis and organogenesis may provide new insights into the treatment and prevention of major birth defects.

▶ Maternal diabetes is associated with a decreased pregnancy rate, an increased pregnancy loss, and a 2 to 3 times increase in the incidence of congenital defects. Diabetic embryopathy appears to be a phenomenon of poor glycemic control during early gestation, and though the tissue effects are widespread, atrioventricular septal defect is the most common. The authors have used as models mice, whole conceptus cultures, and atrioventricular canal explants that can be exposed to increased glucose concentrations. They demonstrate here and in related publications that some changes are early; the vitelline circulation, for example, can only be affected before the arteriovenous bed differentiates. Other processes such as neural tube closure, caudal regression, and cardiac cushion formation can still be affected by glycemic insults later in development. Since VEGF expression is tightly regulated during development, it is a molecular target of prime interest, and the authors document that there is an effect of glycemia on its expression. The specific pathway by which glycemic modification of VEGF affects the developing organs remains to be elucidated, though persistence of PECAM-1 (CD31) expression and failure of MMP-2 induction are documented. These appear to be informative models for studying the process of diabetic-induced malformations.

R. Jaffe, MB, BCh

Neonatal Enteropathies: Defining the Causes of Protracted Diarrhea of Infancy
Sherman PM, Mitchell DJ, Cutz E (Univ of Toronto)
J Pediatr Gastroenterol Nutr 38:16-26, 2004   16–3

Background.—Chronic and prolonged diarrhea has a variety of underlying etiologies. A recent position statement from the American Gastroenterological Association has provided a comprehensive review of the subject in adults. However, a different approach is required for the evaluation of infants and young children with protracted diarrhea. Intractable diarrhea of infancy is a term that describes chronic, unexplained diarrhea in young children. This phrase has been criticized because it describes a symptom complex rather than a discrete disease entity. More recently, the term has been used to describe infants with loose and frequent stools severe enough to require nutritional support, often in the form of parenteral alimentation. The current emphasis on adequate total caloric intake and nutritional rehabilitation has dramatically improved the survival of affected infants and children. The causes of protracted diarrhea beginning early in life can be divided into those entities with a normal villus-crypt and those associated with villus atrophy. The value of identifying an underlying cause of chronic protracted diarrhea is that it allows improved counseling of parents, referring physicians, and other health care providers regarding long-term prognosis and therapeutic options. A number of neonatal enteropathies that cause protracted diarrhea of infancy were reviewed.

Overview.—Microvillus inclusion disease is a severe enteropathy with watery diarrhea that often begins on the first day of life. In this disease, diarrhea can be so watery as to be mistaken for urine. This severe, intractable enteropathy requires total parenteral nutrition and is inevitably fatal without continuous IV nutrition or intestinal transplantation. However, there have been reports of milder variants of the disease in which the prognosis may be better. Tufting enteropathy, or intestinal epithelial dysplasia, presents in the first few months of life with chronic watery diarrhea and impaired growth. The long-term prognosis is variable. Parenteral alimentation is necessary in most patients to ensure a caloric intake sufficient for normal growth and development. Autoimmune enteropathy is characterized by villus atrophy and infiltration of activated T cells into the lamina propria. Children with autoimmune enteropathy frequently have extraintestinal manifestations of autoimmunity and rarely have a family history of unexplained infant diarrhea. The onset of diarrhea frequently begins after the first 8 weeks of life, and there is an apparent clinical response to potent immune suppression. IPEX syndrome is characterized by immune dysregulation, polyendocrinopathy, enteropathy, and X-linkage. There are many intestinal manifestations in IPEX syndrome that are shared by autoimmune enteropathy.

Conclusions.—There is an urgent need to define the molecular bases of microvillus inclusion disease, tufting enteropathy, and autoimmune enteropathy. Such an approach is more likely to provide for rational therapy and appropriate prenatal testing compared with the empiric approach that has been undertaken to date.

▶ Chronic and debilitating diarrhea of the newborn and infant is serious, sometimes fatal, but a clearer understanding of the mixed collection of responsible disorders is coming into focus, and this Toronto group has contributed to this advance. A detailed discussion and color illustrations of microvillus disease and its variants, tufting enteropathy, and the autoimmune enteropathies make this review article a seminal resource.

R. Jaffe, MB, BCh

Amniotic Infection Syndrome: Nosology and Reproducibility of Placental Reaction Patterns

Redline RW, and the Society for Pediatric Pathology, Perinatal Section, Amniotic Fluid Infection Nosology Committee (Case Western Reserve Univ, Cleveland, Ohio; Univ of Alabama, Birmingham; Univ of Medicine and Dentistry of New Jersey-New Jersey Med School, Newark, NJ; et al)
Pediatr Dev Pathol 6:435-448, 2003
16–4

Introduction.—Clinically responsive placental examination is used to provide useful information concerning the etiology, prognosis, and recurrent risk of pregnancy disorders. Questions have been raised regarding the reliability of placental diagnosis, including the ability of expert placental pathologists to agree with each other and with their general pathology colleagues. Because of the renewed interest in the clinical significance of placental pathology, more precision and uniformity should be introduced for placental diagnosis. The Perinatal Section of the Society for Pediatric Pathology undertook to review, define, and validate diagnostic criteria for several different placental reaction patterns. The findings of the Amniotic Fluid Infection Nosology Committee are presented.

Methods.—Twenty cases were obtained from case files. Three slides from each case (umbilical cord, placental membranes, and 1 full-thickness section of placental parenchyma) were chosen. Gestational age and placental weight were recorded for each case. All 20 cases (14 with amniotic fluid infection, 6 normal control cases) were reviewed blindly by 6 pathologists after agreement on a standard set of diagnostic criteria. After examining initial results, criteria were refined, and a second, overlapping set of cases were reviewed. A majority vote acted as the gold standard. Grading and staging of maternal and fetal inflammatory responses were more reproducible using a 2- versus 3-tiered grading system (overall agreement, 81% vs 71%). Placental reaction patterns relevant to amniotic fluid infection were used for assessment. The range for sensitivity, specificity, and efficiency for individual observation was 67% to 100%. Reproducibility was determined using unweighted kappa values and interpreted as less than 0.2, poor; 0.2-0.6, fair/moderate; and more than 0.6, substantial.

Results.—Kappa values for the 12 lesions assessed in the 20 cases were as follows: (1) acute chorioamnionitis/maternal inflammatory response (any, 0.93; severe, 0.76; advanced stage, 0.49); (2) chorioamnionitis, 0.25; (3) acute chorioamnionitis/fetal inflammatory response (any, 0.90; severe, 0.55; advanced stage, 0.52); (4) chorionic vessel thrombi, 0.37; (5) peripheral funisitis, 0.84; (6) acute villitis, 0.90; acute intervillositis/intervillous abscesses, 0.65, and decidual plasma cells, 0.30.

Conclusion.—The adoption of this clearly defined, clinically pertinent, and pathologically reproducible terminology could improve clinicopathologic correlation and contribute a framework for future clinical research.

▶ Placental pathology had the unjustified reputation of being poorly reproducible and often too late to be of clinical utility. The Perinatal Section of the Society for Pediatric Pathology is actively changing that perception. In this publication, the authors define an objective set of morphologic characteristics that are reaction patterns that follow infection of the amniotic fluid. Adoption of the schema outlined in their Table 1 (see Table in original article) will lead to greater reproducibility in placental diagnosis.

R. Jaffe, MB, BCh

Histopathology of Congenital Hyperinsulinism: Retrospective Study With Genotype Correlations

Suchi M, MacMullen C, Thornton PS, et al (Univ of Pennsylvania, Philadelphia)
Pediatr Dev Pathol 6:322-333, 2003   16–5

Introduction.—Most severe cases of congenital hyperinsulinism (HI) are caused by defects in the β-cell adenosine triphosphate (ATP)-sensitive potassium channel and usually necessitate pancreatectomy to control blood sugar levels. In contrast to recent advances in understanding the pathophysiology and genetic bases of HI, the histologic classification of this condition continues to be controversial. A recent proposal to classify the HI pancreata into diffuse and focal forms is of interest because of its relative simplicity and good correlation with genetic abnormalities. Whether this classification scheme could be applied to 38 pancreata resected for HI was retrospectively determined.

Methods.—Leukocyte genomic DNA was obtained from 29 cases. The exons of *ABCC8* and *KCNJ11* genes were screened for the presence of mutations.

Results.—Nineteen cases (50.0%) were histologically characterized as diffuse HI; 14 cases (36.8%) were categorized as focal form. Mutational analysis showed that 14 of 16 diffuse cases examined had either homozygous or compound heterozygous mutations of *ABCC8* or *KCNJ11*. Seven of 10 focal cases demonstrated only the paternally inherited mutations, which was consistent with earlier observations. Two patients (5.3%) had normal pancreatic histology, yet persistent hypoglycemia postoperatively; this left the possibility of residual focal lesion. Three of 38 cases (7.9%) did not match either the diffuse or focal category. Two cases varied from the described pattern for the diffuse form in that the nuclear enlargement was restricted to a single area of the pancreas. The other case had a focal lesion, yet β-cell nuclear enlargement was present in nonadjacent areas. Mutations for typical diffuse or focal HI were not seen in 2 of the 3 equivocal cases.

Conclusion.—About 90% of HI cases can be categorized into either a diffuse or a focal form. A small percentage of cases represents a diagnostic challenge.

▶ "Nesidioblastosis" as a histopathologic diagnosis was for years much abused and misunderstood. Two parallel avenues of advance have changed this. First was the unraveling of the genetic forms of infantile hyperinsulinism. There are dominantly inherited mild forms, more severe recessive forms of hyperinsulinism, and the loss of a maternally imprinted growth inhibitor that is tissue-specific to the pancreas. At least 6 genetic forms are now known. The other advance was the understanding that there were 2 morphologic patterns of expression in the pancreas, a localized endocrine overgrowth or a diffuse hyperplasia, with features that allow for intraoperative distinction in most instances.[1] This article originates from an institution that sees a large volume of hyperinsulinemic infants. The authors seek to make the 2 paths of advance intersect, and correlate the genotype of the hyperinsulinemic defect with the tissue manifestations in the pancreas. They demonstrate that there is validity to the genotypic-phenotypic categorization into a diffuse and a localized form, but also document that almost 10% of cases do not fit neatly, a cautionary point that has been made in other articles too.[2,3]

R. Jaffe, MB, BCh

References

1. Sempoux C, Guiot Y, Lefevre A: Neonatal hyperinsulinemic hypoglycemia: Heterogeneity of the syndrome and keys for differential diagnosis. *J Clin Endocrinol Metab* 83:1455-1461, 1998.
2. Smith VV, Malone M, Risdon RA: Focal or diffuse lesions in persistent hyperinsulinemic hypoglycemia of infancy: Concerns about interpretation of intraoperative frozen sections. *Pediatr Dev Pathol* 4:138-143, 2001.
3. Jack MM, Walker RM, Thomsett MJ, et al: Histologic findings in persistent hyperinsulinemic hypoglycemia of infancy: Australian experience. *Pediatr Dev Pathol* 3:532-547, 2000.

17 Techniques/Molecular

Design and Standardization of PCR Primers and Protocols for Detection of Clonal Immunoglobulin and T-Cell Gene Recombinations in Suspect Lymphoproliferations: Report of the BIOMED-2 Concerted Action BMH4-CT98-3936
van Dongen JJM, Langerak AW, Brüggemann M, et al (Univ Med Ctr Rotterdam, The Netherlands; II Medizinische Klinik des Universitätsklinikums Schleswig-Holstein, Kiel, Germany; Univ of Leeds, England; et al)
Leukemia 17:2257-2317, 2003   17–1

Background.—In most patients with suspected lymphoproliferative disorders, histomorphology or cytomorphology supplemented with immunohistology or flow cytometric immunophenotyping can discriminate malignant from reactive lymphoproliferations. However, the diagnosis is more complex in 5% to 10% of cases. The diagnosis of lymphoid malignancies can be supported by clonality assessment because, in principle, all cells of a malignancy have a common clonal origin. Most lymphoid malignancies belong to the B-cell lineage (90% to 95%), with only a minority being T-cell (5% to 7%) or NK-cell lineage (<2%). Acute lymphoblastic leukemias are of T-cell origin in 15% to 20% of cases, but T-cell malignancies are relatively rare in the group of mature lymphoid leukemias and in non-Hodgkin lymphomas. Currently, there is a significant degree of variability between methodologies used in individual laboratories for the detection of immunoglobulin and T-cell receptor (TCR) gene rearrangements for clonality assessment. Standardized protocols are described that have been developed for the detection of clonally rearranged immunoglobulin (Ig) and TCR genes and the chromosome aberrations t(11;14) and t(14;18).

Overview.—As a result of a European BIOMED-2 collaborative study, multiplex polymerase chain reaction (PCR) assays have been developed and standardized for the detection of clonally rearranged Ig and TCR genes and the chromosome aberrations t(11;14) and t(14;18). The result has been 107 different primers in only 18 multiplex PCR tubes. The detection rate of clonal rearrangements with the BIOMED-2 primer sets is remarkably high, mainly because of the complementarity of the various BIOMED-2 tubes.

Conclusions.—The BIOMED-2 multiplex tubes are now available for use in diagnostic clonality studies as well as for the identification of PCR targets suitable for the detection of minimal residual disease.

▶ Detection of clonal populations with Ig and TCR gene rearrangements is now considered the standard of practice for the diagnosis and follow-up of lymphoproliferative disorders. Unfortunately, there is great variability between methodologies used in individual laboratories for detection of these rearrangements with a PCR approach. This variability is reflected in the detection sensitivity of these assays, which is dependent on a variety of factors that include the specific type of lymphoma/leukemia, the primer design (V, D, and J regions detected), the method of detection, and the experience of the individual interpreting the results. This study reports the results of a large European multi-institutional effort in developing and testing standardized methodologies for Ig and TCR gene rearrangements and recombinations involving the IgH locus (t[11;14] and t[14;18]). Such efforts in standardization are increasingly needed as new molecular techniques make their way into the clinical laboratories. The standardized protocols appear to have an increased detection rate in most B- and T-cell neoplasms than previously reported methods. This is an important achievement, especially in lymphomas that frequently show somatic hypermutation, like those of germinal center origin. However, only a limited number of samples from each diagnostic category were tested, and the detection, false-positive, and false-negative rates need to be validated in larger patient populations. In addition, the implementation of these protocols for routine use in molecular diagnostics laboratories might be difficult because of the unprecedented number of multiplex reactions needed to evaluate a single patient. This could potentially elevate the cost of testing and have a negative impact on the laboratory's budget and reimbursement. The development of testing algorithms for specific clinical scenarios might help to make standardized protocols like these more amenable to routine clinical use.

F. Monzon-Bordonaba, MD

Standardization and Quality Control Studies of 'Real-time' Quantitative Reverse Transcriptase Polymerase Chain Reaction of Fusion Gene Transcripts for Residual Disease Detection in Leukemia: A Europe Against Cancer Program

Gabert J, Beillard E, van der Velden VHJ, et al (Institut Paoli Calmettes, France; Univ Med Ctr Rotterdam, The Netherlands; Applied Biosystems, Foster City, Calif; et al)
Leukemia 17:2318-2357, 2003   17–2

Background.—Current treatment protocols for acute lymphoblastic leukemia, acute myeloid leukemia, and chronic myeloid leukemia are based on prognostic factors, which contribute to stratification of therapy. Key prognostic factors in leukemia that have been identified over the years include pretreatment characteristics such as age, white blood cell count, immunophenotypic profiles, specific chromosomal abnormalities, aberrant fusion genes (FGs), and mutations, such as *FLT3* gene alterations in acute myeloid leukemia. However, patient outcome cannot be reliably predicted from such classic parameters. In recent years, minimal residual disease testing has emerged as a potentially important diagnostic factor for treatment stratification of childhood acute lymphoblastic leukemia, chronic myeloid leukemia, and acute promyelocytic leukemia. This report focused on the accurate quantitative measurement of FG transcripts as can be applied in 35% to 45% of cases of acute lymphoblastic leukemia and acute myeloid leukemia, and in more than 90% of cases of chronic myeloid leukemia.

Methods.—A total of 26 European university laboratories from 10 countries have collaborated to establish a standardized protocol for TaqMan-based real-time quantitative polymerase chain reaction (RQ-PCR) analysis of the main FGs associated with leukemia within the Europe Against Cancer (EAC) program. After final validation of the Europe Against Cancer primer and probe sets, the expression level of the 9 major FG transcripts was evaluated in a large series of stored diagnostic leukemia samples (278 samples).

Results.—After normalization, there was no statistically significant difference in expression level between bone marrow and peripheral blood on paired samples at diagnosis. However, RQ-PCR showed significant differences in FG expression between each of the FG transcripts in leukemic samples at diagnosis, which would account for differential assay sensitivity for each FG.

Conclusions.—The development of standardized protocols for RQ-PCR analysis of FG transcripts is a significant advancement for the molecular determination of minimal residual disease levels. It is likely that the use of these protocols will be invaluable to the management of patients entered into multicenter therapeutic trials.

▶ The advent of quantitative protocols based on the "real-time" PCR platform is the most recent advance in the use of reverse transcriptase PCR for detection of pathogenic translocations in leukemias. These protocols are rapidly changing the approach for patient follow-up, with the detection of minimal residual disease based on quantitative measurements of the fusion transcript in peripheral blood or bone marrow aspirates. In most instances, the fusion transcript measurement is expressed as a ratio of a "housekeeping" gene to correct for sample cellularity (control gene). However, sensitivity of these assays varies widely between laboratories, and the reported results are not always comparable between institutions because of a lack of standardization in the choice of the control gene. This study reports on the efforts of 26 European university laboratories to develop standardized protocols for RQ-PCR for the 9 most common FG transcripts in human leukemias. A well thought out experimental approach, divided in 4 phases, was used for the development of these assays, including steps to maximize sensitivity, minimize false positives and negatives, and ensure reproducibility of the assays across laboratories. Three control genes were evaluated, and the use of the ABL gene showed better correlation with the FG transcripts and improved reproducibility. The choice of control gene, and specifically the choice of ABL as a control gene for detection of bcr-abl fusion transcripts, is a topic of great controversy and continues to be actively discussed in the molecular diagnostics community.

This article represents a good example of the type of concerted efforts that are needed to achieve standardized methodologies across borders. Only efforts like this will allow us to offer better clinical tests to our doctors and ultimately, to our patients. As we await confirmation and validation of the clinical utility of minimal residual disease monitoring with RQ-PCR through clinical trials, efforts to standardize the quantitative methodologies for bcr-abl fusion transcripts in US laboratories are underway.

F. Monzon-Bordonaba, MD

Frequency of Major Molecular Responses to Imatinib or Interferon Alfa Plus Cytarabine in Newly Diagnosed Chronic Myeloid Leukemia
Hughes TP, for the International Randomised Study of Interferon Versus STI571 (IRIS) Study Group (Inst of Med and Veterinary Science, Adelaide, Australia; et al)
N Engl J Med 349:1423-1432, 2003   17–3

Background.—Chronic myeloid leukemia (CML) is a clonal disease of the hematopoietic stem cell in which a reciprocal translocation between chromosomes 9 and 22 forms the Philadelphia chromosome (Ph) with a novel fusion gene, BCR-ABL. An activated tyrosine kinase expressed by the BCR-ABL gene is central to the pathogenesis of CML. Imatinib mesylate is a tyrosine kinase inhibitor that blocks the kinase activity of BCR-ABL, which inhibits the proliferation of Ph-positive progenitors. Imatinib has demonstrated activity against all phases of CML, yet responses have been most durable and substantial in patients in the chronic phase of disease. In a previous study, 1106 patients in the chronic phase of CML were assigned to imatinib or interferon alfa plus cytarabine as initial therapy. Levels of BCR-ABL transcripts were measured in all patients in this trial who had a complete cytogenetic remission.

Methods.—Levels of BCR-ABL transcripts were measured by a quantitative real-time polymerase chain reaction (RT-PCR) assay. The results were expressed in relation to the median level of BCR-ABL transcripts in the blood of 30 patients with untreated CML in the chronic phase.

Results.—In the patients who experienced a complete cytogenic remission, levels of BCR-ABL transcripts had dropped after 12 months of treatment by at least 3 log in 57% of those in the imatinib group and in 24% of patients in the group that received interferon alfa plus cytarabine. An estimated 39% of all patients treated with imatinib but only 2% of all patients given interferon alfa plus cytarabine had a reduction in BCR-ABL transcript levels of at least 3 log. For patients who had a complete cytogenetic remission and a reduction in transcript levels of at least 3 log at 12 months, the probability of remaining progression-free was 100% at 24 months, compared with 95% for patients with a reduction of less than 3

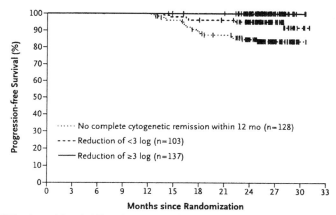

FIGURE 3.—Actuarial probability of progression-free survival among 128 patients who were treated with imatinib for 12 months without a complete cytogenetic remission and 240 patients who had a complete cytogenetic remission and had PCR data available, according to the extent of the reduction from baseline in BCR-ABL transcript levels. $P < .001$ for the overall comparison, $P = .013$ for the comparison of patients without a complete cytogenetic remission with those with a reduction of at least 3 log, and $P = .007$ for the comparison of patients with a reduction of less than 3 log with those with a reduction of at least 3 log. (Reprinted by permission of *The New England Journal of Medicine*, from Hughes TP, for the International Randomised Study of Interferon Versus STI571 [IRIS] Study Group: Frequency of major molecular responses to imatinib or interferon alfa plus cytarabine in newly diagnosed chronic myeloid leukemia. *N Engl J Med* 349:1423-1432, 2003. Copyright 2003, Massachusetts Medical Society. All rights reserved.)

log and 85% for patients who were not in complete cytogenetic remission at 12 months (Fig 3).

Conclusions.—The proportion of patients with chronic myeloid leukemia who had a reduction in BCR-ABL transcript level of at least 3 log after 12 months of therapy was much greater among those treated with imatinib than among those who received interferon alfa plus cytarabine. Patients in the imatinib group who attained this level of molecular response had a negligible risk of disease progression during the subsequent 12 months.

▶ This article explores the role of molecular tests in the management of patients with CML undergoing treatment with 2 different chemotherapeutic regimens. There are 2 important contributions of this work. One is the confirmation that quantitative measurements of transcripts from the BCR-ABL fusion gene can be used for monitoring response to therapy in CML patients with complete cytogenetic response and that a cutoff measurement with a clear prognostic value can be identified. The second is the approach used by the investigators to standardize the molecular tests for BCR-ABL transcripts in multiple laboratories. Efforts to standardize quantitative tests for fusion genes are currently being undertaken worldwide by different professional organizations. However, the use of an external set of reference samples, as reported in this article, is highly contested within the molecular diagnostics community. The validity and reproducibility of this approach needs to be confirmed in future studies.

F. Monzon-Bordonaba, MD

Use of Gene-Expression Profiling to Identify Prognostic Subclasses in Adult Acute Myeloid Leukemia

Bullinger L, Döhner K, Bair E, et al (Stanford Univ, Calif; Univ of Ulm, Germany)
N Engl J Med 350:1605-1616, 2004   17–4

Background.—Acute myeloid leukemia (AML) is the most common form of leukemia in adults. Complete remission is induced in about 70% to 80% of younger patients (age 16 to 60 years) who undergo chemotherapy, but many of them experience a relapse and die of their disease. The presence or absence of recurrent cytogenetic aberrations has been used to identify the appropriate therapy in AML patients, but the classification system currently in use does not fully reflect the molecular heterogeneity of AML and treatment stratification is difficult, particularly in patients with intermediate-risk AML who have a normal karyotype. The molecular variation underlying the biologic and clinical heterogeneity in AML was systematically investigated. This approach has also provided insight into diffuse large B-cell lymphoma and childhood acute lymphoblastic leukemia.

Methods.—Complementary DNA microarrays were used to determine the levels of gene expression in peripheral-blood samples or bone marrow samples from 116 adults with AML (including 45 with a normal karyotype). Unsupervised hierarchical clustering analysis was used to identify molecular subgroups with distinct gene-expression signatures. A training set of samples from 59 patients was used to apply a novel supervised learning algorithm to devise a gene-expression-based clinical-outcome predictor that was then tested with an independent validation group composed of the remaining 57 patients.

Results.—New molecular subtypes of AML were identified through unsupervised analysis, including 2 prognostically relevant subgroups in AML with a normal karyotype. The supervised learning algorithm was then used to construct an optimal 133-gene clinical-outcome predictor, which accurately predicted overall survival among patients in the independent validation group, including the subgroup of patients with AML with a normal karyotype. Multivariate analysis showed that the gene-expression predictor was a strong independent prognostic factor.

Conclusions.—It would appear from these findings that the use of gene-expression profiling improves the molecular classification of AML in adults.

Prognostic Useful Gene-Expression Profiles in Acute Myeloid Leukemia

Valk PJM, Verhaak RGW, Beijen MA, et al (Erasmus Univ, Rotterdam, The Netherlands; Leiden Univ, The Netherlands)
N Engl J Med 350:1617-1628, 2004   17–5

Background.—Acute myeloid leukemia (AML) is a group of neoplasms rather than a single disease, and as such has diverse genetic abnormalities and variable responses to treatment. Cytogenetics and molecular analyses can be used to identify subgroups of AML with different prognoses. However, inconsistencies in the genetic abnormalities that signal poor versus intermediate risk in some patients rather than others and the absence of cytogenetic abnormalities in a significant proportion of patients have made it desirable to refine the classification of AML. Molecular classification on the basis of DNA-expression profiling is a powerful way to distinguish myeloid from lymphoid cancer and subclasses within these 2 diseases, and has the potential to identify distinct subgroups of AML with the use of one comprehensive assay. Gene-expression profiles were used to identify established and novel subclasses of AML and otherwise unrecognized cases of poor-risk AML.

Methods.—Gene-expression profiles were determined for samples of peripheral blood or bone marrow from 285 patients with AML. Data analyses were performed with Omniviz, significance analysis of microarrays, and prediction analysis of microarrays software. Statistical analyses were performed to determine the prognostic significance of cases of AML with specific molecular signatures.

Results.—Unsupervised cluster analyses identified 16 groups of patients with AML on the basis of molecular signatures. Genes that defined these clusters were identified, and the minimal numbers of genes needed to identify prognostically important clusters with high accuracy were determined. The clustering was driven by the presence of chromosomal lesions, particular genetic mutations (*CEBPA*), and abnormal oncogene expression (*EVI1*). Several novel clusters were identified, some of which consisted of specimens with normal karyotypes. A unique cluster with a distinctive gene expression signature included cases of AML with a poor treatment outcome.

Conclusions.—Gene-expression profiling can provide a comprehensive classification of AML that includes previously identified genetically defined subgroups and a novel cluster with an adverse prognosis.

▶ These are 2 recent articles (Abstracts 17–4 and 17–5) evaluating the use of gene profiling for classification and prognostication in AML in large populations. Both groups were able to identify gene expression signatures that separated AML profiles into well-defined groups with different array technologies (complementary DNA [cDNA] vs oligonucleotide arrays). Some of these groups could be identified by the signature profile that reflected the chromosomal translocation present in the patient (eg, inv16, t[15;17], and t[8;21]). Interestingly, profiling with cDNA resulted in a less clear separation of some groups with gene fusions (Abstract 17–4) than the separation achieved with commercial oligonucleotide arrays (Abstract 17–5). Both groups were also able to identify novel groups in patients with no recognizable chromosomal translocations, and derive prognostic classifications for patients with this type of AML. More importantly, Bullinger et al (Abstract 17–4) were able to find an underlying poor prognosis signature for all types of AML, regardless of chromosomal translocation status. Studies to validate the prognostic signatures should be performed with increased numbers of patients in each of the newly identified subgroups. However, these results highlight the diagnostic and prognostic uses of gene expression profiling, and forecast the application of this technology in the diagnosis and management of hematologic malignancies in the not so distant future.

F. Monzon-Bordonaba, MD

Detection of *FLT3* Internal Tandem Duplication and D835 Mutations by a Multiplex Polymerase Chain Reaction and Capillary Electrophoresis Assay

Murphy KM, Levis M, Hafez MJ, et al (Johns Hopkins Univ, Baltimore, Md)
J Mol Diag 5:96-102, 2003   17–6

Background.—FMS-like tyrosine kinase 3 (*FLT3*) is a member of the class III receptor tyrosine kinase family that also includes PDGF-R, KIT, and FMS. *FLT3* is expressed on early hematopoietic progenitor cells and plays an important role in survival and differentiation of stem cells. The first and best-studied *FLT3* mutation is an internal tandem duplication (ITD) mutation. ITDs arise from duplications of the juxtamembrane portion of the gene and result in constitutive activation of the *FLT3* protein. The ITD mutation has been identified in approximately 20% to 30% of patients with acute myeloid leukemia (AML) and appears to be associated with a worse prognosis. Another type of *FLT3* mutation involves missense mutations at aspartic acid residue 835, which occurs in about 7% of patients with AML. These mutations also appear to be activating and to portend a worse prognosis. The identification of *FLT3* mutations is important because it provides prognostic information and may be critical to determining appropriate treatment options. A molecular diagnostic approach was evaluated that is capable of detecting both ITD and D835 mutations of the *FLT3* gene in a single multiplex polymerase chain reaction (PCR) assay.

Methods.—A single multiplex PCR assay was developed to identify both ITD and D835 *FLT3* mutations. This assay was used to evaluate 147 clinical specimens. After amplification, the PCR products were analyzed by capillary electrophoresis for length mutations and resistance to *Eco*RV digestion.

Results.—Most samples tested with this approach have been peripheral blood or bone marrow samples from patients with AML, although some tested samples have come from patients with myelodysplastic syndrome, acute lymphocytic leukemia, myeloproliferative disorders, and biphenotypic leukemia. Of the 110 patients reported to have AML, 22 (20%) were positive for an ITD mutation. Three of these patients (13.6%) were found to have 2 different ITD mutations. Three of 110 patients with AML tested positive for a D835 mutation (2.7%). Overall, the *FLT3* mutation rate was 21.8%.

Conclusions.—The prospective clinical identification of *FLT3* mutations can provide important data on the incidence and natural history of *FLT3* mutations in AML and is likely to become an important factor in the optimization of patient care.

▶ Mutations in *FLT3* have been shown to cause constitutive activation of this tyrosine kinase, and their presence in patients with AML seems to confer a worse prognosis. These authors validated the use of a multiplex PCR assay to detect different types of mutations (tandem duplication and missense) in the same gene with a single assay. This interesting approach allows for efficient use of the sample and a streamlined protocol suitable for use in a clinical laboratory. The method uses a multiplex PCR with fluorescently labeled primers, followed by restriction enzyme digestion (for the single base change) and capillary electrophoresis. This method is easily adaptable to the workflow of most molecular diagnostics laboratories. Confirmation of the clinical utility of *FLT3* mutation detection as a routine prognostic marker or as a therapeutic target is currently underway. Although *FLT3* is a rare example of genes with different types of mutations that have clinical significance, the development of assays that allow for their detection is a welcome addition to the molecular diagnostics armamentarium.

F. Monzon-Bordonaba, MD

Plasma DNA Microsatellite Panel as Sensitive and Tumor-Specific Marker in Lung Cancer Patients
Beau-Faller M, Gaub MP, Schneider A, et al (Hôpitaux Universitaires de Strasbourg, France; Univ of Geneva)
Int J Cancer 105:361-370, 2003   17–7

Background.—Lung cancer is one of the most common tumors in the world. It has been known for many years that the concentration of free circulating DNA in plasma is higher in tumor patients than in healthy persons. It is not known how this plasma DNA is released into the bloodstream, but it has been suggested that analysis of plasma DNA may be useful for prognostic purposes or for early diagnosis, such as the detection of subclinical disease recurrence. However, the detection of mutations in plasma is time-consuming, and the sensitivity of this approach is dependent on the prevalence of these gene alterations in the cancer studied. No studies have investigated the detection of tumor-derived markers for lung cancer in circulating plasma DNA by using a larger panel of genetic markers able to optimize the detection of molecular changes in plasma DNA. The sensitivity and specificity of fluorescent microsatellite analysis for detecting alterations in plasma and tumor DNA were evaluated.

Methods.—The plasma DNA microsatellite panel was used to detect plasma and tumor DNA alterations in 34 patients who underwent bronchoscopy for lung cancer, including 11 with small cell lung cancer (SCLC) and 23 with non–small cell lung cancer (NSCLC), and 20 control subjects. Allelotyping was performed with a selected panel of 12 microsatellites from 9 chromosomal regions—3p21, 3p24, 5q, 9p, 9q, 13q, 17p, 17q, and 20q.

Results.—Plasma DNA allelic imbalance (AI) was found in 88% of patients. The sensitivity of the test was similar for SCLC and NSCLC. In the 24 paired available tumor tissues, 83% presented at least one AI, and among these patients, 85% also presented at least one AI in paired plasma DNA. However, the location of the allelic alterations in the paired plasma and tumor DNA could differ, suggesting the presence of heterogeneous tumor clones. None of the 20 control subjects showed any alterations in plasma or bronchial DNA. A smaller panel of 6 markers showed a sensitivity of 85%. It was also determined that different smaller panels of microsatellites could be used specifically in SCLC and NSCLC patients.

Conclusions.—The use of this targeted microsatellite panel for analysis of plasma DNA could be a valuable noninvasive test and a useful tool for monitoring disease progression in patients with lung cancer without assessing the tumor.

▶ This article explores the use of AI detection in plasma DNA for the diagnosis of lung cancer. Using fluorescent polymerase chain reaction for 12 microsatellite loci, these investigators were able to detect AI in plasma DNA in 88% of the lung cancer patients tested. It is important to mention that the patient cohort tested is heavily biased towards stage III and IV tumors, so the use of this technology for early detection of lung cancer has yet to be explored. As expected, the rate of detection is higher in patients with metastatic disease in comparison with localized tumors, most likely reflecting tumor burden or the presence of tumor cells in circulation. However, these results suggest that assays for AI might be useful in monitoring patients after surgical resection or systemic therapies, as well as an aid in diagnosis through bronchoscopic biopsies. It is intriguing that loci with AI did not show high correlation between plasma and tumor DNA, raising questions about the origin of the plasma DNA and its relationship with the tumor biology. Clinical use of these technologies needs to be validated with larger patient populations and other technologies to detect AI.

F. Monzon-Bordonaba, MD

Measurement of Gene Expression in Archival Paraffin-Embedded Tissues: Development and Performance of a 92-Gene Reverse Transcriptase–Polymerase Chain Reaction Assay
Cronin M, Pho M, Dutta D, et al (Genomic Health Inc, Redwood City, Calif: Providence–St Joseph Med Ctr, Burbank, Calif)
Am J Pathol 164:35-42, 2004   17–8

Background.—It has been shown that messenger RNA levels in formalin-fixed and paraffin-embedded (FPE) tissue specimens can be quantified by reverse transcriptase–polymerase chain reaction (RT-PCR) techniques despite the extensive RNA fragmentation that occurs in tissues preserved in this manner. The ability of gene expression analysis to provide the most useful diagnostic information is dependent on measuring the contributions of multiple genes (dozens or more). Consequently, efforts have been directed toward the development of RT-PCR assays of FPE RNA that measure the expression of many genes at once from small amounts of archival tumor blocks. The results of 48- and 92-gene RT-PCR assays were reported.

Methods.—A 48-gene assay was used to compare gene expression profiles from the same breast cancer tissue that had been either frozen or prepared by FPE. This assay showed very similar expression profiles for the 2 methods after reference gene–based normalization. A 92-gene assay was then performed, using RNA extracted from three 10-μm FPE sections of archival breast cancer specimens dating from 1985 to 2001. This assay yielded analyzable data for these genes in all 62 tested specimens.

Results.—There was significant concordance in the results when estrogen receptor, progesterone receptor, and HER2 receptor status determined by RT-PCR was compared with immunohistochemistry assays for these receptors.

Conclusions.—These findings highlight the advantages of RT-PCR over immunohistochemistry in terms of quantitation and dynamic range, and support the development of RT-PCR analysis of FPE tissue RNA as a platform for multianalytic clinical diagnostic tests.

▶ Extraction of RNA from paraffin-embedded tissues (PET) has been in use in clinical diagnostics laboratories for some time now. The most frequent use of this methodology is the detection of chromosomal translocations by doing RT-PCR of fusion gene transcripts, and is not always successful. The article by Cronin et al describes the use of a commercially available RNA extraction method to assess levels of gene expression in PET. The authors used very stringent criteria for primer design and by using a normalization based on 6 reference genes, they were able to obtain usable data for 92 genes in 62 samples, including samples that were 17 years in storage. Furthermore, when they tested 48 genes in matched frozen and PET samples, they were able to obtain very good concordance in gene expression values. This article represents a step forward in the unlocking of the paraffin tissue archives to analysis of gene expression patterns. Since real-time PCR is already a mainstay technology in the molecular diagnostics laboratories, one can envision this methodology as a framework to translate focused microarray-based gene expression signatures to clinical applications in the short-term. Because of the advantages of real-time RT-PCR in terms of automation and multiplexing, another possible application of this technology is to replace gene expression assays currently done with other methods (ie, immunohistochemistry), if it is shown to be at least as sensitive and specific as current assays.

F. Monzon-Bordonaba, MD

Multi-platform, Multi-site, Microarray-Based Human Tumor Classification

Bloom G, Yang IV, Boulware D, et al (Univ of South Florida, Tampa; Inst for Genomic Research, Rockville, Md)
Am J Pathol 164:9-16, 2004   17–9

Background.—It is preferable to make the correct pathologic diagnosis of a tumor before the start of treatment because cancer therapy is directed mainly by tumor origin. However, it is estimated that up to 5% to 10% of tumors may actually be misclassified with standard pathologic techniques. The introduction of gene expression profiling has resulted in the production of rich human data sets with the potential for determining tumor diagnosis and prognosis and directing therapy. The way in which artificial neural networks (ANNs) can be applied to 2 completely different microarray platforms (complementary DNA [cDNA] and oligonucleotide), or a combination of both, to build tumor classifiers capable of identifying most human cancers was described.

Methods.—Data used to develop diagnostic classifiers were derived from both cDNA and oligonucleotide microarray platforms from up to 7 different performance sites. Metastatic tumors of mixed origin and primary colon tumors derived from brain, liver, and lung and interrogated by cDNA microarrays served as blinded, independent validation sets.

Results.—A total of 78 tumors representing 8 different types of histologically similar adenocarcinoma were evaluated with a 32k cDNA microarray and correctly classified by a cDNA-based ANN, with a mean accuracy of 83%. Oligonucleotide data derived from 6 independent sites, representing 463 tumors and 21 tumor types, were investigated with an oligonucleotide-based ANN, trained on a random fraction of the tumors. This oligonucleotide-based ANN was 88% accurate in predicting the known pathologic origin of the remaining fraction of tumors not exposed to the training algorithm. In the final experiment, a mixed-platform classifier using a combination of both cDNA and oligonucleotide microarray data from 7 performance sites, normalized and scaled from a large and diverse set of 539 tumors, was 85% accurate on independent test sets. Further validation of these ANN classifiers was obtained through prediction, with 84% accuracy, of the known primary site of origin for an independent set of 50 metastatic lesions resected from brain, lung, and liver.

Conclusions.—The cDNA and oligonucleotide-based classifiers provided the first confirmation of the principle that data derived from multiple platforms and performance sites can be exploited to build multitissue tumor classifiers.

▶ Metastatic tumors of unknown primary are a challenging task for pathologists and oncologists in routine clinical practice. Determination of tumor origin by morphology or immunohistochemistry, or both, is not always successful, and this has a major impact on patient management. This article discusses the use of gene expression–based classifiers built with ANNs to determine the organ of origin in primary and metastatic tumors. The authors were able to create a classification algorithm with approximately 85% accuracy that can use data from different gene expression platforms. These results are quite encouraging for the clinical use of array-based classification strategies. However, in the great majority of cases, tumor classification can be achieved with current approaches, with a greater degree of accuracy. Since some of the arrays used for this work do not contain all known transcripts, one can expect further refinement of classifiers with new-generation arrays (representing the whole genome). Also as the gene expression platforms move towards standardization, it is possible that these classifiers will have higher accuracy rates. More importantly, these assays will only reach the clinical laboratory if we are able to prove the clinical utility of array-based classifications in the diagnostic or prognostic setting.

F. Monzon-Bordonaba, MD

The Cost-effectiveness of Screening Blood Donors for Malaria by PCR
Shehata N, Kohli M, Detsky A (Univ of Toronto; Canadian Blood Services, Toronto; Mount Sinai Hosp, Toronto)
Transfusion 44:217-228, 2004   17–10

Background.—Malaria is imported to Canada mainly by immigrants from countries in which malaria is endemic or by travelers who visit these regions. The incidence of malaria in Canada during the past 10 years has ranged from 1.00 to 3.40 per 100,000 persons, which is 5 to 10 times the rate observed in the United States. The number of cases of malaria reported in Canada in 1997 was 1036, a 238% increase over the number of cases since 1994. The risk of transfusion-transmitted malaria in North America is small; however, 11% of recipients of transfusion-transmitted malaria who received infected units in the United States died of their infection. In Canada, the use of the established questionnaire to exclude allogeneic blood donors at risk of malaria is the only available method of decreasing the risk of transmission. The cost-effectiveness of 4 blood donor screening patterns was estimated to determine whether the incidence of transmission of malaria by blood transfusion can be reduced.

Methods.—A decision model analysis was developed to compare 4 strategies: not screening allogeneic blood donors for malaria (strategy 1); using the standard questionnaire (strategy 2); using the standard questionnaire followed by testing blood donors with risk factors for malaria with polymerase chain reaction (PCR) (strategy 3); and screening all blood donors with PCR (strategy 4). The expected costs and the number of cases of malaria for each strategy were compared, and incremental cost-effectiveness ratios were calculated as the cost per case of malaria averted. All costs are in Canadian dollars.

Results.—Strategies 2 and 3 were equally effective but had different costs, with strategy 3 being less costly. In comparison with strategy 1, the incremental cost-effectiveness ratio was $6463 per case of malaria averted for strategy 3. The use of strategy 4 resulted in less transmission of malaria, but the cost, when compared with strategy 3, was $3,972,624 per case of malaria averted.

Conclusions.—The addition of PCR to the standard screening questionnaire is economically attractive in comparison with the standard screening questionnaire currently in use.

▶ The evaluation of cost-effectiveness of introducing a new molecular diagnostic test is seldom performed. Although the case discussed in this article is viewed through a public health perspective, this approach should be encouraged when we consider new diagnostic or prognostic tests in the molecular diagnostics laboratory. We are now performing more molecular tests than ever, and for some of them, especially some genetic polymorphisms, there is no beneficial clinical intervention in case of a positive result. Molecular test utilization should be critically reviewed with cost-effectiveness analysis in order to decrease health care costs and improve patient management.

F. Monzon-Bordonaba, MD

PART II

LABORATORY MEDICINE

Introduction

2003-2004 saw the announcement of the first set of commercially available clinical chemistry analytes for a clinical diagnostic problem that has never before been within the realm of clinical laboratory testing, namely, the differential diagnosis of stroke. Moreover, the process by which these analytes were developed is extraordinary. It heralds the emergence of the new proteomic era, and leads to the confident prediction that clinically correlated studies of the human proteome (the sum of all expressed proteins and peptides in and from the cell, including all post-transitional modifications) will be the source of the majority of truly novel analytes in the years ahead. The year also saw continuing interest in emerging infectious threats like SARS, as well as new views of the fundamentals of infectious agents. All this in addition to the steady progress in our further understanding of the human cancer genome, with all its diagnostic applications. The field of laboratory medicine continues truly to blossom.

Michael G. Bissell, MD, PhD, MPH

18 Laboratory Management and Outcomes

Population-based Study of Repeat Laboratory Testing
van Walraven C, for the Network of Eastern Ontario Medical Laboratories (NEO-MeL) (Ottawa Hosp, Ont, Canada; Queen's Univ, Kingston, Ont, Canada)
Clin Chem 49:1997-2005, 2003   18–1

Background.—Laboratory use has increased throughout the world in the past several decades. There is a perception, though weakly supported by evidence, that inappropriate laboratory use is widely prevalent, which would explain a significant portion of increased laboratory utilization. Repeat testing is one component of laboratory utilization that could be modified. Information technology can decrease repeat testing by presenting previous test results or the probability that a test will be abnormal. However, repeat testing has not been rigorously studied at a population-based level. The prevalence of, and charges associated with, repetition of 8 common laboratory tests were determined.

Methods.—Between September 1999 and September 2000, the incidence of repeating 8 common laboratory tests—hemoglobin, sodium, creatinine, thyrotropin, total cholesterol, high-density lipoprotein cholesterol, ferritin, and hemoglobin A_{1C}—was determined in a cross-sectional study by using high-quality, population-based clinical databases that included adults in Eastern Ontario, Canada. The tests were determined to be potentially redundant if they were repeated within the test's baseline testing interval. For creatinine, sodium, and hemoglobin, only tests repeated in the community were considered. A sensitivity analysis was used to vary the repeat interval by 25%, to exclude tests repeated by different physicians, and to exclude repeats of normal tests.

Results.—Nearly 4 million tests were conducted during the study year. Most of the tests (76%) were conducted on patients in the community. More than one half of the population had at least one laboratory test, with an overall testing rate of 367 tests per 100 persons per year. Repeat testing within 1 month accounted for 30% of all laboratory utilization and was more common in hospitalized patients. Repeat testing varied extensively among tests and was concentrated in a limited number of patients. The charges of potentially redundant repetition in adults for the 8 tests totaled between $13.9 and $35.9 million (Canadian dollars) annually.

Conclusions.—Repetition of laboratory tests is very common and accounts for a significant component of overall test utilization at considerable expense.

▶ This article addresses the issue of laboratory utilization in a way seldom seen in the literature. It looks at the overall ordering of lab tests throughout a geographic region. The analysis includes seldom-encountered information such as the percent of testing carried out on outpatients (76%), in addition to its primary concern with the number of repeat tests, and the number of these that can be considered redundant. A valuable reference for those concerned with lab utilization issues.

M. G. Bissell, MD, PhD, MPH

Physician Use of Genetic Testing for Cancer Susceptibility: Results of a National Survey

Wideroff L, Freedman AN, Olson L, et al (Natl Cancer Inst, Bethesda, Md; Abt Associates, Chicago)
Cancer Epidemiol Biomarkers Prev 12:295-303, 2003   18–2

Background.—Genetic testing is an emerging technology that can be applied to inherited germ line mutations associated with cancer susceptibility. Currently, little is known about physician use of cancer susceptibility tests (CSTs). Results of a national survey were reported.

Methods.—In 1999 and 2000, a nationally representative sample of 1251 US physicians was surveyed to estimate the prevalence of CST use. Demographics, training, practice setting, and practice patterns associated with the use of CST were documented. The stratified random sample of 8 specialty areas included 820 physicians in primary care and 431 in tertiary care. Questionnaires were sent by mail, fax, or the Internet or conducted by phone. The response rate was 71%.

Findings.—In the preceding 12 months, 30.6% of physicians in primary care and 33.4% in tertiary care had ordered CSTs or referred patients elsewhere for risk assessment or testing. More clinicians referred patients than ordered tests themselves. The ordering of tests or referral was associated with practice location in the Northeast, a feeling of qualification to recommend CSTs, receiving CST advertisements, and responding to patients who asked whether they could or should be tested. Lack of knowledge of local testing and counseling facilities was associated with lower CST use.

Conclusion.—Many issues still need to be addressed to ensure appropriate CST use in clinical care. Effective clinical approaches to test use must be established. In addition, physician education regarding CST is needed.

▶ We all know that genetic testing for disease susceptibility is on the way in, but just how far has actual day-to-day medical practice come in terms of utilizing this potentially powerful approach? The current authors surveyed physicians nationwide regarding their use of genetic CSTs, which are surely good markers of the broader trend. Many lab medicine futurists' crystal balls contain images of this testing menu becoming one of our mainstays in the years ahead.

M. G. Bissell, MD, PhD, MPH

Results of a Physician Survey on Ordering Viral Load Testing: Opportunity for Laboratory Consultation
Hofherr LK, Francis DP, Astles JR, et al (San Diego State Univ, Calif; Ctrs for Disease Control and Prevention, Atlanta, Ga)
Arch Pathol Lab Med 127:446-450, 2003   18–3

Background.—AIDS continues to be a serious public health concern. This investigation profiled physician practice, utilization, and understanding of HIV-1 RNA testing as well as the role of the laboratory in such testing.

Methods.—A 34-item self-report survey was mailed to physicians identified as requesting viral load testing. The sample consisted of US physicians specializing in infectious diseases, internal medicine, and family practice. Follow-up mailings were sent to nonresponders. One hundred forty-seven physicians eventually completed the survey, for a response rate of 29.4%.

Findings.—Most of the respondents using viral load findings were infectious disease specialists with urban practices. Seventy-five percent of respondents reported requesting viral load testing for patient follow-up or monitoring, and 62.5% requested such testing to initiate or guide treatment. Interpreting and using viral load findings were reported to present difficulty in patient treatment and in determining what change from baseline was significant clinically. Few respondents said they used the testing laboratory pathologist as a resource for interpreting viral load test results.

Conclusion.—Many physicians have questions about the meaning of viral load tests, how often to monitor viral load, and what change from baseline is significant. In this study, few clinicians took advantage of the expertise available in the laboratory for testing viral loads and interpreting the findings.

▶ Lest we forget, the AIDS epidemic continues, and HIV-1 RNA viral load testing has become a very frequently ordered test. Who exactly orders it and why do they do so? As we know, some degree of interpretation is required to really understand the results. But is it true, as the authors suggest, that there is any kind of a market for the laboratory to provide these interpretations? Perhaps so, if and when it starts being ordered by others than just infectious disease specialists.

M. G. Bissell, MD, PhD, MPH

Down's Syndrome Screening Is Unethical: Views of Today's Research Ethics Committees
Reynolds TM (Queen's Hosp, Staffordshire, England)
J Clin Pathol 56:268-270, 2003   18–4

Background.—Screening for Down syndrome has been part of routine obstetric practice since the late 1980s. However, this screening was introduced at a time when ethical assessment lacked its current prominence, and it was introduced without ethical review. Ethical considerations related to genetic screening constitute a significant part of the workload of research ethics committees. In recent years, there have been discussions about whether screening for Down syndrome is primarily a eugenic exercise.

The human genome project will allow screening programs to be conducted for a wider variety of characteristics, both desirable and undesirable, and will present ethical dilemmas for the future. The attitudes of research ethics committee members toward several conditions of varying clinical severity and prognosis, including Down syndrome, were investigated.

Methods.—A survey was conducted among members of 40 randomly selected research ethics committees. A simple questionnaire comprising 19 clinical scenarios based around 4 clinical conditions was designed to review conditions that were potentially embarrassing, affecting life span (but not mental ability), premature death, and intellectual impairment with a risk of neonatal cardiac defects (Down syndrome). Screening tests with different degrees of effectiveness were described. The diagnostic test descriptions ranged from having no risk to an unaffected fetus to causing spontaneous abortion of 2 normal fetuses for each affected fetus identified. The replies were graded on a scale from 1 to 5.

Results.—Replies were received from 77 members of 28 different research ethics committees. Screening for treatment of a life-threatening condition was supported by 95% of the respondents, but screening for conditions of a slight increase in premature death or of cosmetic features was considered unethical, with only 14% and 10% of respondents, respectively, in favor of screening for those conditions. Views about conditions involving significant shortening of lifespan were more ambiguous (49% in favor). Down syndrome screening was considered more ethical when it was described as a serious condition (56% of respondents in favor) than when clinical features were described (44% in favor). When increased rates of spontaneous abortion on confirmatory testing were added, 79% and 86% of respondents, respectively, stated that screening was unethical (for "serious" and "clinical features" descriptions, respectively).

Conclusion.—There are ethical concerns regarding screening for Down syndrome and regarding genetic testing in general. These concerns must be addressed before the introduction of any prenatal screening test.

▶ So is there a moral "slippery slope" on which genetic screening merges inexorably with eugenics? According to this article, a sampling of research ethics committees (analogues of US institutional review boards) would indicate that a majority of their members think so. Well, if so, can we draw a line? With the products of the human genome project rapidly moving toward potential availability in this context, the prospect of parents utilizing genetic screening for selection of traits that represent aesthetic preferences becomes conceivable. Will this become socially possible and, if so, where will it lead?

M. G. Bissell, MD, PhD, MPH

Algorithm to Determine Cost Savings of Targeting Antimicrobial Therapy Based on Results of Rapid Diagnostic Testing
Oosterheert JJ, Bonten MJM, Buskens E, et al (Univ Med Centre Utrecht, The Netherlands)
J Clin Microbiol 41:4708-4713, 2003   18–5

Background.—Rising costs, in addition to therapeutic efficacy, have become a major concern in the treatment of patients with serious infections. The unnecessary use of broad-spectrum antibiotics is an important factor in the high costs associated with the treatment of these patients. "Streamlining" can target the antimicrobial therapy to isolated pathogens; however, the results of diagnostic procedures such as microbiologic cultures or serologic tests have delays of days to weeks and so are not suitable as guides to therapy in the early stage of disease. However, other diagnostic procedures yield nearly instantaneous results and could be useful in guiding initial antimicrobial therapy. A rapid diagnosis of pneumococcal pneumonia may allow the earlier use of narrow-spectrum antimicrobial therapy. Whether rapid diagnostic testing of patients hospitalized with community-acquired pneumonia lowers costs was determined.

Methods.—An algorithm was designed to calculate the costs associated with the diagnosis and treatment of community-acquired pneumonia. The algorithm was applied to clinical data for 122 consecutively hospitalized patients with community-acquired pneumonia whose sputum samples were Gram stained and whose urine was tested for *Streptococcus pneumoniae* antigen. The costs of personnel, initial antimicrobial therapy, and materials were measured.

Results.—In comparison with the most expensive empirical regimen, rapid diagnostic testing would result in cost savings per patient of (Euro) 3.51 for Gram staining and (Euro)8.11 for urinary pneumococcal antigen testing (1 Euro equal to $1.13 in 2000). Compared with the cheapest regimen, Gram staining would increase the cost by (Euro)2.25 per patient, and urinary antigen testing would increase the cost by (Euro)24.26 per patient.

Conclusions.—In this setting, rapid diagnostic testing would not lower costs. However, costs savings are dependent on the differences of prices of the different antibiotics chosen and the proportion of evaluable and positive samples.

▶ The problem: can we save money by using rapid diagnostic testing to narrow the spectrum of antibiotic coverage used in the initial treatment of community-acquired pneumococcal pneumonia? In this case the answer was no, but that "no" depended on the details. The larger point illustrated by this article is that decision analysis is relevant and useful in getting the answers to questions like these that arise in the course of managing and deploying limited laboratory resources. We should use it more often.

M. G. Bissell, MD, PhD, MPH

Microbiological Testing and Outcome of Patients With Severe Community-Acquired Pneumonia
Rello J, Bodi M, Mariscal D, et al (Joan XXIII Univ Hosp, Tarragona, Spain; Hosp de Sabadell, Barcelona)
Chest 123:174-180, 2003   18–6

Introduction.—Both the Infectious Disease Society of America and the American Thoracic Society agree that severe community-acquired pneumonia (SCAP) forms an etiologically differentiated subgroup that necessitates a specific therapeutic approach. The recommendations of both societies concerning the role of the microbiology laboratory in the diagnosis of lower respiratory tract infections are controversial. The impact of microbiological investigations on therapeutic decisions and outcome was examined in patients with SCAP in a retrospective analysis of prospectively collected data.

Methods.—Between January 1, 1993 and January 1, 2000, 204 consecutive patients admitted to the ICU with SCAP were evaluated. The medical management was similar for all participants. Blood samples were routinely obtained for cultures and serologic investigation at hospital admission. Blood samples for follow-up serologic testing were obtained from most patients.

Results.—Of 204 patients with SCAP, 106 needed intubation and 98 did not. Of the latter, 81 were managed with noninvasive mechanical ventilation. A microbiological diagnosis was determined in 57.3% of patients. The most frequently observed pathogens were *Streptococcus pneumoniae*, *Legionella pneumophila*, and *Haemophilus influenzae*. In patients who were intubated, *Pseudomonas* (6.6% vs 1.0%; $P < .05$) and *Legionella* (15.1% vs 7.1%; $P < .05$) were most commonly documented.

The overall mortality rate was 23.5% (44.3% in intubated patients). The most lethal pathogens were *S pneumoniae*, *Pseudomonas aeruginosa*, and *L pneumophila* in 7, 7, and 5 patients, respectively. Antibiotic prescriptions were changed in 41.6% of patients because of bacteriological investigation, including 11 patients (5%) for whom the initial treatment was not effective against microbial isolates. The most common reason for changes was simplification of therapy in 65 episodes (31.8%).

Conclusion.—Microbiological testing is fully justified in patients with SCAP. Identifying the causative agent and adjusting treatment are important in patient outcome. It is recommended that intubated patients be empirically treated for *Pseudomonas* and *Legionella* until bacterial results are ready.

▶ What is the value of the microbiology lab in the workup and treatment of severe community-acquired pneumonia? This article seeks to provide population-based outcomes data to support its role. As studies of this kind, teasing out the marginal contribution of the lab to patient outcomes, are still regrettably rare, this contribution has value for our overall understanding of the deployment and appropriate utilization of lab resources.

M. G. Bissell, MD, PhD, MPH

Surge Capacity for Response to Bioterrorism in Hospital Clinical Microbiology Laboratories
Shapiro DS (Boston Univ)
J Clin Microbiol 41:5372-5376, 2003   18–7

Background.—"Surge capacity" is a term used to describe the ability to rapidly respond to a sudden and dramatic increase in needs. Surge capacity has historically been addressed in the military as one component of readiness. In the civilian emergency preparedness setting, it pertains to response to the needs of the population after a natural disaster. Today there is a need to expand the concept of surge capacity to include the setting of a terrorist event. In the setting of a bioterrorism event, plans already in place have increased the surge capacity of the public health and emergency medical system to deal with the diverse needs of the population.

Although large amounts of federal funding have been allocated to public health laboratories, little funding has been directed toward hospital microbiology laboratories. There are concerns that hospital laboratories may have inadequate surge capacities for responding to a significant bioterrorism incident. The surge capacity of 1 clinical microbiology laboratory in an urban medical center in a major urban area was evaluated.

Methods.—A workflow analysis was conducted for the clinical microbiology laboratory of Boston Medical Center to identify barriers to surge capacity in the case of a bioterrorism event and to identify solutions to accompanying problems (Fig 1).

Results.—Among the barriers identified were a national shortage of trained medical technologists; the inability of clinical laboratories to deal with a dramatic increase in the number of blood cultures; delays in the production, transport, and delivery of critical products to clinical laboratories while manufacturers "ramp up" their production; and a shortage of class II biological safety cabinets.

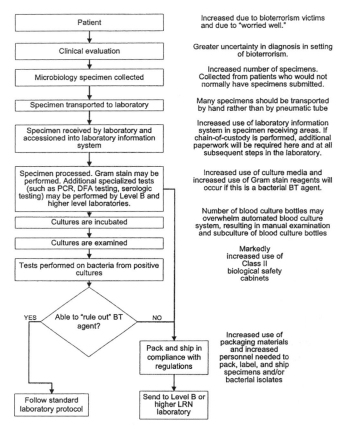

The flowchart (left to right):

Patient → Increased due to bioterrorism victims and due to "worried well."

Clinical evaluation → Greater uncertainty in diagnosis in setting of bioterrorism.

Microbiology specimen collected → Increased number of specimens. Collected from patients who would not normally have specimens submitted.

Specimen transported to laboratory → Many specimens should be transported by hand rather than by pneumatic tube

Specimen received by laboratory and accessioned into laboratory information system → Increased use of laboratory information system in specimen receiving areas. If chain-of-custody is performed, additional paperwork will be required here and at all subsequent steps in the laboratory.

Specimen processed. Gram stain may be performed. Additional specialized tests (such as PCR, DFA testing, serologic testing) may be performed by Level B and higher level laboratories. → Increased use of culture media and increased use of Gram stain reagents will occur if this is a bacterial BT agent.

Cultures are incubated → Number of blood culture bottles may overwhelm automated blood culture system, resulting in manual examination and subculture of blood culture bottles

Cultures are examined

Tests performed on bacteria from positive cultures → Markedly increased use of Class II biological safety cabinets

Able to "rule out" BT agent? YES / NO

Pack and ship in compliance with regulations → Increased use of packaging materials and increased personnel needed to pack, label, and ship specimens and/or bacterial isolates

Follow standard laboratory protocol

Send to Level B or higher LRN laboratory

FIGURE 1.—Analysis of steps in the process of specimen collection and culture during a bioterrorism event. *Abbreviations*: *PCR*, Polymerase chain reaction; *DFA*, direct fluorescent antibody; *BT*, bioterrorism; *LRN*, Laboratory Response Network. (Courtesy of Shapiro DS: Surge capacity for response to bioterrorism in hospital clinical microbiology laboratories. *J Clin Microbiol* 41:5372-5376, 2003. Copyright American Society for Microbiology.)

Conclusion.—Increased federal funding is needed to ensure that hospital clinical microbiology laboratories have sufficient surge capacity to respond to a bioterrorism event. Increased funding could remedy staffing shortages by raising the salary of medical technologists to parity with similarly educated health care professionals and providing financial incentives for students to enroll in clinical laboratory science programs. It is recommended that blood culture bottles and possibly continuous-monitoring blood culture instruments be added to the national antibiotic stockpile.

It is also recommended that federal support ensure that manufacturers of essential laboratory supplies are able to rapidly increase production. Hospitals must provide increased numbers of biological safety cabinets and more space dedicated to clinical microbiology laboratories. Laboratories are encouraged to initiate limited cross-training of technologists, ensure the availability of sufficient packaging supplies, and be able to move to a 4-day blood culture protocol.

▶ Laboratorians are not used to being in the spotlight. But the world is changing and so must this attitude. In an era of ever-present concern over the possibility of bioterrorist attack, hospital microbiology laboratories should, as the author suggests, plan for the day when they will find themselves in the middle of the action. They are a scarce community resource that may or may not be adequate to cope.

M. G. Bissell, MD, PhD, MPH

Implementation of a Point-of-Care Satellite Laboratory in the Emergency Department of an Academic Medical Center: Impact on Test Turnaround Time and Patient Emergency Department Length of Stay
Lee-Lewandrowski E, Corboy D, Lewandrowski K, et al (Harvard Med School, Boston; Massachusetts Gen Hosp, Boston)
Arch Pathol Lab Med 127:456-460, 2003   18–8

Background.—The problem of overcrowding in emergency departments (EDs) in the United States, particularly in urban areas, has reached crisis proportions. Many hospitals are working to identify process re-engineering efforts to reduce crowding and patient length of stay in the ED. The impact of a point-of-care testing (POCT) satellite laboratory in the ED of a large academic medical center was investigated.

Methods.—The study was conducted in the ED of a large urban hospital. Physician satisfaction, turnaround time, and ED length of stay were evaluated before and after the implementation of the POCT laboratory. ED length of stay was measured by patient chart audits. Turnaround time was assessed by manual and computer audits. Clinician satisfaction surveys were used to measure satisfaction with test turnaround time and test accuracy.

Results.—Blood glucose, urine human chorionic gonadotropin, urine dipstick, creatine kinase–MB, and troponin tests were performed in the ED POCT laboratory. Test turnaround time declined by an average of 87% after the initiation of POCT. The ED length of stay decreased for patients who received pregnancy testing, urine dipstick, and cardiac markers. The differences were not significant for individual tests; however, when the tests were combined, the decreased length of stay was an average of 41.3 minutes.

Surveys of clinician satisfaction showed equivalent satisfaction with test accuracy between the central laboratory and the POCT laboratory. These surveys also documented dissatisfaction with central laboratory turnaround time and increased satisfaction with the turnaround time of the POCT program.

Conclusion.—Institution of a point-of-care satellite laboratory decreased test turnaround time and length of stay in the ED. Excellent satisfaction with test accuracy and turnaround time was documented.

▶ Here is one of those perennial quandaries of laboratory management: to centralize or decentralize? The tension between the ED's seemingly endless need for ever-decreasing turnaround time above all else versus the central clinical laboratory's regulatory responsibility for maintenance and control of quality leads to inbuilt tension in most academic medical centers. So what, you're asking yourself, do they do about this at Massachusetts General? The article is the answer.

M. G. Bissell, MD, PhD, MPH

Critique of the *Guide to the Expression of Uncertainty in Measurement* Method of Estimating and Reporting Uncertainty in Diagnostic Assays
Krouwer JS (Krouwer Consulting, Sherborn, Mass)
Clin Chem 49:1818-1821, 2003   18–9

Background.—Inaccuracy in clinical chemistry is the result of random and systematic errors. The Guide to the Uncertainty of Measurement (GUM) provides instruction for constructing uncertainty intervals for a measurement. GUM is usually reserved for reference materials but has recently been proposed as a method for expression of uncertainty for commercial diagnostic assays. The applicability of GUM to commercial diagnostic assays was investigated.

Methods.—The official GUM standard and the published applications of GUM to commercial diagnostic assays were used to determine whether applying GUM to commercial diagnostic assays is warranted.

Results.—Some important assays, such as troponin I, would not be candidates for GUM because troponin I is not a well-defined physical quantity. While definitive methods attempt the detection and elimination of all systematic error sources, commercial assays often trade features such as ease of use and cost with accuracy and allow the presence of systematic errors as long as the overall accuracy meets the medical need goal.

Laboratories have difficulty in preparing GUM models because the knowledge required to specify some systematic errors is often available only to manufacturers. Some non-GUM methods for estimating uncertainty rely on observed data, which include both known and unknown sources of error. It is not unusual for large, unknown errors to occur in assays in routine use (eg, outliers) because diagnostic assays must be chemically specific in the presence of thousands of potential interfering substances. GUM has no provision for dealing with unexplained outliers, which may result in uncertainty intervals that are not sufficiently wide.

Conclusion.—Evaluations for accuracy on the basis of description of the distribution of result differences between commercial assays and reference methods have indicated that some assays have a few results with large differences, or outliers, which leads to a wide accuracy interval. It is unlikely that GUM would be capable of predicting these wide intervals, particularly because there is little or no provision for outlier treatment in GUM. The modeling used by practitioners of the GUM method has the potential to be useful in improving quality, but commercial diagnostic assays are not prepared for GUM uncertainty statements.

▶ It has been a long-held desire of some clinical chemists and other laboratorians to be able to provide to the clinician not only an analytical result and reference range, but also an estimate of the degree of uncertainty the result represents. This would be analogous to what we are used to hearing on the nightly weather report, eg, "The forecast for tomorrow in the greater metropolitan area is for light rain, and the probability of this is 65%." The question is, on what theoretical basis could the clinical laboratory provide such an estimate? One source of a possible answer is the approach outlined in the International Organization for Standardization standards document *Guide to the Expression of Uncertainty in Measurement.*[1] Here Dr Krouwer explains why he feels this approach is not yet ready for "prime time."

M. G. Bissell, MD, PhD, MPH

Reference

1. International Organization for Standardization. *Guide to the expression of uncertainty in measurement.* Geneva, ISO, 1995, 101 pp.

The *Guide to Expression of Uncertainty in Measurement* Approach for Estimating Uncertainity: An Appraisal
Kristiansen J (Natl Inst of Occupational Health, Copenhagen)
Clin Chem 49:1822-1829, 2003   18–10

Background.—The *Guide to Expression of Uncertainty in Measurement* (GUM) is intended to harmonize the different practices for estimation and reporting of uncertainty of measurement. The GUM uncertainty has been criticized, and it has been concluded by some authors that although GUM may be suitable for values assigned to reference materials, the application of the GUM approach to commercial diagnostic assays is unwarranted. However, it is argued in this report that although there are clear advantages to a common approach for the evaluation of uncertainty, application of the GUM approach to chemistry measurements is not straightforward. Some of the arguments against the application of the GUM approach to diagnostic assays were evaluated.

Methods.—A review was conducted of some of the arguments against the application of the GUM approach to diagnostic assays. Sodium measurements were modeled mathematically to demonstrate the GUM approach to uncertainty. A standardized uncertainty evaluation process was presented.

Results.—Modeling of sodium measurements demonstrates how the GUM uncertainty interval reflects the treatment of a bias. The width of the uncertainty interval varied, depending on whether a correction for a calibrator lot bias was applied, but in both cases it was consistent with the distribution of measurement results (Fig 2).

A Using uncertainty statement on certificate

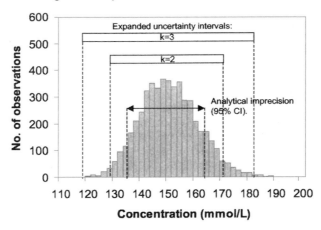

B Estimating bias and adjusting the calibrator value

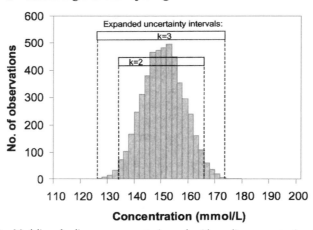

FIGURE 2.—Modeling of sodium measurements. A sample with a sodium concentration of 150 mmol/L was measured 5000 times, each time with a different calibrator lot. The histograms show the distribution of individual results. The horizontal bars represent expanded standard uncertainty intervals ($k = 2$ and 3). Calculation of the uncertainty was as follows: **A**, No estimation of bias. The uncertainty of the calibrator lot was combined with the analytical imprecision to yield the uncertainty of the result. The *horizontal double arrow* indicates the 95% confidence interval calculated from the analytical imprecision. **B**, Estimation of bias. The uncertainty of the bias estimate was combined with CV_A in the calculation of the uncertainty of results. (Courtesy of Kristiansen J: Counterpoint: The *Guide to Expression of Uncertainty in Measurement* approach for estimating uncertainty: An appraisal. *Clin Chem* 49:1822-1829, 2003. ©2003 The American Association for Clinical Chemistry (1-800-892-1400.)

Conclusion.—It is argued in this report that the GUM uncertainty should be applied to measurements in laboratory medicine because it may support the forces that drive the work to improve the quality of measurement procedures. However, it is important that the uncertainty evaluation procedure be standardized as much as possible to make the GUM approach more manageable. It is essential that attention be given to the traceability and uncertainty of calibrators and reagents supplied by assay manufacturers. There is a need for information about uncertainty in the evaluation of the uncertainty associated with manufacturers' measurement procedures. This may compel manufacturers to further improve the metrologic and analytical quality of their products.

▶ Here Dr Kristiansen argues in favor of implementing the International Organization for Standardization approach to uncertainty in laboratory medicine. In contrast to Dr Krouwer's position, he feels that it may represent the best leverage consumers (laboratorians, clinicians, and, ultimately, patients) may have on the situation. He argues that its use may force in vitro diagnostics manufacturers to standardize their approach to assuring and reporting the traceability and uncertainty of calibrators and reagents.

M. G. Bissell, MD, PhD, MPH

19 Transfusion Medicine and Coagulation

Ethnic Differences in Markers of Thrombophilia: Implications for the Investigation of Ischemic Stroke in Multiethnic Populations: The South London Ethnicity and Stroke Study
Jerrard-Dunne P, Evans A, McGovern R, et al (St George's Hosp, London; King's College, London)
Stroke 34:1821-1827, 2003   19–1

Background.—The incidence of ischemic stroke is higher among persons of African and African-Caribbean descent compared with whites, and strokes occur at a younger age. The prevalence of inherited thrombophilic states has shown significant interethnic variation, and the role of thrombophilia in the pathogenesis of ischemic stroke in blacks is not known. The factor V Leiden mutation is rare in blacks, but deficiencies of both protein S and C and in lupus anticoagulant have been reported to be more common in persons of African descent who have ischemic stroke. However, data on normal reference ranges in the black community are not available. Ethnic-specific reference ranges were estimated in a community population to determine the prevalence of thrombophilic states in a multiethnic stroke population.

Methods.—The study group was composed of 130 consecutive patients aged 65 years or older with ischemic stroke. The patients included 50 black Caribbeans, 30 black Africans, and 50 whites. A control group of 130 stroke-free persons from the community, matched 1:1 for age, sex, and self-declared ethnicity, was also recruited. Free protein S, protein C, antithrombin III, activated protein C resistance, IgG anticardiolipin antibodies, and lupus anticoagulant were assayed in patients and controls.

Results.—Protein C and protein S levels were significantly lower in black Africans in the control group compared with white control subjects, and they showed a trend toward lower antithrombin III levels compared with their white counterparts. Black African and Caribbean control subjects had higher diluted Russell's viper venom time ratios compared with white controls. The application of ethnic-specific reference ranges showed that 8 control subjects (6.3%) and 11 patients (8.5%) had thrombophilia abnormalities. Odds ratios were 0.96 for whites, 1.57 for black Carribeans, and 2.07 for black Africans.

Conclusions.—The failure to account for ethnic differences in the normal reference ranges for thrombophilia markers may result in inappropriate diagnosis and investigation of hypercoagulable states in black individuals. Deficiencies in proteins S and C and in lupus anticoagulant may be contributing factors to the risk of stroke in a minority of black cases, but they are unlikely to be major contributors to the excess risk of stroke that is observed in young persons of African and African-Caribbean descent.

▶ It is well known that hypertension in the black population has a number of unique characteristics. This article reinforces the case for having separately defined reference ranges for different ethnic groups when relevant. In this instance, applying white reference ranges for thrombophilia markers to black populations has inadvertently biased studies of hyercoagulable states and stroke risk. When the right reference ranges are used, hypercoagulation does not have a disproportionate impact on prevalence of stroke in this population.

M. G. Bissell, MD, PhD, MPH

DNA Microsatellite and Linkage Analysis Supports the Inclusion of LOCR in the Rh Blood Group System
Coghlan G, Zelinski T (Univ of Manitoba, Winnipeg, Canada)
Transfusion 43:440-444, 2003
19–2

Background.—A new red blood cell low-incidence antigen, called LOCR, was described in 1994. It was established that red blood cells expressing LOCR had altered expression of Rh antigens (c or e). Unfortunately, because of an insufficient number of informative families, it was not possible to formally assign LOCR to the Rh blood group solely on the basis of serologic findings. Through the performance of molecular genetic studies, conclusive evidence was provided to support the assignment of LOCR to the Rh blood group system.

Methods.—Genomic DNA from a total of 18 families (including 72 children) of diverse ethnic backgrounds was analyzed. DNA from the members of 3 families (13 children) segregating for *LOCR* was analyzed for repeat polymorphisms of the chromosome 1p microsatellite markers *D1S1612*, *D1S1597*, *D1S552*, *D1S247*, and *D1S2134*.

Results.—There was no observable evidence of recombination, in either paternal or maternal meioses, between *LOCR* and *D1S1597*, *D1S552*, or *D1S247*. Peak lods for combined paternal and maternal meioses were 2.41 for either *LOCR:D1S552* or *LOCR:D1S247*. Lods for linkage between *LOCR* and *D1S1597* peaked at 1.81 for maternal meioses alone.

Conclusions.—In previous studies in which serologic methods were used, a peak lod of 2.107 was determined between *LOCR* and *RH*. In this study, DNA analysis of the only informative family (with 7 children) not segregating for *RH* yielded a peak lod of 1.81 between *LOCR* and *D1S1597-D1S552-D1S247*. By combining the results produced by each approach (lods of 3.917), evidence has been provided that supports the placement of LOCR in the Rh blood group system.

▶ Here's a case where molecular genetics comes to the rescue in the placement of a new low-incidence red blood cell marker LOCR. Although associated with altered Rh expression, serologic evidence alone was insufficient to allow it to be correctly assigned. With the more fundamental analysis provided by microsatellite and linkage studies, the assignment to the Rh group can now definitely be made.

M. G. Bissell, MD, PhD, MPH

Pseudoplatelets: A Retrospective Study of Their Incidence and Interference With Platelet Counting
van der Meer W, MacKenzie MA, Dinnissen JWB, et al (Univ Med Centre, Nijmegen, The Netherlands)
J Clin Pathol 56:772-774, 2003   19–3

Introduction.—Spurious platelet counts caused by the fragmentation of blood cells can be seen in acute leukemias. Microscopic examination of a blood smear should be performed to identify the presence of these so-called pseudoplatelets. When present, the platelet count should be corrected because of the important clinical consequences that a lower platelet count can have in these patients. To determine the bleeding tendency of patients with leukemia and pseudoplatelets, a study was done.

Methods.—The study included 169 patients with leukemia, both de novo diagnosed and relapsed, who were classified into a risk group for bleeding disorders after correction of the automated platelet count. Blood samples were obtained, anticoagulated with K_3EDTA, and measured on an automatic blood cell counter. A blood smear was performed and stained according to the May Grünwald-Giemsa method for microscopic observation. A 500 cell/particle differentiation was done, and the automated platelet count was corrected.

Results.—Pseudoplatelets were identified in 43 (25.4%) patients. Seven (4.1%) patients were reclassified as having a major bleeding risk (platelet count < 15 × 10^9/L).

Conclusion.—Platelets should be evaluated morphologically in patients with acute leukemia. A routine screening method for the identification of pseudoplatelets should be created.

▶ Patients with acute leukemia sometimes have serious problems with bleeding, in addition to all the other manifestations of their disease. This is due to thrombocytopenia that is nearly always present, but frequently unnoticed because of the phenomenon of the so-called pseudoplatelet, the subject of this study.

M. G. Bissell, MD, PhD, MPH

Thrombin-Activable Fibrinolysis Inhibitor Levels in the Acute Phase of Ischemic Stroke

Montaner J, Ribó M, Monasterio J, et al (Vall d'Hebron Hosp, Barcelona, Spain)
Stroke 34:1038-1040, 2003   19–4

Introduction.—Thrombin-activable fibrinolysis inhibitor (TAFI) is a recently recognized fibrinolysis inhibitor in plasma. The TAFI levels were prospectively evaluated in the acute phase of ischemic stroke, and their association with stroke evolution was investigated.

Methods.—The TAFI plasma levels were determined via enzyme-linked immunosorbent assay (percentage of the pooled reference kit expressed as mean ± SD) in 30 consecutive patients with ischemic stroke and compared with those of 30 healthy control subjects. All samples were obtained within the first 24 hours after symptom onset (mean, 4.6 hours) and before any treatment was initiated.

Results.—The TAFI plasma concentration was significantly greater in patients with stroke, compared with that of the control subjects (158.4% vs 105.6%; $P < .001$). The highest mean TAFI levels were observed in cases of neurologic deterioration (worsening, 198.1%; stability, 130.5%; improvement, 173.9%; $P = .057$).

Conclusion.—High levels of TAFI are present in the acute phase of ischemic stroke.

▶ Procarboxypeptidase B or TAFI is a proenzyme, which, when activated, cleaves the plasminogen binding sites from fibrin, inhibiting fibrinolysis. Elevated TAFI levels have been reported in cases of acute coronary syndrome and deep vein thrombosis. This is the first time it has been looked at in stroke.

M. G. Bissell, MD, PhD, MPH

Effects of X-ray Radiation on the Rheologic Properties of Platelets and Lymphocytes

Thomas S, Bolch W, Kao KJ, et al (Univ of Florida, Gainesville)
Transfusion 43:502-508, 2003   19–5

Background.—Irradiation of blood components has been performed since the early 1960s in order to prevent a potentially fatal complication of transfusion-associated graft-versus-host disease in severely compromised patients. However, the effects of this radiation exposure on the structure and function of blood cells has not been fully studied, and there is only limited information available on the effects of radiation on the mechanical properties of cells. The effects of x-ray radiation on platelet and lymphocyte rheology were evaluated because the ability of these blood cells to deform is vital to their flow throughout the microvascular system.

Methods.—Seven 4.5-mL fresh blood samples were obtained from healthy human volunteer donors, and each was anticoagulated with 0.5 mL of 3.8% sodium citrate anticoagulant. Micropipetted aspiration experiments were conducted on platelets and lymphocytes exposed to x-ray radiation. Four samples were exposed to x-ray radiation with the use of a stereotactic linear accelerator, with 2 of the samples exposed to 25-Gy x-ray radiation and 2 samples exposed to 50-Gy x-ray radiation. The remaining 3 control samples were not irradiated.

Results.—There was a significant increase in the Young modulus of elasticity between control platelets and irradiated platelets at 25 Gy and at 50 Gy. The percentage of cell activation was significantly increased in 25-Gy irradiated platelets. In addition, lymphocytes irradiated at 25 Gy were found to have a higher viscosity than controls. A significantly larger number of activated cells were found in the 50-Gy irradiated lymphocyte population.

Conclusion.—The alterations in the deformability and activation of irradiated platelets and lymphocytes may cause a reduction in local blood flow, leading to intermittent blockage that may cause a change in blood flow in microvasculatures.

▶ Many of our advances in medicine come from the recognition, understanding, and subsequent modification of the previously unforeseen consequences of our interventions. Here, the authors teach us something about an unforeseen consequence of blood irradiation for the prevention of graft-versus-host disease. Irradiated lymphocytes and platelets with stiffer membranes flow less freely through the microvasculature, but what this fully means remains to be understood.

M. G. Bissell, MD, PhD, MPH

Tissue Plasminogen Activator Plasma Level as a Potential Diagnostic Aid in Acute Pulmonary Embolism
Flores J, García-Avello A, Flores VM, et al (Hosp Universitario "Príncipe de Asturias," Madrid; Hosp Universitario "Ramón y Cajal," Madrid; Universidad Complutense de Madrid, Madrid)
Arch Pathol Lab Med 127:310-315, 2003   19–6

Background.—Pulmonary embolism (PE) is a potentially fatal and frequent complication of deep venous thrombosis. However, the most reliable techniques for the diagnosis of PE are not universally available, and all have some limitations. The purpose of this study was to determine the efficacy of 4 different fibrinolysis system parameters: tissue plasminogen activator (tPA), tissue plasminogen activator inhibitor type 1 (PAI-1), plasmin-antiplasmin complexes (PAP), and D-dimer, in the diagnosis of acute PE.

Methods.—The setting for this study was a 350-bed university hospital in an urban area of Spain. The study group was composed of 66 consecutive outpatients with clinically suspected PE. The diagnosis was based on ventilation-perfusion lung scan in combination with clinical assessment, lower limb study, and (as needed) pulmonary angiography. At the moment of clinical suspicion, a sample of venous blood was obtained to measure levels of tPA, PAI-1, PAP, and D-dimer using an enzyme-linked immunosorbent assay method.

Results.—Of the 66 patients studied, 27 (41%) were classified as PE-positive and 39 patients (59%) were classified as PE-negative. The sensitivity/negative predictive value for tPA using a cutoff of 8.5 ng/mL and PAI-1 using a cutoff of 15 ng/mL were 100%/100% and 100%/100%, respectively. A tPA level lower than 15 ng/mL was present in 13 (19.7%; all PE-negative) of 66 patients with suspected PE, and PAI-1 levels were lower than 15 ng/mL in 9 (13.6%; all PE-negative) of 66 patients with suspected PE. The D-dimer, using a cutoff of 500 ng/mL, showed a sensitivity and negative predictive value of 92.6% and 87.5%, respectively.

Conclusion.—These findings indicate the potential value of tPA and PAI-1 levels in excluding PE, although tPA would appear to be a better parameter. The sensitivity levels and negative predictive values for the rapid enzyme-linked immunosorbent assay for D-dimer used in this investigation were low in comparison with previous studies using the same test.

▶ Angiography, a gold standard diagnostic modality, is not universally available for ruling out PE in the emergency department, and D-dimer alone does not have a sufficiently high negative predictive value. Proposed answer: a test panel approach incorporating other known fibrinolytic parameters: tPA and PAI-1.

M. G. Bissell, MD, PhD, MPH

A Simple and Reproducible Method to Reliably Assess Platelet Activation
Nickels RM, Seyfert UT, Wenzel E, et al (Univ of Saarland, Homburg/Saar, Germany; Univ of Rostock, Germany)
Thromb Res 110:53-56, 2003   19–7

Background.—The activation of platelets is an essential component of the pathophysiologic process of thrombosis and hemostasis. The development of a simple and reproducible method for the assessment of different degrees of platelet activation has for many years been a primary focus of research on the evaluation of platelet responses both in vitro and in vivo. The purpose of this report was to present a simple, economical, and reproducible method for assessment of platelet activation that comprises the adhesion and retention of platelets passing an athrombogenic filter via centrifugal force (retention test Homburg [RT-H]). RT-H was compared with conventional measures of platelet activation, such as flow cytometric analysis of P-selectin expression and assessment of platelet shape on spreading.

Methods.—Blood from healthy volunteers was drawn from the left cubital vein with a 21-gauge needle. After centrifugation for 15 minutes at 110 × g and room temperature, platelet-rich plasma was transferred in a separate tube. Platelet count was assessed with a Coulter ACT diff Analyzer (Coulter Electronics, Luton, England).

Aliquots of platelet-rich plasma were either used as unstimulated negative controls or activated to serve as positive controls. Flow cytometric analysis was performed to assess surface expression of P-selectin, which is a reliable indicator of cell activation. The RT-H and spreading analysis test were performed. Platelet activation was performed using adenosine diphosphate and thrombin receptor activating peptide (TRAP) as agonists.

Results.—Flow cytometry showed that a fraction of less than 5% of platelets from PRP expressed P-selectin. After exposure to adenosine diphosphate (ADP), the fraction of P-selectin expressing platelets increased by 5- to 6-fold to approximately 17%, regardless of the dose of ADP used. TRAP was found to be a stronger platelet agonist, causing membrane translocation of P-selectin in almost half of the PRP platelets. Stimulation with ADP and TRAP caused about 85% of all types of platelets to spread to small, but mostly to large, forms, while the fraction of transition or spider forms decreased to 15%. The presence of pronounced agglutination and aggregation provided additional evidence of ADP- and TRAP-exposed platelets.

Conclusion.—The RT-H is capable of directly reflecting activation of platelets from platelet-rich plasma and therefore may be an ideal adjunctive method for refining the tools for assessment of platelet response in physiology and pathophysiology.

▶ Platelet activation represents a complex sequence of cellular and metabolic events essential for hemostasis and key to the pathogenesis of a number of important disease states and conditions. The authors describe a simple and inexpensive approach to the in vitro monitoring of platelet activation based on platelet adhesion to surfaces.

M. G. Bissell, MD, PhD, MPH

Molecular Bases of the Antigens of the Lutheran Blood Group System
Crew VK, Green C, Daniels G (Bristol Inst for Tranfusion Sciences, England)
Transfusion 43:1729-1737, 2003   19–8

Background.—The Lutheran blood group is a complex blood group system that comprises 18 identified antigens. There are 4 pairs of allelic antigens in the Lutheran group, whereas others are independently expressed antigens of a high frequency. Lutheran antigens are carried by the Lutheran glycoproteins, which are a product of the *LU* gene. Two *LU* transcripts have been isolated, differing as a result of the alternative splicing of intron 13. This study utilized data from a previous study by Parsons et al on the predicted IgSF domain placement of Lutheran antigens to select relevant *LU* exons for sequencing to determine the molecular bases of other Lutheran antigens.

Methods.—Genomic DNA was obtained from 21 persons representing 12 Lutheran phenotypes. This material was used for polymerase chain reaction of selected *LU* exons that were directly sequenced and compared with control DNA of a common Lutheran phenotype.

Results.—Lutheran phenotypes were caused mainly by single-nucleotide polymorphisms within *LU*, resulting in single amino acid changes (Fig 2). The mutations derived were LU:−4; G524A, Arg175Gin; in LU:−5, G326A, Arg109His; in LU:−6,9; C824T, Ser275Phe; in LU:−8,14, T611A, Met204Lys; in LU:−13; three point mutations (C1340T, Ser447Leu, C1671T silent mutation for Ser557 and A1742T, Gin581Leu); in LU:−16, C679T, Arg227Cys; in LU:−17, G340A, Glu114Lys; and in LU:−20, C905T, Thr302Met. Differing results were obtained in 2 LU:−12 samples; 1 person

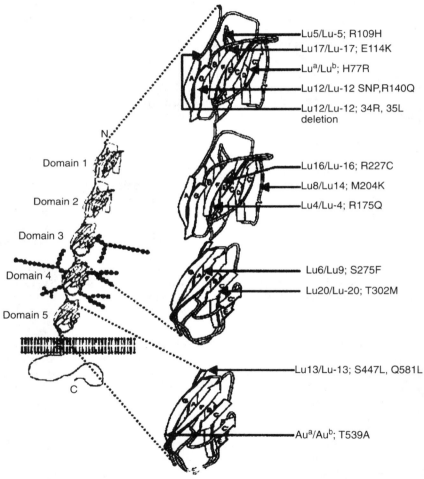

FIGURE 2.—The predicted structure of the Lu-glycoprotein with 5 extracellular IgSF domains (domains 1-3 and domain 5 enlarged) and potential glycolyzation sites. The spatial positioning of examined Lutheran antigens and the related mutations are shown on the enlarged domains. (Published with permission from *Transfusion* courtesy of Crew VK, Green C, Daniels G: Molecular bases of the antigens of the Lutheran blood group system. *Transfusion* 43:1729-1737, 2003. Reprinted by permission on Blackwell Publishing.)

had a deletion 99GCGCTT, Arg34, and Leu35, and the second person had a point mutation G419A, Arg140Gin.

Conclusion.—These findings provided evidence of the genetic background of 11 antigens in the Lutheran blood group system. It is suggested that these antigens be placed on the Lutheran glycoprotein.

▶ The Lutheran blood group system consists of 18 antigens (LU1-LU20, with LU10 and LU15 designated as obsolete). The Lutheran antigens are carried by the Lutheran glycoproteins, all the product of the single gene *LU*. Four pairs of the Lutheran antigen genes are allelic and polymorphic, and the remaining 10 are very high frequency. This report outlines further delineation of the molecular genetics of this complex system.

M. G. Bissell, MD, PhD, MPH

Management of Patients Refractory to Platelet Transfusion
Sacher RA, Kickler TS, Schiffer CA, et al (Univ of Cincinnati, Ohio; Johns Hopkins Univ, Baltimore, Md; Wayne State Univ, Detroit; et al)
Arch Pathol Lab Med 127:409-414, 2003   19–9

Background.—Platelet transfusions, either as platelets from whole blood or platelet pheresis concentrates, are usually indicated for prophylaxis against major bleeding for patients with severe thrombocytopenia or therapeutically for bleeding patients with thrombocytopenia or platelet dysfunctional states. However, platelet transfusions are relatively contraindicated for patients with thrombotic thrombocytopenic purpura. The management of these patients, and of other patients who are unresponsive to platelet transfusions, can be extremely difficult. A current assessment of and practical approach to the diagnosis and management of patients who are refractory to platelet transfusions was presented.

Methods.—A task force was convened by the College of American Pathologists to outline current concepts in the definition and diagnosis of patients who are refractory to platelet transfusions and for the selection of the optimal platelet component for these patients. A literature review and dialogue were conducted among members of the task force.

Results.—The report presents a contemporary approach to the diagnosis and management of patients who are refractory to platelet transfusions. The selection process for platelet transfusion in alloimmunized patients has been the subject of continuing investigation. The paradigm used in red cell compatibility testing has been advocated for platelet transfusion. In this paradigm, antigen typing is first determined and, if alloantibodies are present, a crossmatch is done. With the availability of standardized platelet crossmatch techniques, many blood centers now routinely perform platelet crossmatching.

Crossmatching can also be performed on available apheresis patients, making a compatible transfusion available in a few hours rather than several days. Alternative methods for the treatment of patients who are refractory to platelets and have thrombocytopenic bleeding include the use of IV immunoglobulin or anti-D in patients who are Rh-positive. WinRho SDF, a human immune IV gamma globulin highly enriched for antibodies to the Rh_0 (D) and licensed for the treatment of immune thrombocytopenic purpura in Rh-positive persons, has been shown to be safe and to have an efficacy similar to high-dose IV immunoglobulin in the treatment of immune thrombocytopenic purpura.

Use of a novel technique to reduce human leukocyte antigen antigenicity has demonstrated that human leukocyte antigens can be at least partially eluted from the platelet membrane without apparent impairment of platelet function. However, success has been limited in the small group of patients who have been treated with these modified platelets.

Conclusion.—This report was prepared in an effort to provide a resource and a practical approach to the issue of diagnosis and management of patients who are refractory to platelet transfusion.

▶ Platelets, supplied either as single-donor units or from random pools, are usually given as prophylaxis against major bleeding. They are contraindicated in certain platelet consumptive states like thrombotic thrombocytopenic purpura. The clinical management of these and other patients who fail to respond to platelet transfusions can be a serious diagnostic and therapeutic challenge. This article offers the results of consensus seeking among College of American Pathologists resource experts in the area.

M. G. Bissell, MD, PhD, MPH

Aggregates of Endothelial Microparticles and Platelets Circulate in Peripheral Blood: Variations During Stable Coronary Disease and Acute Myocardial Infarction
Héloire F, Weill B, Weber S, et al (Université René Descartes, Paris)
Thromb Res 110:173-180, 2003   19–10

Background.—Thrombus formation on the surface of disrupted atherosclerotic plaques is a fundamental component of the progression of coronary disease and in the development of acute coronary syndromes. Activated endothelial cells can shed fragments of their plasma membranes, called microparticles (MPs), into the extracellular space. MPs have been detected in the peripheral blood of normal subjects and, at higher levels, in patients with acute coronary syndromes and lupus anticoagulant. Whether circulating endothelial MPs could bind platelets, form aggregates, and be involved in the formation of thrombus during acute myocardial infarction (AMI) was investigated.

Methods.—This prospective study included 44 patients with angiographic documentation of coronary disease. Twenty patients had stable coronary disease without ongoing myocardial ischemia at rest nor at exercise during the time of the study. The remaining 24 patients had AMI and were directly admitted to the catheterization laboratory within 6 hours after the onset of symptoms. In addition, a group of 20 healthy volunteers with no cardiac disease were studied as control subjects.

The in vitro formation of aggregates comprising endothelial MPs and platelets was assessed by incubating supernatants of activated endothelial cells in culture with freshly isolated platelets. Endothelial MP–platelet (EMP-P) aggregates were characterized by flow cytometry using antibodies to specific markers of endothelial cells and of platelets.

Results.—Identical EMP-P aggregates were detected in vivo in the peripheral blood of healthy control subjects, patients with stable coronary disease, and patients with AMI. The levels of EMP-P aggregates were significantly higher in patients with stable coronary disease than in control subjects; however, the levels of EMP-P aggregates in the first hours of AMI were significantly lower than in the control group and in patients with stable coronary disease, both before primary angioplasty and at 2 hours after reperfusion. However, by 48 hours after onset of AMI, the levels of EMP-P aggregates

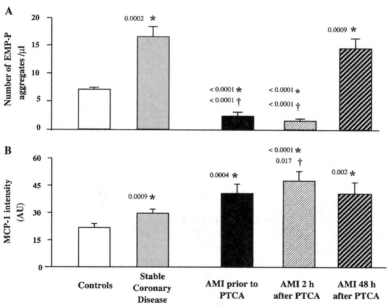

FIGURE 4.—A, Enumeration of endothelial microparticle–platelet (*EMP-P*) aggregates in the whole blood of healthy control subjects (*white bar*), patients with stable coronary disease (*shaded bar*), and patients with acute myocardial infarction (*AMI*) within 6 hours of the onset of symptoms (*black bar*) and 2 hours (*lightly striped bar*) and 48 hours (*heavily striped bar*) after percutaneous transluminal coronary angioplasty (*PTCA*). B, Expression of macrophage chemotactic protein 1 (*MCP-1*) by EMP-P aggregates in the whole blood of control patients, those with stable coronary disease, and those with AMI. Statistical significance was calculated by the nonparametric Mann and Whitney test. *Asterisk* indicates *P* versus healthy control subjects; *dagger* indicates *P* versus stable coronary disease. (Reprinted from *Thrombosis Research* courtesy of Héloire F, Weill B, Weber S, et al: Aggregates of endothelial microparticles and platelets circulate in peripheral blood: Variations during stable coronary disease and acute myocardial infarction. *Thromb Res* 110:173-180, 2003. Copyright 2003 with kind permission from Elsevier Science Ltd, The Boulevard, Langford Lane, Kidlington OX5 1GB, UK.)

had returned to values near those observed in patients with stable coronary disease (Fig 4).

Conclusion.—These findings support the concept that EMPs can bind to platelets and form aggregates. There were significant differences in the enumeration of those aggregates in the peripheral blood of the 3 groups of patients tested. The new test described here can aid in the evaluation of the level of endothelial cell activation and the damages created by chronic atherosclerosis.

▶ Though we know that tears forming in the endothelial surface of atherosclerotic plaques play a major role in the pathogenesis of the acute coronary syndrome, there are many biochemical details that remain obscure. The little chunks of endothelial cells known as EMPs are known to result from such endothelial wear and tear as may occur in normal subjects, as well as those with coronary artery syndrome. The fact is, these MPs have the potential to act as potent procoagulants and thus may play a critical role.

M. G. Bissell, MD, PhD, MPH

Antibodies to High-Frequency Antigens May Decrease the Quality of Transfusion Support: An Observational Study
Seltsam A, Wagner FF, Salama A, et al (Hannover Med School, Germany; Univ Hosp Ulm, Germany; Inst for Clinical Transfusion Medicine and Immunogenetics Ulm, Germany; et al)
Transfusion 43:1563-1566, 2003   19–11

Background.—High-frequency red blood cell (RBC) antigens occur at frequencies of over 99%. Immunization against these antigens therefore occurs in isolated cases only. Blood donors lacking these antigens are therefore rare and go unrecognized as long as donor typing for high-frequency antigens is not performed. It can be difficult to provide transfusion support for these patients because of the scarcity of compatible units, high transport and storage requirements, and the inexperience of many physicians in the treatment of these patients. Little information is available on the transfusion support of patients with antibodies to high-frequency RBC antigens. The quality of transfusion support provided to patients with antibodies against high-frequency antigens was assessed.

Methods.—All immunohematologic reference laboratories and blood banks in Germany, Switzerland, and Austria were asked to report all patients with clinically significant antibodies to high-frequency antigens (other than anti-k) who were hospitalized during a 20-month period from May 2000 to December 2001. An antibody was assumed to be clinically significant if the specificity involved had been implicated in hemolytic transfusion reactions or HDN. The patients were followed up until discharge or until no additional data were available.

Results.—A total of 52 patients with antibodies to high-frequency antigens were treated in hospitals. Of these patients, 22 received 104 antigen-negative RBCs. In 23 patients, a deviation from the standard transfusion policy—eg, transfusion of antigen-incompatible units—occurred. Institutions in the different countries varied in the use of frozen or fresh units, but this variation did not affect the rate of deviation from protocol. Approximately 20% of all units were supplied internationally. Four antibody specificities (anti-Kp^b, anti-Vel, anti-Lu^b, and anti-Yt^a) were found in two thirds of the patients.

Conclusion.—This survey of references laboratories and transfusion services in 3 European countries—Germany, Austria, and Switzerland—found that transfusion support was unsatisfactory in about one third of the hospitalized patients with antibodies to high-frequency antigens. Maintenance of a rapidly accessible stock of just 4 types of rare blood units would ensure adequate transfusion support for the majority of these patients.

▶ Blood banking is all about supply and demand. The rare patient who presents with an antibody to one of the high-frequency antigens to which more than 99% of the rest of us are exposed presents us with one of these "blood economics" problems. The authors document that all too often such problems are not well solved. They suggest that access to supplies of just 4 of these rare blood units would allow us to deal with the bulk of the problem.

M. G. Bissell, MD, PhD, MPH

20 Clinical Microbiology

A Novel Coronavirus Associated With Severe Acute Respiratory Syndrome
Ksiazek TG, Erdman D, Goldsmith CS, et al (Ctrs for Disease Control and Prevention, Atlanta, Ga; World Health Organization, Hanoi, Vietnam; Queen Mary Hosp, Hong Kong; et al)
N Engl J Med 348:1953-1966, 2003   20–1

Introduction.—A worldwide outbreak of severe acute respiratory syndrome (SARS) has been linked with exposures originating from a single ill health care worker from Guangdong Province, China. The etiologic agent of this outbreak was examined.

Methods.—Clinical specimens were received from patients in 7 countries and were tested with virus isolation techniques, electron microscopic and histologic studies, and molecular and serologic assays to detect a wide range of potential pathogens.

Results.—None of the previously described respiratory pathogens were consistently detected. A novel coronavirus was isolated from patients who fulfilled the case definition of SARS. Cytopathologic characteristics were identified in Vero E6 cells inoculated with a throat swab specimen (Fig 2). Electron microscopic examination showed ultrastructural features that were characteristic of coronaviruses. Immunohistochemical and immunofluorescence staining demonstrated reactivity with group I coronavirus polyclonal antibodies. Consensus coronavirus primers designed to amplify a fragment of the polymerase gene by reverse transcription–polymerase chain reaction (RT-PCR) were used to determine a sequence that clearly identified the isolate as a unique coronavirus only distantly associated with previously sequenced coronaviruses. With the use of specific diagnostic RT-PCR primers, several identical nucleotide sequences were identified in 12 patients from several locations. This finding was consistent with a point-source outbreak. Indirect fluorescence antibody tests and enzyme-linked immunosorbent assays made with the new isolate have been used to illustrate a virus-specific serologic response. This virus may never have been previously circulated in the US population.

Conclusion.—A novel coronavirus is linked with the worldwide outbreak of SARS, with evidence suggesting that this virus has an etiologic role in SARS.

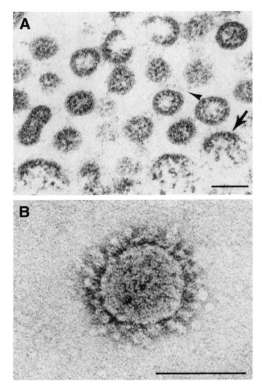

FIGURE 2.—Ultrastructural characteristics of SARS-associated coronavirus grown in Vero E6 cells. **A,** A thin-section electron-microscopical view of viral nucleocapsids aligned along the membrane of the rough endoplasmic reticulum (*arrow*) as particles bud into the cisternae. Enveloped virions have surface projections (*arrowhead*) and an electron-lucent center. Directly under the viral envelope lies a characteristic ring formed by the helical nucleocapsid, often seen in cross section. **B,** Negative-stain electron microscopy shows a stain-penetrated coronavirus particle with an internal helical nucleocapsid-like structure and club-shaped surface projections surrounding the periphery of the particle, a finding typical of coronaviruses (methylamine tungstate stain). The *bars* represent 100 nm. (Reprinted by permission of *The New England Journal of Medicine*, courtesy of Ksiazek TG, and the SARS Working Group: A novel coronavirus associated with severe acute respiratory syndrome. *N Engl J Med* 348:1953-1966, 2003. Copyright 2003, Massachusetts Medical Society. All rights reserved.)

▶ There are various ways that individuals' names can come to be associated with a disease, syndrome, or finding in medicine. Unfortunately, one of these is illustrated in this now-famous report of the new variant coronavirus associated with SARS. The authors chose to name the first isolate the Urbani strain in honor of one of them, Dr Carlo Urbani of the World Health Organization (Vietnam), who died of SARS in the course of this investigation.

M. G. Bissell, MD, PhD, MPH

Identification of a Novel Coronavirus in Patients With Severe Acute Respiratory Syndrome

Drosten C, Günther S, Preiser W, et al (Natl Reference Ctr for Tropical Infectious Diseases, Hamburg, Germany; Johann Wolfgang Goethe Univ, Frankfurt am Main, Germany; Philipps Univ, Marburg, Germany; et al)
N Engl J Med 348:1967-1976, 2003   20–2

Introduction.—The World Health Organization (WHO) has created a network of international laboratories to facilitate the identification of the causative agent of severe acute respiratory syndrome (SARS). As a function of this network, a novel coronavirus was identified and characterized in patients with SARS.

Methods.—The study included 49 specimens from 18 patients with suspected or probable SARS, according to the WHO case definition, and specimens from 21 healthy control subjects, which were sampled between March 5, and March 27, 2003 during the SARS epidemic in Hanoi, Vietnam. Fifty-four samples from patients in Germany were used as control specimens. Respiratory and blood specimens from patients in Frankfurt were analyzed. Specimens were searched for unknown viruses with the use of cell cultures and molecular techniques.

Results.—A novel coronavirus was identified in the specimens from patients with SARS. The virus was isolated in cell cultures. A sequence 300 nucleotides in length was obtained via a polymerase-chain-reaction (PCR)-based random-amplification procedure. Genetic characterization indicated that the virus is only distantly associated with known coronaviruses (identical in 50% to 60% of the nucleotide sequence). On the basis of the obtained sequence, conventional and real-time PCR assays for specific and sensitive identification of the novel viruses were established. The virus was seen in a variety of clinical specimens from patients with SARS; it was not found in control specimens. High concentrations of viral RNA of up to 100×10^6 molecules/mL were detected in sputum. The viral RNA was also seen in extremely low concentrations in plasma during the acute phase and in feces during the late convalescent phase. Infected patients demonstrated seroconversion on the Vero cells in which the virus was isolated.

Conclusion.—A novel coronavirus that may play a role in causing SARS has been found in patients with SARS. Patients with SARS are acutely infected with this virus, since virus-specific IgG seroconversion occurs.

▶ One measure of the real and novel power that genomic methods have conferred on medicine and public health is the speed by which some newly-emerging agents can be identified, classified, and tested for. The SARS story is a clear example of this new reality. It sets a standard that the public has now come to expect, if not, to take for granted.

M. G. Bissell, MD, PhD, MPH

Viable but Nonculturable Bacteria Are Present in Mouse and Human Urine Specimens

Anderson M, Bollinger D, Hagler A, et al (Univ of North Carolina, Charlotte)
J Clin Microbiol 42:753-758, 2004   20–3

Background.—Up to 50% of women are affected by urinary tract infection (UTIs) at least once during their lifetime, and 25% of women who acquire a UTI will have another infection within the following 6 months. One method of diagnosing a UTI is by culture of urine specimens. However, this is not an absolute indicator, as both asymptomatic bacteriuria and patients with UTI symptoms having no culturable urine bacteria have been reported. Urine within the urinary tract is generally considered sterile, a conclusion based on a lack of culturable cells present in urine specimens obtained via clean-catch and catheterization methods. The presence of viable bacteria in the urine specimens of healthy patients would affect hypotheses to explain recurrent UTIs as well as diagnostic procedures. Most recurrent UTIs result from reinfection; however, a higher percentage than would be expected by chance are caused by the index strain. The physical location and physiologic status of index strain cells that remain after successful antibiotic therapy are unknown. It has been proposed that the bladder epithelium can act as a persistent reservoir for "quiescent" uropathogenic *Escherichia coli* bacteria, which can result in infection when reentering an active replicative state. The physiologic status of bacteria found in clean-catch urine specimens from humans and mice was characterized.

Methods.—Urine specimens were obtained for culture from women infected with a UTI, and bladder-isolated urine specimens were obtained from BALB/c mice.

Results.—The urine specimens obtained from the women volunteers were found to contain significantly more viable than culturable forms of bacteria. Examination of the bladder-isolated urine specimens from the mice provided additional support for the presence of viable but nonculturable cells in urine specimens considered sterile. Because the viability assay used to study the viable but nonculturable condition is growth independent and therefore indirect, the accuracy of this assay was investigated. More than 95% of *E coli* cells exposed to lethal doses of ultraviolet radiation were found to lose the integrity of their membrane within 1 day, which is similar to the time frame used to examine urine specimens.

Conclusions.—Viable but nonculturable cells can occur within regions of the urinary tract that have previously been considered sterile.

▶ There is a metabolic state of quiescence that certain bacteria (particularly gram-negatives) may enter in response to certain environmental stresses, such as lack of nutrients, temperature shifts, and exposure to metals. This state is one in which the bacterial cells retain detectable metabolic activity but cannot be cultured on nonselective media. Since it is culturability that has been the defining factor in declaring parts of the urinary tract normally sterile heretofore, a question naturally arises. Could a reservoir of these viable but nonculturable bacterial cells, present in various parts of the urinary tract, account for recurrent UTIs?

M. G. Bissell, MD, PhD, MPH

Nonvalue of Culturing Cerebrospinal Fluid for Fungi
Barenfanger J, Lawhorn J, Drake C (Mem Med Ctr, Springfield, Ill)
J Clin Microbiol 42:236-238, 2004   20–4

Background.—Studies have addressed the efficacy of performing mycobacterial cultures on CSF, but no studies have evaluated the efficacy of culturing CSF for fungi. In some laboratories, the criteria used for rejection of cultures on CSF for fungi may actually be similar to those established for the rejection of mycobacterial cultures. However, actual data to provide evidence for this process are lacking. The efficacy of routinely performing fungal cultures specifically for recovery of fungi on CSF has been questioned because *Cryptococcus* and *Candida* species grow well in media used for routine bacterial cultures and because cryptococcal antigen tests are commonly ordered. The clinical utility of routinely performing fungal cultures on CSF was determined.

Methods.—Data were examined from 1225 samples of CSF that had been cultured for both bacteria and fungi.

Results.—Fungi were present in 12 specimens, 10 from fungal cultures and 8 from bacterial cultures. *Cryptococcus neoformans* was found in 10 specimens, *Candida albicans* was found in 1 specimen, and *Cladosporium* species was found in 1 case. Of the 12 positive specimens, 8 had concordant culture results. Among the discordant culture results, 1 specimen was bacterial culture positive but fungal culture negative, and 3 specimens were fungal culture positive but bacterial culture negative. Of the 3 discordant fungal culture–positive specimens, 1 had fungal contamination only, and the other 2 were positive for cryptococcal antigen. Thus, the omission of the fungal cultures on these specimens would not adversely affect patients. When both bacterial cultures and cryptococcal antigen tests are ordered routinely, the elimination of fungal cultures on CSF would have had no adverse effect on the patients in this study.

Conclusions.—All the clinically significant fungi were detected by the cryptococcal antigen test or bacterial culture, or both. The combined use of the cryptococcal antigen test and bacterial culture of the CSF could, with a few exceptions, replace routine fungal cultures of CSF. The exceptions would include settings in which fungal pathogens other than *Cryptococcus* and *Candida* could be important causes of meningitis.

▶ It is good to have a definite evidence basis for determinations of when not to do things that have always routinely been done. This report documents for us that routinely ordering fungal cultures on CSF specimens being worked up on patients with suspected meningitis falls into this category. Between the fact that most suspect fungi grow on bacterial cultures and the fact that cryptococcal antigen testing is now routine, fungal cultures are redundant and unlikely to yield value.

M. G. Bissell, MD, PhD, MPH

Accuracy of Screening for Inhalational Anthrax After a Bioterrorist Attack
Hupert N, Bearman GML, Mushlin AI, et al (Cornell Univ, New York)
Ann Intern Med 139:337-345, 2003   20–5

Introduction.—The 2001 anthrax attacks in the United States, in which 11 people had the inhalation form of the disease and 5 died, demonstrated a weakness in the US medical response to bioterrorism. Physicians were largely unprepared to identify the early symptoms and signs of this extremely rare and rapidly progressive infection. Mass screening to identify early inhalation anthrax may enhance both the management of individual cases and the efficiency of health resource usage. Review, compilation, and data extraction from English-language case reports of inhalation anthrax and epidemiologic studies of influenza and other viral respiratory infections were performed to develop an evidence base for outpatient anthrax screening protocols. Differences in clinical presentation between inhalation anthrax and common viral respiratory tract infections were also determined.

Methods.—Data from 13 reports of 28 cases of inhalation anthrax from 1920 to 2001 and from 5 trials reporting the clinical characteristics of 2762 cases of influenza and 1932 cases of noninfluenza viral respiratory disease were reviewed. The presenting clinical symptoms in anthrax and viral disease were characterized. Likelihood ratios were calculated for the presence of selected clinical features.

Results.—Fever and cough do not reliably differentiate between inhalation anthrax and viral respiratory tract infection. Characteristics suggestive of anthrax include the presence of nonheadache neurologic symptoms (positive likelihood ratio cannot be calculated), dyspnea (positive likelihood ratio, 5.3 [95% confidence interval [CI], 3.7-7.4]), nausea or vomiting (positive likelihood ratio, 5.1 [95% CI, 3.0-8.5]), and finding of any abnormality on lung auscultation or lung auscultation (positive likelihood ratio, 8.1 [CI, 5.3-12.5]). Rhinorrhea (positive likelihood ratio, 0.2 [95% CI, 0.1-0.4]) and sore throat (positive likelihood ratio, 0.2 [95% CI, 0.1-0.5]) are more indicative of viral respiratory tract infection.

Conclusion.—Inhalation anthrax has characteristic clinical features that are different from those observed in common viral respiratory tract infections. Screening protocols based on these characteristics may enhance the rapid identification of patients with presumptive inhalation anthrax in the setting of a large-scale anthrax attack.

▶ As the 11 cases and 5 deaths from inhalational anthrax occurring in the United States during the bioterrorism incidents of 2001 illustrate, community-wide perceptions can drive enormous laboratory usage. For every death, literally hundreds of thousands of specimens were processed by clinical and public health laboratories. Clearly then, anything that would serve as a reliable guide to "rule out" prelaboratory order would favorably impact this state of affairs. The degree to which the clinical criteria presented here prove to be effective remains to be seen.

M. G. Bissell, MD, PhD, MPH

Visualizing Infection of Individual Influenza Viruses

Lakadamyali M, Rust MJ, Babcock HP, et al (Harvard Univ, Cambridge, Mass)
Proc Natl Acad Sci U S A 100:9280-9285, 2003   20–6

Introduction.—As an opportunistic pathogen exploiting the cellular endocytic machinery, influenza also acts as a valuable model system for exploring the cell's constitutive endocytic pathway. The transport, acidification, and fusion of single influenza viruses in living cells were analyzed via real-time fluorescence microscopy. Individual stages of the viral entry pathway were examined.

Findings.—The movement of individual viruses demonstrated a notable 3-stage active transport process that preceded viral fusion with endosomes, beginning with an actin-dependent movement in the cell periphery, then followed by a rapid-dynein-directed translocation to the perinuclear region,

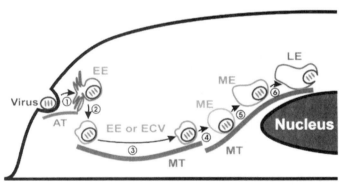

FIGURE 5.—A model of the endocytic pathway toward late endosomes. (1) The virus is internalized and transported to the early endosome (EE) in an actin (AT)-dependent way (stage I movement). (2) The virus-containing endocytic compartment leaves the EE, still at the extracellular pH. This may occur either through a virus-bearing endocytic carrier vesicle (ECV) budding from the EE or the membrane-rich tubular region of the EE recycling to leave a more vesicular EE that contains the virus. (3) The ECV or vesicular EE is transported to the perinuclear region via a dynein-directed movement on a microtubule (MT) (stage II movement). (4) The ECV or vesicular EE matures into a maturing endosome (ME) by changing the membrane-bound motor protein activity (transition from stage II to stage III movement). (5) The endosome further matures by changing its pH from the extracellular value to pH ≈6 (initial acidification as indicated by the change in fluorescence ratio between CypHer 5 and Cy3 conjugated to viruses). (6) Further acidification brings the pH of the endosome to the late endosomal (LE) value, pH ≈5 (second acidification as indicated by viral fusion). (Courtesy of Lakadamyali M, Rust MJ, Babcock HP, et al: Visualizing infection of individual influenza viruses. *Proc Natl Acad Sci U S A* 100:9280-9285, 2003. Copyright 2003, National Academy of Sciences, U.S.A.)

and finally, an intermittent movement involving both plus- and minus-end-directed microtubule-based motilities in the perinuclear regions (Fig 5).

Conclusion.—Surprisingly, most viruses experience their initial acidification in the perinuclear region immediately after the dynein-directed rapid translocation step. This finding indicates a previously undescribed scenario of the endocytic pathway toward late endosomes: endosome maturation, including initial acidification, mainly occurs in the perinuclear region.

▶ Those of us who use science findings mainly as consumers can be the conceptual victims of other peoples' cartoons, that is, conceptual simplifications made graphic. This graphic thinking in our basic science background can lead us to believe that certain cellular processes, for example, proceed in ways that are intuitive. The mechanisms underlying these processes, in fact, may not be at all well understood. This article helps us with a better mechanistic understanding of 1 of these basic cellular processes underlying viral infection of cells. Note the accompanying cartoon.

M. G. Bissell, MD, PhD, MPH

Discovery of Gene Function by Expression Profiling of the Malaria Parasite Life Cycle
Le Roch KG, Zhou Y, Blair PL, et al (Scripps Research Inst, La Jolla, Calif; Genomics Inst of the Novartis Research Found, San Diego, Calif; Naval Med Research Ctr, Silver Spring, Md; et al)
Science 301:1503-1508, 2003   20–7

Background.—The completion of the genome sequence for *Plasmodium falciparum*, which is responsible for most human deaths from malaria, has the potential to reveal hundreds of new drug targets and proteins involved in the pathogenesis of malaria. However, only approximately 35% of the genes code for proteins with an identifiable function. The absence of routine genetic tools for the study of *Plasmodium* parasites suggests a lack of rapid change in this number if conventional serial methods are used for characterizations of encoded proteins. Expression profiles of human and mosquito stages of the malaria parasite's life cycle were generated.

Methods.—Nine different stages of development were examined: mosquito salivary gland sporozoites, which infect humans; seven periodic erythrocytic asexual time points, from early ring forms through mature schizonts to free merozoites, the stages responsible for the pathologic manifestations of malaria; and the sexual stage gametocytes, from which the parasite is transmitted from humans to mosquitoes. A high-density oligonucleotide array was used to characterize encoded proteins.

Results.—By means of a probability function based on a gene's expression level and its probe signal distribution, it was determined that 4557 genes (88% of the predicted genes) were expressed in at least 1 stage of the mosquito life cycle. The proportion of expression for different functional classes for different states is evidence of the shift in transcriptional energy from protein synthesis to cell surface structures within the life cycle. Among the most highly expressed genes (2%) were many that encode ribosomal proteins, histones, or actin and genes involved in glucose metabolism.

Conclusion.—This study presented a description of a custom-made, high-density oligonucleotide array that was designed by using the *P falciparum* genome nucleotide sequence to determine the relative level and temporal pattern of expression of over 95% of the predicted *P falciparum* genes through the course of the mosquito's life cycle. These data, when combined with sequence data, should be viewed as starting points for investigators interested in the validation of some of the thousands of proteins identified as new drug or vaccine targets in the *P falciparum* genome sequencing projects.

▶ Identifying new biomarkers and drug targets for the various stages of the malaria parasite life cycle will lead to progress against a real scourge of mankind. The authors of his article make the case that that will only happen with the aid of efficient, high-throughput gene expression profiling analysis.

M. G. Bissell, MD, PhD, MPH

Early Diagnosis of Typhoid Fever by the Detection of Salivary IgA
Herath HMTU (Univ of London)
J Clin Pathol 56:694-698, 2003

20–8

Background.—Typhoid fever is an endemic disease that continues to be a significant public health problem in the developing countries of Southeast Asia, the Indian subcontinent, parts of Central and South America, and in much of sub-Saharan Africa. The diagnosis of typhoid is based on a combination of the clinical picture, the isolation of *Salmonella typhi* from body fluids, and the Wildt test. The most widely used serological assay for typhoid is the Widal test. This test has some disadvantages when used in endemic areas and has low sensitivity and specificity. The utility of the enzyme-linked immunosorbent assay (ELISA) in the diagnosis of typhoid fever has been determined by various investigations using serum and urine.

It has been determined that the ELISA using serum and urine has greater sensivity and specificity than the Widal test. This study set out to develop an ELISA with greater sensitivity and specificity for the detection of salivary immunoglobulin A for early diagnosis of typhoid fever.

Methods.—The ELISA was developed and evaluated in 29 patients with hemocultures positive for *S typhi*, 51 patients with hemocultures negative for *S typhi*, and 125 healthy control subjects who were blood donors and volunteers. A sequential study of patients with culture-confirmed typhoid was also performed to determine the time of maximum sensitivity.

Results.—The ELISA was able to successfully detect anti–*S typhi* lipopolysaccharide salivary immunoglobulin A antibodies. A 6-month follow-up study of patients with culture-confirmed typhoid fever demonstrated that the ELISA was at maximum efficiency during the second and third weeks of fever and facilitated detection of the acute infection during the early phase.

Conclusion.—The ELISA has the capacity for detection of typhoid fever during the early phase of infection and is most efficient in the second and third weeks of fever, when patients are typically first seen for treatment. This test will be useful for the diagnosis of acute infection because the sensitivity of the assay is greatly reduced after the second and third weeks of fever.

► Saliva is a potentially very useful noninvasive specimen for testing in field conditions and for epidemiologic studies. With the variation in presentation shown by typhoid fever in recent years and its high third world incidence, this development of a saliva-based assay for immunoglobulin A anti-typhoid lipo-polysaccharide antibodies is timely.

M. G. Bissell, MD, PhD, MPH

Transmission of West Nile Virus Through Blood Transfusion in the United States in 2002
Pealer LN, for the West Nile Virus Transmission Investigation Team (Ctrs for Disease Control and Prevention, Atlanta, Ga and Fort Collins, Colo; et al)
N Engl J Med 349:1236-1245, 2003   20–9

Introduction.—During the 2002 West Nile virus epidemic in the United States, some patients had a West Nile virus illness that was temporarily linked with the receipt of transfused blood and blood components. The findings from recipients suspected of acquiring West Nile virus through transfusion of blood components are reported in a study that also investigated the transfusion donors.

Methods.—Patients with laboratory evidence of recent West Nile virus infection within 4 weeks after receipt of a blood component from a donor with viremia were considered to have a confirmed transfusion-associated infection. Donors of the components were interviewed about whether they had symptoms compatible with the presence of a viral illness before or after their donation. Blood specimens retained from the time of donation and collected at follow-up were analyzed for West Nile virus.

Results.—Twenty-three patients were verified to have acquired West Nile virus through transfused leukoreduced and nonleukoreduced red cells, platelets, or fresh-frozen plasma. Of the 23 recipients, 10 (43%) were immunocompromised because of transplantation or cancer. Eight patients (35%) were 70 years or older. Immunocompromised recipients tended to have longer incubation periods than did nonimmunocompromised recipients and infected individuals in mosquito-borne community outbreaks. Sixteen donors with evidence of viremia at donation were linked to the 23 recipients with West Nile virus infection. Of these, 9 donors reported viral symptoms before or after donation, 5 were asymptomatic, and 2 were lost to follow-up. Fevers, new rashes, and painful eyes were independently linked with being a donor with viremia rather than a donor without viremia. All 16 donors had negative test results for West Nile virus-specific IgM antibody at donation.

Conclusion.—It is possible for transfused red cells, platelets, and fresh-frozen plasma to transmit West Nile virus. Screening of potential donors with the use of nucleic acid–based assays for West Nile virus may decrease this risk.

▶ The societal concern associated with the appearance or emergence of a new blood-borne pathogen is always a very great one. This concern however is multiplied instantaneously by verifying the presence of the organism in the nation's blood supply. With each new threat that must be averted through screening, the cost of blood, already high, inevitably increases, adding insult to injury, as it were.

M. G. Bissell, MD, PhD, MPH

Relationships Between Patient- and Institution-Specific Variables and Decreased Antimicrobial Susceptibility of Gram-Negative Pathogens
Bhavnani SM, Hammel JP, Forrest A, et al (Cognigen Corp, Buffalo, NY; Univ at Buffalo, New York; JONES Group/JMI Labs, North Liberty, Iowa; et al)
Clin Infect Dis 37:344-350, 2003   20–10

Background.—Antimicrobial resistance is a problem throughout the world. The pharmaceutical industry has recently shifted its focus away from the development of antibiotics, particularly those for the treatment of patients infected with antibiotic-resistant bacteria. As various organizations in this country engage in discussions of issues and strategies for maintaining high standards for the clinical study of new antimicrobial agents, it has become clear that there is a need for more-complete information to identify patients who have serious infections associated with antibiotic-resistant organisms.

The identification of patients who are infected with antibiotic-resistant strains of bacteria for inclusion in clinical trials has become a serious challenge to the future development of agents to combat these infections. This study provided an overview of the Antimicrobial Resistance Rate Epidemiology Study (ARREST), a collaborative effort to use surveillance data and analytic techniques to more fully understand the factors predictive of antimicrobial resistance. The utility of these analytical techniques was also discussed.

Methods.—Five years (1997-2001) of North American surveillance data were analyzed to identify patient- and institution-specific factors predictive of reduced susceptibility of *Enterobacter* species, *Pseudomonas aeruginosa*, and *Klebsiella pneumoniae* to cefepime, ciprofloxacin, and piperacillin-tazobactam. The relationship between minimum inhibitory concentration (MIC) values for each organism-agent pair and patient- and institution-specific variables was analyzed with multivariable general linear modeling.

Results.—The variables most commonly associated with decreases in susceptibility were duration of hospital stay before pathogen isolation, hospital size, primary diagnosis, and medical service. Combinations of these variables were associated with increases in observed MIC_{90} values of as much as 16- to 32-fold.

Conclusion.—A relationship between MIC and certain patient- and institution-specific variables is demonstrated by these findings. These data should be considered in the design of clinical trials directed toward the study of resistant pathogens.

▶ There are a great deal of data around the world on antimicrobial susceptibility patterns of pathogenic microorganisms in inpatient settings. The authors here suggest an approach to utilizing the demographic information associated with these data to guide the design of some very badly needed multicentric clinical trials by the pharmaceutical industry. With recent de-emphasis on the problem by the pharmaceutical industry, the need to take up and more deeply understand the problem of antibiotic resistance has never been greater.

M. G. Bissell, MD, PhD, MPH

Classification of Transmission Risk in the National HIV/AIDS Surveillance System
Lee LM, McKenna MT, Janssen RS (Ctrs for Disease Control and Prevention, Atlanta, Ga)
Public Health Rep 118:400-407, 2003   20–11

Background.—AIDS has been a reportable condition since the early 1980s in all 50 states, the District of Columbia, and all US possessions and dependencies. The primary goals of the national HIV/AIDS surveillance system are to monitor the epidemic by counting cases and estimating the incidence and prevalence and to determine the epidemiology of HIV by answering questions related to person, place, and time. The ultimate purpose of these data collection efforts is to guide public health programs and practice, to prevent new HIV infections, and to prevent morbidity and mortality in persons already infected with AIDS.

Risk behavior information is an essential component of the appropriate allocation of resources and development of effective HIV prevention strategies. However, over time, transmission risk information on HIV/AIDS cases has been less likely to be reported to the national surveillance system. As a result, a consultation group was convened by the Centers for Disease Control and Prevention (CDC) to generate recommendations on how to deal with the lack of risk data. The utility of these recommended changes was assessed.

Methods.—A consultation was conducted in December 2001 among approximately 30 experts in HIV/AIDS and behavioral research from state and local health departments, academia, community-based organizations, and the CDC. The group was given the task of providing recommendations on methods for classifying and reporting risk information and for identifying methods and sources for improving the ascertainment of transmission risk behaviors for individuals infected with HIV.

Results.—The committee has recommended 2 changes in how the CDC presents HIV/AIDS transmission risk data. First, it was recommended that a probable heterosexual contact category be added to the list of current modes of exposure. The second recommended change was the discontinuation of use of the hierarchy of most probable mode of transmission and reporting of mutually exclusive categories of all risk behaviors.

Conclusion.—A scientific approach using a standard definition of high-risk heterosexual behavior has been recommended over the presumption that patients having heterosexual partners and no other reported risk factor be designated as presumed heterosexual contact. The effective surveillance of HIV risk behaviors among persons with newly diagnosed HIV will require a variety of data collection strategies and statistical approaches.

▶ Systematically collected information on behavioral characteristics associated with increased risk of HIV transmission remains essential to combating the AIDS epidemic. This information has been less frequently collected in recent years, and this article represents an attempt to glean the thoughts of some of the best experts in the field on how to revise our approaches to risk classification and reporting. This is intended to address this critical issue.

M. G. Bissell, MD, PhD, MPH

21 Clinical Immunology and Hematology

Elimination of Instrument-Driven Reflex Manual Differential Leukocyte Counts: Optimization of Manual Blood Smear Review Criteria in a High-Volume Automated Hematology Laboratory
Lantis KL, Harris RJ, Davis G, et al (Univ of Michigan, Ann Arbor)
Am J Clin Pathol 119:656-662, 2003   21–1

Background.—The use of automated peripheral blood leukocyte differential counts (LDCs) is widely accepted in routine practice. However, many laboratories still reflexively perform manual LDCs that are based solely on abnormal automated results or instrument "flags," before any manual triage step is taken. The transition at one institution to a procedure in which manual methods are used to validate, rather than to replace, automated LDCs was described.

Methods.—Before the implementation of a revised manual review policy, the standard procedure at the study institution included instrument criteria by which blood smears should be microscopically scanned before determining the appropriateness of a manual LDC and instrument criteria by which a manual LDC should be ordered reflexively, without initial microscopic scan (Fig 1). In the revised system, criteria for the instrument-driven reflexive performance of manual differential counts were eliminated, except when the instrument was unable to issue any differential result because of marked interference (the so-called dot-out results). The arbitrary limit of greater than 2 immature granulocytes discovered on scanning was selected for the performance of a manual differential count. The finding of even a single promyelocyte or a single blast on scanning triggered the ordering of a manual LDC. After implementation of the new policy, the performance of the new system was analyzed by a series of audits that involved a total of 204 cases for which manual scans were performed but for which the automated LDC was released. Quantitative comparisons between automated and manual LDCs were made with the Student *t* test and Pearson correlation coefficients.

Results.—The revised policy reduced manual LDCs by more than 70%. These results were validated by a manual retrospective audit.

Conclusions.—Laboratory operations and patient care can be improved by the use of manual microscopic examination as a validation procedure

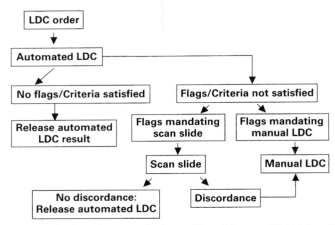

FIGURE 1.—Algorithm for performance of leukocyte differential counts (*LDCs*) before elimination of reflex manual differential counts based on instrument criteria. (Courtesy of Lantis KL, Harris RJ, Davis G, et al: Elimination of instrument-driven reflex manual differential leukocyte counts: Optimization of manual blood smear review criteria in a high-volume automated hematology laboratory. *Am J Clin Pathol* 119:656-662, 2003. Copyright 2003 by the American Society for Clinical Pathology. Reprinted with permission.)

rather than as a reflexive substitute for automated methods. No clinical rationale exists for reflex performance of manual LDCs based solely on instrument warnings.

▶ This issue of whether and/or when to reflexly perform manual "diffs" in response to instrument flags has waxed heated at various times and in various places. The current authors have apparently successfully reduced utilization of the manual diff in their institution by redefining it to be a validation of the instrument count, rather than a replacement for it. The question going forward will be just how widely and rapidly their example can be emulated.

M. G. Bissell, MD, PhD, MPH

Gene Expression Profiling During All-*trans* Retinoic Acid–Induced Cell Differentiation of Acute Promyelocytic Leukemia Cells

Yang L, Zhao H, Li S-W, et al (Univ of Florida, Gainesville; Med College of Georgia, Augusta)
J Mol Diag 5:212-221, 2003   21–2

Background.—Acute promyelocytic leukemia (APL), a subtype of acute myeloid leukemia, is characterized by the accumulation of cells arrested at the promyelocytic stage of myeloid differentiation. APL cells are extremely sensitive to all-*trans* retinoic acid (ATRA), which induces APL cell differentiation into mature granulocytes and leads to cell apoptosis. The use of ATRA in addition to chemotherapy has provided a high rate of complete remission and long-term survival. It is generally believed that ATRA-induced differentiation of APL cells to a mature state is mediated, at least partially, by the regulation of gene transcription. The transcription events that occur in the ATRA-induced cell differentiation process in APL cells were determined.

Methods.—The expression of 12,288 genes in the human APL NB4 cell line was analyzed after 12 hours, 24 hours, 48 hours, 72 hours, and 96 hours of exposure to ATRA by means of complementary DNA (cDNA) microassays.

Results.—A total of 168 upregulated genes and 179 downregulated genes were identified. Most of these genes have not previously been reported. Many of the altered genes were observed to encode products that participate in signaling pathways, cell differentiation, programmed cell death, transcription regulation, and production of cytokines and chemokines. An interesting finding was that the CD52 and protein kinase A regulatory subunit α (PKA-R1α) genes, the products of which are being used as therapeutic targets for certain human neoplasias in current clinical trials, were among the genes observed to be significantly upregulated after ATRA treatment.

Conclusions.—This study provides valuable data to further elucidate the mechanism of ATRA-induced APL cell differentiation and suggests potential therapeutic alternatives for APL.

▶ This article is another example of the value of cDNA microarray analysis profiling of gene expression patterns. Among the upregulated genes, the authors found CD52 and PKA-R1α, both known drug targets for the drug differentiation of PML that takes place with ATRA treatment.

M. G. Bissell, MD, PhD, MPH

Parallel Detection of Autoantibodies With Microarrays in Rheumatoid Diseases
Feng Y, Ke X, Ma R, et al (Shangai HealthDigit Co Ltd, China)
Clin Chem 50:416-422, 2004   21–3

Introduction.—Clinical needs frequently govern testing for several autoantibodies in a single patient with evidence of autoimmune disease. A microarray system was developed containing 15 autoantigens for identification of autoantibodies in the rheumatic autoimmune diseases.

Methods.—Recombinant centromere protein B, cytokeratin 19, SSA 52-kDa antigen, SSA 60-kDa antigen, SSB antigen, and Jo-1 antigen were synthesized, and antinuclear antibody antigens were prepared. Cyclic citrullinated peptide, histone, goat IgG for identification of rheumatoid factor, double-stranded DNA, and single-stranded DNA were obtained, as were recombinant small nuclear ribonucleoprotein U1, topoisomerase I, and Smith antigen (Sm). All 15 antigens were of human origin, with the exception of calf thymus Sm. The proteins were printed on polystyrene. The arrays were incubated using serum samples, then with horseradish peroxidase-conjugated secondary antibodies and chemiluminescent substrates. Light signals were captured via a charge-coupled device camera-based chip reader. Antibodies were quantified via use of calibration curves. Positive samples were verified by commercially available methods.

Results.—The detection limit of the microarray system was 20 pg of IgG, which was printed on the polystyrene support. More than 85% of the verified positive sera were so identified on the basis of cutoff values instituted with the microarray system. The imprecision (CV) of the microarrays was less than 15% for all 15 autoantibody assays, except for single-stranded DNA within and between batches (18% and 23%, respectively). Characteristic autoantibody patterns were seen in 83 patients with clinical diagnoses of rheumatoid arthritis, 71 with systemic lupus erythematosus, 36 with systemic sclerosis, 38 with polymyositis, and 20 with Sjögren syndrome.

Conclusion.—The described microarray system provides results similar to those of conventional methods. Evaluation of the diagnostic accuracy of the system needs to be performed.

▶ Let's face it, autoimmune diseases have always been just plain hard to test for. The need for a variety of immunologic laboratory methods, including relatively nonspecific morphologic ones, have contributed to an impression that this group of diseases is ill-defined. This study suggests that all of this may partly be a bioinformatics problem, approachable by the creation of microarrays providing numerous simultaneous serologic results interpretable as a pattern.

M. G. Bissell, MD, PhD, MPH

Acanthocytes in the Urine: Useful Tool to Differentiate Diabetic Nephropathy From Glomerulonephritis?

Heine GH, Girndt M, Sester U, et al (Univ of Homburg, Germany)
Diabetes Care 27:190-194, 2004   21–4

Introduction.—It has been suggested that microscopic hematuria in patients with diabetes is indicative of nondiabetic glomerulopathy. Hematuria is often found in patients with biopsy-verified diabetic glomerulosclerosis without nondiabetic nephropathy. Urine microscopy provides discrimination of glomerular hematuria, which is defined as acanthocyturia (urinary excretion of acanthocytes, which are dysmorphic erythrocytes with vesicle-like protrusions), from nonglomerular hematuria. The prevalences of hematuria and acanthocyturia in patients with clinically diagnosed diabetic nephropathy and in patients with biopsy-verified glomerulonephritis were investigated to determine whether acanthocyturia occurs with both glomerular lesions or whether it is specific for glomerulonephritis.

Methods.—Urine samples of 68 patients with diabetic nephropathy, 43 patients with biopsy-confirmed glomerulonephritis, and 20 age-matched healthy control subjects were analyzed via phase-contrast microscopy for the presence of hematuria (≥ 8 erythrocytes/μL) and acanthocyturia. Acanthocyturia of 5% or more (5 acanthocytes among 100 excreted eryth-

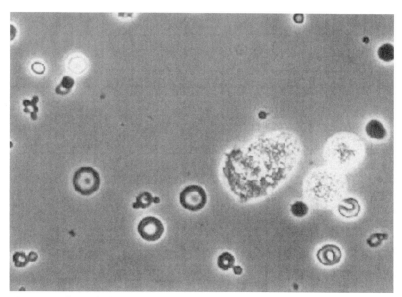

FIGURE 1.—Glomerular hematuria characterized by the presence of 5% or more acanthocytes (ring-formed erythrocytes with vesicle-shaped protrusions) among all erythrocytes excreted (phase-contrast microscopy). (Courtesy of Heine GH, Girndt M, Sester U, et al: Acanthocytes in the urine: Useful tool to differentiate diabetic nephropathy from glomerulonephritis? *Diabetes Care* 27:190-194, 2004. Reprinted with permission from The American Diabetes Association.)

rocytes) was categorized as glomerular hematuria (Fig 1); acanthocyturia of 2% to 4% was categorized as suspected glomerular hematuria.

Results.—Hematuria was detected in 62% of patients with the clinical diagnosis of diabetic nephropathy, in 84% of those diagnosed with glomerulonephritis, and in 20% of the healthy control subjects on a single urine examination. Glomerular hematuria was observed in 4% of patients with diabetic nephropathy and in 40% of those with glomerulonephritis ($P < .001$).

Conclusion.—In contrast to hematuria, acanthocyturia is not common in patients with diabetic nephropathy. In patients with diabetes and proteinuria, the presence of acanthocyturia indicates nondiabetic glomerulopathies, and a renal biopsy is recommended.

▶ Urinary red blood cells indicate glomerular damage, but the specific morphology of these cells conveys additional information. This study is an important addition to the evidence base for interpretation of microscopic urinalysis in the context of diabetes: urinary acanthocytes indicate nondiabetic nephropathy superimposed on the diabetes.

M. G. Bissell, MD, PhD, MPH

Noninvasive Monitoring of Hemoglobin: The Effects of WBC Counts on Measurement

Saigo K, Imoto S, Hashimoto M, et al (Kobe Univ, Japan; Kakogawa Municipal Hosp, Japan; Hyogo Red Cross Blood Ctr, Kobe, Japan; et al)

Am J Clin Pathol 121:51-55, 2004   21–5

Background.—Noninvasive monitoring with near-infrared radiation has gained wide clinical use. In 1999, a Japanese company developed a device for monitoring hemoglobin levels by using the principle of near-infrared spectroscopy in combination with analysis of optical images taken by a charge-coupled device camera located at the opposite side of light sources (Fig 1). The utility of this device for the monitoring of hemoglobin levels in patients with hematologic disorders was investigated.

Methods.—The efficacy of a noninvasive hemoglobin monitoring device was evaluated in 97 healthy volunteers and in 49 patients with hematologic

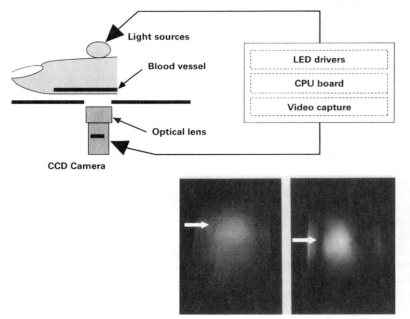

FIGURE 1.—Principles of measuring and sample imaging. Incident near-infrared light is transmitted from light sources (light-emitting diode [*LED*]) to a charge-coupled device (*CCD*) camera, accompanied by absorption and scattering in the human finger. Absorption is due mainly to hemoglobin in blood and scattering to tissue in the finger. The optical image of the transmitted lights taken by the CCD camera can visualize the peripheral blood vessels in the finger. Hemoglobin levels are calculated by examining the optical image of blood vessels in the finger. Sample optical images are shown on the **bottom**. The **bottom left panel** shows an image of the finger of an anemic volunteer with a hemoglobin level of 10.7 g/dL (107 g/L) featuring low contrast between the blood vessel (*arrow*) and the surrounding tissue. On the **bottom right** is an image of the finger of a healthy volunteer with a hemoglobin level of 17.1 g/dL (171 g/L) featuring high contrast between the blood vessel (*arrow*) and the surrounding tissue. *Abbreviation: CPU,* Central processing unit. (Courtesy of Saigo K, Imoto S, Hashimoto M, et al: Noninvasive monitoring of hemoglobin: The effects of WBC counts on measurement. *Am J Clin Pathol* 121:51-55, 2004. Copyright 2004 by the American Society of Clinical Pathologists. Reprinted with permission.)

disorders. Concurrently, the effects of white blood cell counts on noninvasive monitoring were studied by clinical evaluation and ex vivo experiments. Comparisons were made between the hemoglobin levels determined by the device (Ast-Hb) and a conventional analyzer (T-Hb).

Results.—The coefficient of correlation between the findings with the Ast-Hb and the T-Hb was $r = 0.626$ for healthy volunteers compared with a coefficient of $r = 0.762$ for patients with hematologic disorders. Comparison of the ratios of measurement errors in hemoglobin levels by Ast-Hb and T-Hb indicated that the number of white blood cells had no effect on hemoglobin monitoring. The results were confirmed in ex vivo studies on isolated white blood cells and an optical model imitative of blood vessels and tissue in human fingers.

Conclusions.—These findings support the utility of this new hemoglobin monitoring device for continuous monitoring of hemoglobin.

▶ Near-infrared spectroscopy is a practical approach to noninvasive hemoglobin monitoring that correlates reasonably well (although not perfectly) with central lab values. In this study, the authors investigate the effect of white blood cell count and hypergammaglobulinemia on the hemoglobin values produced by the Sysmex Astrim near-infrared instrument.

M. G. Bissell, MD, PhD, MPH

Monocytes With Altered Phenotypes in Posttrauma Patients
Kampalath B, Cleveland RP, Chang C-C, et al (Med College of Wisconsin, Milwaukee; Case Western Reserve Univ, Cleveland, Ohio)
Arch Pathol Lab Med 127:1580-1585, 2003   21–6

Background.—Posttrauma patients are extremely susceptible to life-threatening infections, and posttrauma sepsis is a major cause of morbidity and mortality in the United States. Studies have shown that monocytes in posttrauma patients can express decreased human leukocyte antigen (HLA)-DR and that the induction of HLA-DR with interferon-γ does not reduce the susceptibility of these patients to infection. That finding suggests the presence of additional factors that may be involved in the impaired immune responsiveness.

CD4 has a central role in most of the functions of HLA-DR. A previous study found a concomitant reduction of CD4 on monocytes with decreased HLA expression. Monocytes in posttrauma patients were evaluated for morphology, co-expression of CD4 and HLA-DR, and activity of α-naphthyl butyrate esterase.

Methods.—Monocyte morphology; expression of CD4, CD11b, CD13, CD16, and HLA-DR by 3-color flow cytometry; and analysis of α-naphthyl butyrate esterase activity by cytochemical staining were investigated in 27 posttrauma patients and 20 control subjects.

Results.—There were significant differences in several characteristics of monocytes of posttrauma patients compared with those of control subjects, including an increase in subsets displaying the CD4⁻/CD14+/HLA-DR⁻ and CD⁻/CD14+/CD16⁻ phenotypes; decrease in mean fluorescence intensity of CD4 and HLA-DR expression in monocytes that were positive for these markers; decrease in α-naphthyl butyrate esterase activity; and decrease in the amount of cytoplasm and cytoplasmic vacuoles.

Conclusion.—These findings suggest that in posttrauma patients, as in newborns, there is a significant increase in monocytes and decreased expression of CD4 and HLA-DR as well as decreased α-naphthyl butyrate esterase activity. It is possible that a concomitant reduction in CD4 and HLA-DR expression on monocytes may be involved in the impairment of the immune response in posttrauma patients.

▶ In seeking to better understand the relative immune suppression associated with the posttrauma state, the current authors compare it to the immune status of the normal newborn. Specifically, monocyte subsets with altered phenotypic profiles appear to be characteristic of both states.

M. G. Bissell, MD, PhD, MPH

β-Thalassemia Microelectronic Chip: A Fast and Accurate Method for Mutation Detection
Foglieni B, Cremonesi L, Travi M, et al (Ospedale San Raffaele, Milan, Italy; Istituti Clinici di Perfezionamento, Milan, Italy; Università di Ferrara, Italy; et al)
Clin Chem 50:73-79, 2004   21–7

Background.—Over 200 causative molecular defects have been described in the β-globin gene that causes β-thalassemia, one of the most common human genetic diseases. A previous study demonstrated the feasibility of performing single-nucleotide polymorphism/mutation analysis in a clinical setting with the use of a commercially available microelectronic platform.

The purpose of this study was to further develop this technology for fast and reliable detection of the 9 most frequent mutations that cause more than 95% of the β-thalassemia alleles in the Mediterranean region. Ultimately, it is expected that further development of this technology will provide a system that covers all or most of the common β-thalassemia–associated mutations that can be easily applied to the analysis of other common diseases.

Methods.—A microchip-based assay identified the 9 most frequent mutations in the β-globin gene by use of the Nanogen Workstation. The biotinylated amplicon was electronically addressed on the chip to selected pads and remained embedded through interaction with streptavidin in the permeation layer. The DNA at each test site was then hybridized to a mixture of fluorescently labeled wild-type or mutant probes.

Results.—Assay conditions were established on the basis of an analysis of 700 DNA samples from compound heterozygotes for the 9 mutations. The assays were blindly validated on 250 mDNA samples previously genotyped by other methods, with complete concordance of results. An exploration of alternative multiplexed formats showed that the combination of multiplex polymerase chain reaction with multiple addressing and/or hybridization allowed analysis of all 9 mutations in the same sample on 1 test site of the chip.

Conclusion.—The open flexible platform represented by the β-thalassemia microelectronic chip can be designed by the user according to the local prevalence of mutations in each geographic area. The results of these experiments demonstrated that this platform can be rapidly extended to include the remaining mutations that are responsible for β-thalassemia in other parts of the world.

▶ What do you do when you have an extremely common genetic condition with clinical consequences and very complex underlying genetics? These days the answer increasingly is: You develop a gene chip assay. The current authors, in addressing the screening/diagnostic problem in β-thalassemia, used the principle of hybridization of probes to DNA molecules electronically immobilized on microchips that target numerous mutations.

M. G. Bissell, MD, PhD, MPH

Novel Translocation in Acute Megakaryoblastic Leukemia (AML-M7)
Toretsky JA, Everly EM, Padilla-Nash HM, et al (Univ of Maryland, Baltimore; NIH, Bethesda, Md; MD Anderson Cancer Ctr, Houston; et al)
J Pediatr Hematol Oncol 25:396-402, 2003   21–8

Background.—Chromosome abnormalities have aided determination of the prognosis of patients with acute megakaryoblastic leukemia (AML). AML subtype M7 is a relatively rare form of leukemia that is found in 7% to 10% of all pediatric patients with AML. There are now well-established immunohistochemical identification criteria for the diagnosis of AML-M7, but its cytogenetic evaluation is still evolving. AML-M7 has a younger age of onset than other subtypes of AML and is poorly responsive to therapy. It is a rare diagnosis in children without Down syndrome, and there is a need for more information to assess the prognosis. A novel karyotype for a patient with AML-M7 who died 18 months after diagnosis was presented.

Case Report.—Girl, 22 months, was referred for evaluation of new-onset rash and bruising. No overt bleeding was reported. A distant cousin of the child had been given a diagnosis of leukemia, but there was no family history of malignancy diagnosed at an unusually young age, and no family history of bleeding disorders. Initial review of the peripheral smear showed no abnormal white cells, and other laboratory studies were normal. The patient appeared to have immune thrombocytopenia purpura, but a bone marrow aspirate was performed because the patient appeared mildly ischemic, and the biopsy showed cells suspicious for malignancy.

Follow-up bone marrow aspirates and core biopsies were performed and evaluated for histology, immunophenotype, and cytogenetic studies, including special karyotyping. After repeated bone marrow aspirations, the patient was given a diagnosis of AML-M7. She underwent induction chemotherapy and later underwent an allogeneic marrow graft.

The patient experienced grade 2 graft-versus-host disease of the skin, which was treated with a pulse of high-dose steroid followed by taper. Sepsis subsequently developed and the girl died with relapsed disease after bone marrow transplantation. Tumor cells were evaluated by cytogenetics (including spectral karyotyping), immunohistochemistry, and flow cytometry. The patient was found to have a previously unreported complex translocation as follows: 50,XX,der(1) t(1;5)(p36?.1;p15?.1),del(5)(p15?.1),+6,+der(6;7)(?;?),der(7) t(6;7)(?;p22)[2],der(9)t(6;9)(?;p21)t(9;14)(q34;q11.2-q13), +10.t(12;16)(p13;q24),-14[2],del(14)(q13)[2],+der(19)t(1; 19) (?;p13.3),+22[cp 4].

Conclusion.—Acute megakaryoblastic leukemia subtype M7 is a rare condition in children without Down syndrome, and improved diagnostic markers are required.

▶ Megakaryoblastic leukemia is a subtype of AML representing 7% to 10% of pediatric cases and first described in 1931. Immunophenotypic criteria are now well established, but the cytogenetics are not as well characterized. Therapeutic stratification of other forms of AML have greatly benefited from cytogenetic analysis; hopefully, this one (AML-M7) will as well.

M. G. Bissell, MD, PhD, MPH

Multiplex RT-PCR for the Detection of Leukemia-Associated Translocations: Validation and Application to Routine Molecular Diagnostic Practice
Salto-Tellez M, Shelat SG, Benoit B, et al (Natl Univ of Singapore; Univ of Pennsylvania, Philadelphia)
J Mol Diag 5:231-236, 2003   21–9

Background.—The pathologic approach to the diagnosis of acute leukemia is multifaceted, involving morphology; cytochemistry; immunophenotyping; and cytogenetic, molecular, and diagnostic studies. Although each of these components is crucial to appropriate diagnostic evaluation, there is increasing evidence that major disease-defining, prognostically relevant, and therapy-determining data are provided by the cytogenetic and molecular diagnostic studies.

Conventional cytogenetic studies have long been the cornerstone of genetic testing, but molecular-based technologies have recently emerged as a most useful tool for the detection of disease-defining genetic lesions. The purpose of this study was to validate the use of a commercially available multiplex reverse transcription–polymerase chain reaction assay for the 7 most common leukemia translocations for routine molecular diagnostic hematopathology practice.

Methods.—A total of 98 adult patient samples, comprising 4 groups, were evaluated. Group 1 comprised 16 diagnostic samples molecularly positive by existing laboratory-developed assays for *PML-RARα/t* (15;17) or *BCR-ABL/t* (9;22). Group 2 comprised 51 diagnostic samples negative by laboratory-developed assays for *PML-RARα/t* (15;17) or *BCR-ABL/t* (9;22). Group 3 was composed of 21 prospectively analyzed diagnostic cases without prior molecular studies, and group 4 was composed of 10 minimal residual disease samples.

Results.—Analysis of groups 1 and 2 (the 2 previously studied groups) confirmed the diagnostic sensitivity and specificity of the multiplex assay in regard to these 2 translocations. However, assay of the "negative" group (group 2) also revealed 3 unexpected translocations (*CBFβ-MYH11*, *BCR-ABL*, and *MLL-AF4*), 2 of which were confirmed on cytogenetic studies. Analysis of the prospective cohort showed that the assay was cost effective and amenable to standard laboratory practice. Virtually all of the results were consistent with the phenotype and karyotype by conventional methods.

Conclusion.—The utility of a kit-based reverse transcriptase–polymerase chain reaction assay for the molecular diagnosis and monitoring of leukemias was demonstrated by this study. The findings also reinforced the complementary roles of molecular testing and cytogenetics in diagnostic hematopathology.

▶ The use of conventional cytogenetics for the identification of the translocations associated with leukemia involves the need to have a sample of dividing cells, may miss certain "cryptic" translocations, and lacks sensitive markers for subsequent testing for minimal residual disease. The authors propose and demonstrate an approach to screening for the 7 most common of these leukemic translocations by using a commercially available multiplex reverse transcriptase–polymerase chain reaction on an automated platform, thus making this task more like other routine lab work.

M. G. Bissell, MD, PhD, MPH

Antimyelin Antibodies as a Predictor of Clinically Definite Multiple Sclerosis After a First Demyelinating Event

Berger T, Rubner P, Schautzer F, et al (Univ of Innsbruck, Austria; County Hosp, Villach, Austria)
N Engl J Med 349:139-145, 2003   21–10

Background.—In most patients with multiple sclerosis, the initial presentation is that of a clinically isolated syndrome. Clinically definite multiple sclerosis will develop in up to 80% of these patients, but the course of the disease is unpredictable at its onset and requires long-term observation or repeated MRI. The purpose of this study was to determine whether the presence of serum antibodies against myelin oligodendrocyte glycoprotein (MOG) and myelin basic protein (MBP) in patients with a clinically isolated syndrome is predictive of the interval to conversion to clinically definite multiple sclerosis.

Methods.—The study group was composed of 103 patients with a clinically isolated syndrome, positive findings on cerebral MRI, and oligoclonal bands in the CSF. At baseline, serum samples were collected for testing for anti-MOG and anti-MBP antibodies with Western blot analysis, and the lesions detected by cerebral MRI were quantified. All of the patients underwent neurologic examinations for assessment of relapse or progression of disease at baseline and every 3 months after the initial examination. Disease progression was defined as conversion to clinically definite multiple sclerosis.

Results.—Patients with anti-MOG and anti-MBP antibodies had relapses more often and earlier than patients without anti-MOG and anti-MBP antibodies. Of the 39 antibody-seronegative patients, only 9 (23%) had a relapse; the mean (± standard deviation) time to relapse was 45.1 ± 13.7 months. However, 21 of 22 patients (95%) with antibodies against both MOG and MBP had a relapse within a mean of 7.5 ± 4.4 months, and 35 of 42 patients (83%) with only anti-MOG antibodies had a relapse within 14.6 ± 9.6 months (Fig 1). The adjusted hazard ratio for the development of clinically definite multiple sclerosis was 76.5 among the patients who were seropositive for both antibodies and 31.6 among the patients who were seropositive only for anti-MOG antibodies, as compared with seronegative patients.

Conclusion.—These results support the analysis of antibodies against MOG and MBP in patients with a clinically isolated syndrome suspicious for multiple sclerosis. The analysis is rapid, inexpensive, and precise for the prediction of early conversion to clinically definite multiple sclerosis. The find-

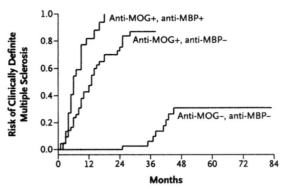

FIGURE 1.—Kaplan-Meier estimates of the risk of clinically definite multiple sclerosis, according to antibody status. *P* <.001 for the comparison between the patients who were seronegative for antibodies against both myelin oligodendrocyte glycoprotein (*MOG*) and myelin basic protein (*MBP*) and the patients who were seropositive only for anti-MOG antibodies or for both anti-MOG and anti-MBP antibodies. *Plus signs* denote seropositive, and *minus signs* denote seronegative. (Reprinted by permission of Berger T, Rubner P, Schautzer F, et al: Antimyelin antibodies as a predictor of clinically definite multiple sclerosis after a first demyelinating event. *N Engl J Med* 349:139-145, 2003. ©2003, Massachusetts Medical Society. All rights reserved.)

ings may have important implications for the counseling and care of patients with a first demyelinating event suggestive of multiple sclerosis.

▶ Like other chronic diseases of presumed autoimmune etiology, multiple sclerosis often presents clinically with a temporally isolated set of symptoms that are not unequivocal in pattern. If it would be possible to risk stratify patients presenting in this way, regarding their likely prognosis for reoccurrence and or progression of symptoms, it would be a great practical benefit to their management. The authors here present an approach to this problem based on the use of the lab assays for antibodies against anti-MOG and anti-MBP

M. G. Bissell, MD, PhD, MPH

22 Molecular Pathology and Cytogenetics

Bioelectronic Sensor Technology for Detection of Cystic Fibrosis and Hereditary Hemochromatosis Mutations
Bernacki SH, Farkas DH, Shi W, et al (Duke Univ, Durham, NC; Motorola Life Sciences, Pasadena, Calif; Coriell Inst, Camden, NJ; et al)
Arch Pathol Lab Med 127:1565-1572, 2003   22–1

Background.—Bioelectronic sensors are an emerging technology in clinical diagnostic testing and combine microchip and biologic components. An electronic detection platform using DNA biochip technology (eSensor) for molecular diagnostic applications is under development. Thus far, there have been limited demonstrations of the successful use of these devices in practical diagnostic applications. The performance of the eSensor bioelectronic method was assessed in the validation of 6 Epstein-Barr virus–transformed blood lymphocyte cell lines with clinically important mutations for use as sources of genetic material for positive controls in clinical molecular genetic testing. Two of these cell lines are carriers of mutations in the *CFTR* gene (cystic fibrosis), and the remaining cell lines carry mutations in the *HFE* gene (hereditary hemochromatosis).

Methods.—Samples from each cell line were analyzed for genotype determination by 6 different molecular genetic testing facilities, including the laboratory that developed the DNA biochips. In addition to the bioelectronic method, at least 3 different molecular diagnostic methods were used in the analysis of each cell line. Detailed data were obtained from the DNA biochip output, and the genetic results were compared with results obtained by the more established methods.

Results.—Two applications of the bioelectronic platform were successful, one for detection of *CFTR* mutations and the other for detection of *HFE* mutations. In all cases, the results obtained with the DNA biochip were in concordance with results reported for the other methods. The electronic signal output from the DNA biochips was found to clearly differentiate between mutated and wild-type alleles.

Conclusions.—Bioelectronic sensors for the detection of disease-causing mutations performed well in the "real-life" situation in this study, the first reported use of the cystic fibrosis detection platform. The results provide evidence of the practical potential of emerging bioelectronic DNA detection technologies for use in current molecular diagnostic applications.

▶ With this report, routine (potentially automatable) DNA testing moves another step closer. Biosensors (analytic detection devices incorporating biomolecules as intrinsic components) have been with us for some time now, the earliest examples being the glucose electrodes that capitalized on the extreme environmental stability of the enzyme glucose oxidase. Well, of course, DNA is another of those environmentally stable molecules, and making DNA-based biosensors robust enough for routine lab work has also been a work in progress for some time.

M. G. Bissell, MD, PhD, MPH

Array-Based Comparative Genomic Hybridization for the Genomewide Detection of Submicroscopic Chromosomal Abnormalities
Vissers LELM, de Vries BBA, Osoegawa K, et al (Univ Med Ctr Nijmegen, The Netherlands; Children's Hosp, Oakland, Calif)
Am J Hum Genet 73:1261-1270, 2003   22–2

Background.—In the general population, the incidence of mental retardation, with or without additional malformations, is 2% to 3%. Much of this incidence is attributable to the presence of gross chromosomal abnormalities or other factors, such as metabolic or neurologic abnormalities; however, the cause of mental retardation is unexplained in about 50% of patients. Microdeletions and microduplications, not visible by routine chromosomal analysis, are responsible for up to 5% of the previously unexplained cases. Novel high-resolution, whole-genomic technologies have the potential to improve the diagnostic detection rate of these small chromosomal abnormalities. Array-based comparative genomic hybridization is a technology that allows high-resolution screening by hybridizing differentially labeled test and reference DNAs to arrays that consist of thousands of genomic clones. The diagnostic capacity of this technology was tested by using approximately 3500 fluorescent in situ hybridization–verified clones selected to cover the genome, with an average of 1 clone per megabase (Mb).

Methods.—The sensitivity and specificity of array-based comparative genomic hybridization were tested in normal-versus-normal control experi-

---

FIGURE 1.—ArrayCGH genomic profile of validation experiments. Arrays contained 3,343 human autosomal clones (indicated by *small circles* representing the mean log_2-transformed and Lowess-normalized T/R intensity ratios), ordered in **A** and **C** from 1pter to 22qter on the basis of the physical mapping positions obtained from the November 2002 freeze of the UCSC genome browser. In panels A and C, chromosome boundaries are indicated by *vertical lines*. Panel A shows the result of a normal-versus-normal hybridization (control 3 vs. control 1). Nearly all clones fall within the a priori thresholds for copy-number gain (log_2 T/R value 0.3) and copy-number loss (log_2 T/R value −0.3) indicated by the *horizontal lines*. One clone on chromosome 2 shows an intensity ratio outside these thresholds and might represent a false-positive result. **Panel B** shows the result of the combined analysis of the two hybridizations performed with control 1 (X-axis: control 1 vs. control 2; Y-axis: control 3 vs. control 1). The *ellipse* represents the border of the reference regions containing 99.999% of the data points; the thresholds for copy-number gain and loss are also integrated into this figure

FIGURE 1

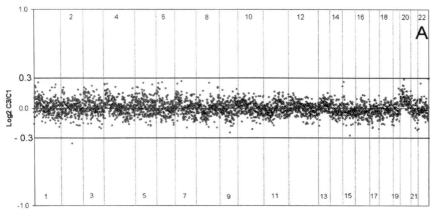

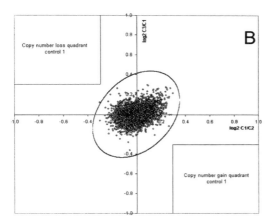

(see the "Patients and Methods" section for details). As can be seen, there is only one clone outside the reference region; however, this clone does not pass the thresholds for copy-number loss in both experiments and can therefore be discarded from further analyses. The clone on chromosome 2 that fell outside the threshold for copy-number loss in **panel A** is clearly within the normal reference region and can therefore also be discarded for further analyses. **Panel C** shows the result of the hybridization of DNA from a patient with trichorhinophalangeal syndrome (TRPS) against DNA from a patient with Prader-Willi syndrome (PWS). A total of four clones, spanning 2.7 Mb of genomic sequence on 8q23.3-q24.11, showed $\log_2$ TRPS-over-PWS intensity ratios below the threshold for copy-number loss, confirming the presence of a deletion of this genomic region in the TRPS patient. In addition, five clones, spanning 2.9 Mb of sequence on 15q11.2, show $\log_2$ intensity ratios above the (reverse) threshold for copy-number gain, indicating a deletion of this genomic region in the PWS patient. No clones outside these target genomic regions show potential false-positive results. The combined results of two experiments involving the PWS patient are shown in **panel D**. The five target clones on 15q11.2 are reproducibly deleted in both experiments and fall outside the bivariate normal distribution reference region ($P = .99999$) and within the copy-number loss quadrant in the **upper left quadrant**. (Courtesy of Vissers LELM, de Vries BBA, Osoegawa K, et al: Array-based comparative genomic hybridization for the genomewide detection of submicroscopic chromosomal abnormalities. *Am J Hum Genet* 73:1261-1270, 2003. Reprinted with permission of the University of Chicago Press.)

(*Continued*)

FIGURE 1 (cont.)

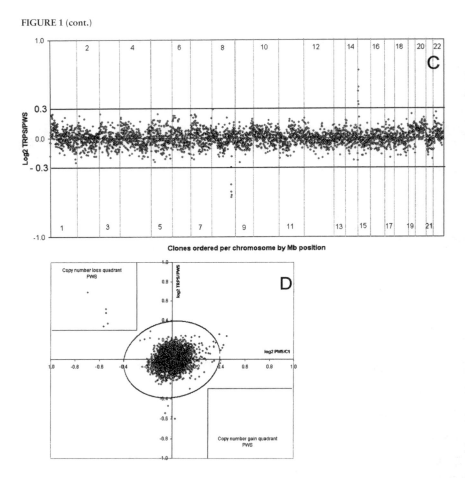

ments and through the screening of patients with known microdeletion syndromes (Fig 1). In the second phase of the study, a series of 20 cytogenetically normal patients with mental retardation and dysmorphisms suggestive of a chromosomal abnormality were analyzed.

Results.—In this series, 3 microdeletions and 2 microduplications were identified and validated. Two of these genomic changes were also identified in one of the parents, indicating that these are large-scale genomic polymorphisms. Deletions and duplications of just 1 Mb could be reliably detected by this approach. The percentage of false-positive results was minimized by the use of a dye-swap-replicate analysis, which virtually eliminated the need for the labor-intensive validation experiments and facilitated the implementation of a routine diagnostic setting.

Conclusions.—The high-resolution assay will facilitate the identification of novel genes involved in human mental retardation and malformation syndromes, and will provide greater insight into the plasticity and flexibility of the human genome.

▶ About 2% to 3% of the population is mentally retarded, and in about half of these cases, the etiology is not known. This is the need that motivated the current authors to develop their approach to genome-wide screening for chromosomal abnormalities too small to be seen under the microscope. Using their array-based genomic hybridization technology, they were able to successfully identify microdeletions and microduplications at resolutions of 1 Mb in cytogenetically normal retarded individuals. The approach holds great promise.

M. G. Bissell, MD, PhD, MPH

Detection of Cystic Fibrosis Mutations by Peptide Mass Signature Genotyping
Malehorn DE, Telmer CA, McEwen SB, et al (Univ of Pittsburgh, Pa)
Clin Chem 49:1318-1330, 2003   22–3

Introduction.—The range of genetic mutations and polymorphisms necessitates the development of practical identification approaches capable of evaluating more than 1 patient per 1 nucleotide position per analysis. Peptic mass signature genotyping (PMSG) is a newly developed technology in which target DNA sequences are translated to create peptide analytes of suitable size in the cystic fibrosis transmembrane conductance regulator (*CFTR*) gene.

Methods.—Exons of the gene were amplified, cloned, and expressed in *Escherichia coli* as peptide fusions, in natural and unnatural reading frames. Peptide analytes were purified via immobilized metal affinity chromatography and analyzed by matrix-assisted, laser desorption/ionization time-of-flight mass spectrometry (MALDI-TOF MS). Synthetic and natural DNA samples with the 25 mutations recommended for *CFTR* carrier screening were evaluated using the PMSG test for the *CFTR* gene.

Results.—Peptide analytes were between 6278 to 17,454 Da and varied 30-fold in expression. Highly expressing peptides were seen via electron microscopy to accumulate as inclusion bodies. Peptides were reliably recovered from whole-cell lysates via a simple purification process. The *CFTR* mutations produced identifiable alterations in resulting mass spectrometry profiles, of which more than 95% were reliably identified in blinded testing of replicate synthetic heterozygous DNA samples. Mutation identification was possible using both sample pooling and multiplexing. The PMSG *CFTR* test was used to ascertain compound heterozygous mutations in DNA samples from patients with cystic fibrosis, which were verified via direct DNA sequencing.

Conclusion.—The PMSG test of the *CFTR* gene has unique capabilities for determining the sequence status of a DNA target by sensitively monitoring the mass of peptides, natural or unnatural, produced from that target.

▶ Here's a new method for detecting the multiple mutations of cystic fibrosis in which genomics lifts a page from proteomics. The pattern of expressed peptide products can be interpreted in a reverse fashion to enable inference of the mutations involved in their synthesis. The new forms of mass spectroscopy, such as MALDI-TOF described here, make this possible.

M. G. Bissell, MD, PhD, MPH

Genomic DNA Extraction From Small Amounts of Serum to Be Used for α_1-Antitrypsin Genotype Analysis
Andolfatto S, Namour F, Garnier A-L, et al (Univ Hosp of Nancy-Brabois, France)
Eur Respir J 21:215-219, 2003   22–4

Introduction.—The α_1-antiprotease inhibitor (Pi), or α_1-antitrypsin (α_1-AT) is the primary serum inhibitor of lysosomal proteases. Since the laboratory diagnosis of α_1-AT deficiency is typically based on its phenotype identification by isoelectric focusing, α_1-PiS and PiZ genotypes can also be ascertained by DNA-based methods. Recently, several techniques have been described for preparing genomic DNA from serum. Forty-three venous blood samples obtained from patients hospitalized for respiratory diseases were evaluated to determine the Pi allele from serum-extracted DNA by polymerase chain reaction (PCR) and to compare these findings with those obtained with whole-blood extracted DNA.

Methods.—Serum α_1-AT concentration and phenotypic detection were systematically performed in the 43 hospitalized patients. The genomic DNA was simultaneously purified from both whole blood and serum. The mutation detection was observed via a PCR-mediated site-directed mutagenesis technique.

Results.—Thirty-seven serum α_1-AT concentrations were regarded as normal or increased, 4 were diminished with the reference values used (91-182 mg/DL), and 6 were less than 91 mg/dL. Twenty-nine patients with MM homozygotes, 11 were heterozygous for S (MS = 7) or Z (MZ = 4), and 3 had a ZZ phenotype. Genotyping analyses produced identical results using serum- and whole–blood-extracted DNA. All results were in agreement with the phenotypic findings.

Conclusion.—A DNA-based test is a reliable tool for detection of α_1-AT deficiency and may be an alternative for the labor-intensive α_1-AT determination via isoelectric focusing. The approach yields good quality DNA from serum, equal to that extracted from whole blood. It can be useful in retrospective investigations of multiple genetic markers.

▶ The standard method for $\alpha_1$1-AT deficiency genotyping is isoelectric focusing of the serum α_1-AT protein. This method is time-consuming and labor intensive. This study makes use of circulating serum DNA, an entity known since about 1948, to detect the genotype directly using PCR. The authors show that this specimen is as good as circulating blood cells for this purpose.

M. G. Bissell, MD, PhD, MPH

Size Distributions of Maternal and Fetal DNA in Maternal Plasma
Chan KCA, Zhang J, Hui ABY, et al (Chinese Univ of Hong Kong, China)
Clin Chem 50:88-92, 2004   22–5

Background.—The existence of fetal-derived DNA in maternal plasma was reported in 1997. Later it was shown that fetal DNA accounted for a mean of 3.4% and 6.2% of the total DNA in maternal plasma in early and late gestation, respectively. These discoveries have facilitated the development of an approach for noninvasive prenatal diagnosis. In spite of the rapid expansion in clinical applications, the molecular characteristics of plasma DNA in pregnant women have not been fully elucidated. The size distributions of maternal and fetal DNA in maternal plasma were investigated.

Methods.—The size distribution of plasma DNA was investigated in 34 nonpregnant women and 31 pregnant women by means of a panel of quantitative polymerase chain reaction assays with different amplicon sizes targeting the leptin gene. The size distribution of fetal DNA in maternal plasma was also determined by targeting the *SRY* gene.

Results.—The median percentages of plasma DNA with size greater than 201 base pair (bp) were 57% and 14% for pregnant and nonpregnant women, respectively. The median percentages of fetal-derived DNA with sizes greater than 193 bp and greater than 313 bp were 20% and 0%, respectively, in maternal plasma.

Conclusion.—Although plasma DNA molecules are mainly short DNA fragments, the DNA fragments in the plasma of pregnant women are significantly longer than those found in the plasma of nonpregnant women. In addition, the maternal-derived DNA molecules are longer than the fetal-derived DNA molecules.

▶ Here we have an exploration of one aspect of the clinical pathologist's dream: a potential opportunity to replace a difficult and sometimes controversial invasive method of sampling (amniocentesis and/or chorionic villus sampling) with a simpler blood test (analysis of maternally circulating fetal DNA). It all starts with characterizing the DNA sample this represents.

M. G. Bissell, MD, PhD, MPH

Genetic Testing for Hereditary Nonpolyposis Colorectal Cancer

Hoedema R, Monroe T, Bos C, et al (Spectrum Health/MSU, Grand Rapids, Mich)
Am Surg 69:387-391, 2003   22–6

Introduction.—About 80% of patients with colorectal cancer have sporadic disease and the remaining 20% appear to have a genetic component. Hereditary nonpolyposis colorectal cancer (HNPCC) is the most frequently occurring autosomal dominant hereditary syndrome predisposing to colorectal cancer (accounts for 1%-6% of all cases of colorectal cancer). Several methods have been described for screening HNPCC and for directly testing for mismatch repair gene mutations. The initial results were assessed concerning (1) microsatellite instability (MSI) and immunohistochemistry (IHC) staining of tumors, and (2) genetic sequencing for mismatch repair gene mutations in patients with suspected HNPCC.

Methods.—Appropriate patients for HNPCC testing were identified from the registry of a high-risk colorectal cancer clinic. Among all patients screened, only those who met Amsterdam criteria for HNPCC or were young age onset (YAO) (<40 years of age) were eligible for evaluation. The tumors underwent testing for MSI; IHC was performed in patients with available tumor specimens. The 5 markers approved by the National Institutes of Health consensus conference underwent MSI testing; MSI-High (MSI-H) was considered to be 2 or more unstable markers. IHC was performed with commercially available stains for MLH1 and MSH2. All patients underwent sequencing of the MLH1 and MSH2 genes to search for mutations. Genetic counseling was provided.

Results.—Fourteen patients were members of kindreds that met Amsterdam criteria. An additional 10 patients were younger than 40 when colorectal cancer was diagnosed, yet they lacked a family history. Testing for both MSI and IHC was performed on available tissue blocks. Among patients who met Amsterdam criteria, 5 had MSH2 mutations and 2 had MLH1 variants. Of 5 patients with MSH2 mutations, 3 of 4 had MSI-H tumors; all 4 had loss of expression of MSH2 on IHC. Of MLH1 variants, 1 had MSI-H tumor and lacked expression of MLH-1 on IHC. Among patients with no mutation, 3 of 6 had MSI-H tumors. Among YAO patients, no genetic mutations were seen. Two of 7 patients had MSI-H tumors.

Conclusion.—Genetic testing for HNPCC, even in patients fulfilling Amsterdam criteria, yielded mutations in 5 of 14 patients; variants of unknown significance were observed in an additional 2 patients. Only 1 MSH2 variant of unknown significance was found in the 10 YAO patients, indicating that screening in this group of patients with MSI, IHC, or both, would be appropriate.

▶ This study represents a proposal to utilize molecular genetic methods (MSI) to screen for HNPCC, the most common condition among the 20% of colorectal cancer cases that currently have identifiable genetics. The authors suggest that this would be a generally viable approach.

M. G. Bissell, MD, PhD, MPH

DNA Integrity as a Potential Marker for Stool-Based Detection of Colorectal Cancer
Boynton KA, Summerhayes IC, Ahlquist DA, et al (EXACT Sciences Corp, Maynard, Mass; Lahey Clinic, Burlington, Mass; Mayo Clinic, Rochester, Minn)
Clin Chem 49:1058-1065, 2003   22–7

Background.—Colorectal cancer is responsible for 10% of all cancer deaths and is second only to lung cancer as a leading cause of cancer-related deaths in industrialized nations. Stool-testing methods are noninvasive and do not require cathartic preparation of the bowel, and they can be performed at a centralized testing facility. However, the promise of these tests has not been fully realized. Molecular genetic analysis of DNA in patient stools have been proposed for screening of colorectal cancer.

Nonapoptotic cells shed from tumors may contain DNA that is less degraded than DNA fragments from healthy colonic mucosa. Therefore, the purpose of this study was to demonstrate that DNA fragments isolated from stools of patients with colorectal cancer had higher integrity than DNA isolated from stools of patients with healthy colonic mucosa.

Methods.—DNA from the stools of a colonoscopy-negative control group and from patients with colorectal cancer was purified. The relationship between long DNA fragments and clinical status was examined by determining the stool DNA integrity, using oligonucleotide-based hybrid captures with specific target sequences in increasingly long polymerase chain reaction reactions (200 bp, 400 bp, 800 bp, 1.3 kb, 1.8 kb, 24 kb). DNA fragments obtained from patients with colorectal cancer were compared with fragments from colonoscopy-negative individuals for length and integrity.

Results.—The DNA fragments isolated from patients with colorectal cancer were found to be of higher molecular weight (more than 18 bands detected of a total of 24 possible bands) than fragments isolated from fecal DNA of the colonoscopy-negative control group.

Conclusion.—It appears that the presence of long DNA fragments in stool is associated with colorectal cancer and may be related to disease-associated differences in the regulation of proliferation and apoptosis. The outcomes in this study support an assay of fecal DNA integrity as a potentially useful biomarker for the detection of colorectal cancer.

▶ Early-stage colorectal cancer is only poorly diagnosed by fecal occult blood screening. The molecular approach involves sampling the genetic composition of the colonic mucosa which is exfoliated into the colon. The authors have observed an association between the efficiency of polymerase chain reaction amplification and the presence of higher molecular weight DNA fragments in stool which is associated with cancer. They suggest that DNA integrity may thus serve as a biomarker for colorectal cancer in stool.

M. G. Bissell, MD, PhD, MPH

Quantitative Analysis of Circulating Mitochondrial DNA in Plasma
Chiu RWK, Chan LYS, Lam NYL, et al (Chinese Univ of Hong Kong, Shatin, New Territories, Hong Kong SAR)
Clin Chem 49:719-726, 2003   22–8

Background.—Recent studies have demonstrated the existence of circulating mitochondrial DNA in plasma and serum. This discovery has demonstrated the potential for noninvasive diagnosis and monitoring of a wide variety of diseases and conditions. Tumor-, fetus-, and donor-derived DNA sequences have been detected in the plasma and serum of cancer patients, pregnant women, and transplant recipients, respectively. However, the concentrations and physical characteristics of circulating mitochondrial DNA are unknown. An assay was developed for use in quantification of mitochondrial DNA in the plasma of healthy persons.

Methods.—A real-time quantitative polymerase chain reaction approach was developed, and the specificity of this assay for detection of mitochondrial DNA with a cell line (ρ^0) devoid of mitochondria was evaluated. Three modules were constructed for experimental investigation of the concentrations and physical characteristics of circulating mitochondrial DNA. The evaluation in module 1 involved the concentrations of mitochondrial DNA in plasma aliquots derived from 4 blood-processing protocols. The evaluation in module 2 investigated the existence of both particle-associated and free forms of mitochondrial DNA in plasma by subjecting plasma to filtration and ultracentrifugation. In the third module, filters with different pore sizes were used to investigate the size characteristics of the particle-associated fraction of circulating mitochondrial DNA.

Results.—The mitochondrial DNA–specific, real-time quantitative polymerase chain reaction method used had a dynamic range of 5 orders of magnitude and a sensitivity that allowed detection of 1 copy of mitochondrial DNA in plasma. In module 1, significant differences in the amounts of circulating mitochondrial DNA were found among plasma aliquots processed by different methods. Data from module 2 showed that a significant fraction of mitochondrial DNA in plasma was filterable or pelletable by ultracentrifugation. In module 3, it was shown that filters with different pore sizes removed mitochondrial DNA from plasma to varying degrees.

Conclusion.—This quantitative analysis of circulating DNA in plasma revealed that both particle-associated and free mitochondrial DNA are present in plasma, and the concentrations of these factors are affected by the process used to harvest plasma from whole blood. These findings may have important implications for the design of future studies on circulating mitochondrial DNA measured in different disease conditions.

► Mutations in the mitochondrial genome are associated with a number of diseases, and the maternal inheritance of mitochondrial DNA has been associated with aging, degenerative diseases, and malignancies (including breast, colon, liver, head and neck, lung, and other cancers). Most analyses of mitochondrial DNA in plasma have been merely qualitative in nature. The authors here undertook to specifically quantify copy numbers of mitochondrial DNA mutations.

M. G. Bissell, MD, PhD, MPH

Genomewide Distribution of High-Frequency, Completely Mismatching SNP Haplotype Pairs Observed to Be Common Across Human Populations
Zhang J, Rowe WL, Clark AG, et al (NIH, Bethesda, Md; Cornell Univ, Ithaca, NY)
Am J Hum Genet 73:1073-1081, 2003   22–9

Background.—The availability of millions of genetic variation markers, or single-nucleotide polymorphisms (SNPs), in the human genome has raised many questions about the use of multi-SNP linkage disequilibrium in genomewide association studies for the identification of genetic risk factors attributed to complex diseases. Knowledge of human haplotype structure has important implications for strategies of disease gene mapping and for understanding of the evolutionary history of humans. Many attributes of SNPs and haplotypes appear to exhibit highly nonrandom behavior, which suggests past operation of selection or other nonneutral forces. Previous work on an algorithm to identify haplocyte-tagging SNPs using human chromosome 21 haplotype blocks found that 42% of the blocks—identified as regions with limited haplotype diversity—have at least 1 pair of high-frequency haplotypes (yin-yang haplotypes) composed of completely mismatching SNP alleles.

Methods.—Genotype data were obtained for the 62 genomic regions in the Altshuler data set. An analysis was conducted of common haplotypes in these random genomic loci and in 85 gene-coding regions in humans.

Results.—The proportion of the genome spanned by yin yang haplotypes was 75% to 85% in the 62 random genomic loci and 85 human gene-coding regions. Population data for 28 genomic loci in Drosophila melanogaster showed a similar pattern.

Conclusion.—The high recurrence of these haplotype patterns (85% or greater) in 4 distinct human populations lends support to the hypothesis that the yin yang haplotypes likely predate the African diaspora. It first appeared to suggest deep population splitting or maintenance of ancient lineages by selection. However, coalescent simulation demonstrated that the yin yang phenomenon can be explained by strictly neutral evolution in a well-mixed population.

▶ The word coinages of investigators in naming and describing new findings become the basis for further communication both within and between fields. The current authors' coinage of the term "yin yang haplotypes" for their discovery of the genetic signature represented by regions with limited haplotype diversity, such that the nucleotides differ at every SNP in the haplotype pair, strikes me as a particularly felicitous one. It may also prove to be a particularly meaningful one.

M. G. Bissell, MD, PhD, MPH

A 3.9-Centimorgan-Resolution Human Single-Nucleotide Polymorphism Linkage Map and Screening Set
Matise TC, Sachidanandam R, Clark AG, et al (Rutgers Univ, Piscataway, NJ; Cold Spring Harbor Lab, NY; Cornell Univ, Ithaca, NY; et al)
Am J Hum Genet 73:271-284, 2003   22–10

Background.—There have been several major advances in the methods and technologies used for linkage analysis of human diseases since restriction fragment length polymorphisms were first used as genetic markers. At the present time, the primary sources for linkage analysis are robust and highly informative microsatellite markers. However, the ability to scale up the typing of microsatellite markers to very high throughput is limited because electrophoretic separation must be performed to accurately determine fragment sizes. Recent advances in technologies for high-throughput single-nucleotide polymorphism (SNP)–based genotyping have improved efficiency and cost to such a degree that it is becoming feasible to consider the use of SNPs for genomewide linkage analysis.

However, as yet there have been no descriptions of a suitable screening set of SNPs and a corresponding linkage map. The first descriptions of such a screening set and a resource for fast genome scanning for disease genes were provided by this study.

Methods.—Evaluations were conducted of 6297 SNPs in a diversity panel composed of European Americans, African Americans, and Asians. The markers were assessed for assay robustness, suitable allele frequencies, and informativeness of multi-SNP clusters. For map construction, persons from 56 Centre d'Etude du Polymorphisme Humain pedigrees, with more than 770 potentially informative meioses, were genotyped with a subset of 2988 SNPs. Extensive genotyping error analysis was performed.

Results.—The resulting SNP linkage map has an average map resolution of 3.9 cM, with map positions containing either a single SNP or several tightly linked SNPs (Table 1). The order of markers on this map was found to compare favorably with several other linkage and physical maps. A comparison was made of map distances between the SNP linkage map and the interpolated SNP linkage map constructed by the deCode Genetics group. In

TABLE 1.—Description of the Single-Nucleotide Polymorphism Linkage Maps

Chromosome	No. of SNPs in Linkage Group	No. of Map Positions*	No. of SNPs on Map†	No. of Clusters	Map Length (cM)‡			Map Resolution (cM)§	Physical Length (Mb)	cM/Mb Ratio
					Sex Averaged	Female	Male			
1	242	93	204	69	277.7	353.8	191.4	3.0	239.74	1.16
2	210	81	176	58	259.9	337.9	175.2	3.2	237.39	1.09
3	185	77	156	50	220.7	203.2	160.9	2.9	197.40	1.12
4	159	57	124	42	216.0	275.1	159.7	3.9	190.04	1.14
5	162	64	130	43	211.3	255.0	164.3	3.4	179.99	1.17
6	155	57	126	43	193.1	235.5	142.5	3.4	169.69	1.14
7	138	56	118	38	182.6	226.1	140.0	3.3	153.76	1.19
8	141	57	113	31	160.1	210.8	109.8	2.9	138.82	1.15
9	130	47	96	32	158.4	190.8	130.9	3.4	131.04	1.21
10	136	54	116	37	176.3	211.1	131.9	3.3	133.36	1.32
11	107	43	87	31	152.6	187.3	116.5	3.6	130.66	1.17
12	127	47	97	29	170.6	210.5	126.3	3.7	131.48	1.30
13	85	36	69	20	121.5	149.3	97.2	3.5	94.08	1.29
14	100	33	82	28	115.3	126.1	86.3	3.6	81.48	1.42
15	84	29	59	17	120.5	143.0	93.5	4.3	75.95	1.59
16	99	34	78	25	137.6	168.8	105.8	4.2	90.08	1.53
17	90	28	65	19	126.8	157.2	94.8	4.7	79.99	1.59
18	99	37	81	27	124.8	149.4	91.0	3.5	75.56	1.65
19	67	25	43	14	120.5	128.1	114.6	5.0	57.89	2.08
20	81	31	74	24	106.4	128.8	85.0	3.5	58.43	1.82
21	51	18	44	11	66.6	79.9	51.2	3.9	31.86	2.09
22	55	22	50	18	78.9	78.2	72.8	3.8	32.01	2.46
X	68	22	35	10	208.6	208.6	...	9.9	144.61	1.44
Overall	2,771	1,048	2,223	716	3,706.8	4,414.5	2,641.6	3.9	2,855.31	1.4

*A map position may consist of a single-nucleotide polymorphism (*SNP*) or a cluster of SNPs.
†These SNPs have single map positions; the remaining SNPs are localized to bins.
‡Assuming zero recombination within clusters.
§Sex-averaged map length divided by the number of map positions.
(Courtesy of Matise TC, Sachidanandam R, Clark AG, et al: A 3.9-centimorgan-resolution human single-nucleotide polymorphism linkage map and screening set. *Am J Hum Genet* 73:271-284, 2003. Published by the University of Chicago Press.)

addition, cM/Mb distance ratios were compared for females and males, along each chromosome, showing broadly defined regions of increased and decreased rates of recombination.

Conclusion.—The SNP screening set described in this report is more informative than the Marshfield Clinic's commonly used microsatellite-based screening set.

▶ SNPs can potentially be used for linkage-based whole genome scans. This approach will, of course, require that such linkages be mapped. Here, to a resolution of 3.9 centimorgans, is the authors' effort in filling this need, which they believe is more informative than the currently commonly used approach based on microsatellites.

M. G. Bissell, MD, PhD, MPH

First-Trimester Screening for Trisomies 21 and 18
Wapner R, for the First Trimester Maternal Serum Biochemistry and Fetal Nuchal Translucency Screening (BUN) Study Group (Drexel Univ, Philadelphia; et al)
N Engl J Med 349:1405-1413, 2003   22–11

Background.—Screening for fetal aneuploidy is usually performed in the second trimester and is based on maternal age plus levels of α-fetoprotein, human chorionic gonadotropin, and unconjugated estriol. This screening approach identifies approximately 65% of fetuses with Down syndrome, with a false-positive rate of approximately 5%. Prenatal diagnosis can also be performed during the first trimester by invasive chorionic-villus sampling. The use of maternal age, maternal levels of free β human chorionic gonadotropin and pregnancy-associated plasma protein A, and US assessment of fetal nuchal translucency to screen for fetal aneuploidy in the first trimester were examined.

Study Design.—The study group consisted of patients with a singleton pregnancy between 74 and 97 days of gestation who had prenatal screening for trisomies 18 and 21. This screening was based on maternal age, maternal levels of free β human chorionic gonadotropin and pregnancy-associated plasma protein A, and US assessment of fetal nuchal translucency (Fig 2). Fetal chromosome status was determined by karyotype analysis. Patient-specific risks were calculated for biochemical assessments alone, for US assessment alone, and for the combination. The sensitivity, specificity, and false-positive and false-negative rates for first trimester screening were calculated.

Findings.—Screening was completed in 8514 patients, of whom 102 had a previous pregnancy affected by aneuploidy and were analyzed separately. The first-trimester screening method identified over 85% of the 61 cases of Down syndrome, with a 9.4% false-positive rate. At a false-positive rate of 5%, the detection rate was 79%. Screening also identified 91% of the 11 cases of trisomy 18, with a 2% false-positive rate. Among women older than

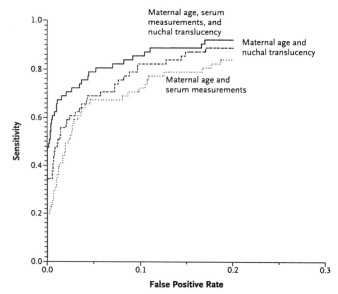

FIGURE 2.—Receiver operating characteristic curves for prediction of trisomy 21 with use of combined approach to screening, screening based on maternal age and nuchal translucency, and screening based on maternal age and serum measurements. (Courtesy Wapner R, for the First Trimester Maternal Serum Biochemistry and Fetal Nuchal Translucency Screening: First-trimester screening for trisomies 21 and 18. *N Engl J Med* 349:1405-1413, 2003. Copyright Massachusetts Medical Society, all rights reserved.)

35 years, first-trimester screening identified 90% of fetuses with trisomy 21, with a false-positive rate of 15%. It also identified 100% of the fetuses with trisomy 18 in this maternal age group.

Conclusions.—This prospective, cohort study demonstrated that first-trimester screening, consisting of maternal age, levels of pregnancy-associated plasma protein A and free β human chorionic gonadotropin, and nuchal translucency thickness, is accurate in clinical practice. First-trimester screening offers patients more privacy, earlier results, and safer alternatives than second-trimester screening.

▶ The earlier trisomies 18 and 21 can be diagnosed, the better. A first-trimester screen would have great potential clinical utility, but none has been adequately evaluated before now. The authors present the results of a multi-center trial of a screening approach based on maternal age, US, and 2 laboratory values. It appears to be effective.

M. G. Bissell, MD, PhD, MPH

23 Clinical Chemistry

Impact of DNA Polymerases and Their Buffer Systems on Quantitative Real-Time PCR
Wolffs P, Grage H, Hagberg O, et al (Lund Univ, Sweden)
J Clin Microbiol 42:408-411, 2004   23–1

Background.—The introduction of real-time polymerase chain reaction (PCR) technology has greatly improved sequence-specific nucleic acid quantification in areas such as diagnostic PCR and molecular biology. This technology has great potential for accurate and sensitive quantification, but further studies addressing the quantification aspect of this technology are required before it can be widely implemented. Previous reports have indicated that DNA polymerases and their buffer systems affect the performance of PCR by altering the detection window and linear range of amplification. The effect of 5 DNA polymerase buffer systems on absolute quantification was determined with the LightCycler instrument.

Methods.—Standard curves for each polymerase buffer system were obtained by using independent triplicates of 10-fold dilutions of *Yersinia enterocolitica* DNA, from 1 mg/mL to 1 fg/mL. After amplification, results from the melting curve were analyzed, and the crossing point values (ROMs) of all samples that gave a positive specific product peak between 88°C and 92°C were plotted against the log of the initial DNA concentration. From the triplicate analysis, a detection probability graph was created that showed the number of detectable points at each DNA concentration (Fig 2).

Results.—The effect of the DNA polymerase buffer system on DNA quantification was demonstrated by quantifying 4 standardized DNA samples. *Taq* and LCTaq generated less-accurate quantification data. The main reason for this is the narrower detection window and the greater deviations in the standard curve. The effects of buffer components on the amplification efficiency and detection window were determined for *Taq* and *Tth*. It is apparent from the data that at least for *Tth*, the buffer composition affects the detection window, since the detection window becomes wider with increasing complexity of the buffer. A comparison of data between *Taq* and *Tth* showed that for all buffers, the use of *Tth* improves the PCR performance, which implies that both buffer composition and DNA polymerase can influence the results.

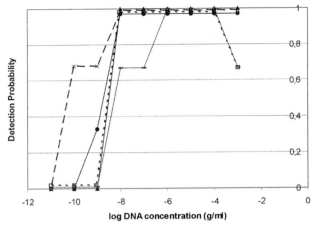

FIGURE 2.—Detection probability using different DNA polymerase-buffer systems. The detection probability for each DNA concentration was determined by checking the amount of data points/total amount of analysis. Data were determined after independent triplicate experiments. *Solid line with solid circle*, DyNazyme II; *dashed line with open square*, LCTaq; *solid line with solid triangle*, rTth; *solid line with solid rectangle*, Taq; and *dashed line with X*, Tth. (Courtesy of Wolffs P, Grage H, Hagberg O, et al: Impact of DNA polymerases and their buffer systems on quantitative real-time PCR. *J Clin Microbiol* 42:408-411, 2004. Copyright American Society for Microbiology.)

Conclusions.—Basing quantitative measurements on single data-set standard curves can result in significant errors when using DNA polymerase buffer systems on real-time PCR.

▶ There is a certain tendency to forget that, at base, molecular assays like PCR are biochemical assays. Just like blood urea nitrogen, parathyroid hormone, or glycated hemoglobin, they have reagents and reaction conditions that vary from assay to assay, and this variation has potential consequences for the results, as described in detail in this article.

M. G. Bissell, MD, PhD, MPH

Relationship Between Sex Hormone–Binding Globulin Levels and Features of the Metabolic Syndrome
Hajamor S, Després J-P, Couillard C, et al (Laval Univ, Québec; Québec Heart Inst; Univ of Ottawa, Canada)
Metabolism 52:724-730, 2003   23–2

Background.—Low plasma levels of sex hormone–binding globulin (SHBG) have been associated with alterations in several components of the metabolic syndrome in both men and women. SHBG levels have been shown to be significant predictors of diabetes development and cardiovascular disease in some but not all prospective studies. However, no study has examined whether SHBG level could be a global predictor of the metabolic syndrome. Whether plasma SHBG level is a significant predictor of the features of the metabolic syndrome was determined.

Methods.—The study group was composed of 203 men and 219 women from the Quebec Family Study for whom detailed measures of body composition and body fat distribution, as well as measures of the metabolic profile and SHBG concentrations, were available.

Results.—Low SHBG levels were associated with increased total and abdominal adiposity in men and in premenopausal and postmenopausal women. Low levels of SHBG were also associated with an altered metabolic profile, especially in premenopausal women. The study participants were subdivided according to the presence of 0, 1 to 2, or 3 or more features of the metabolic syndrome. One quarter of the men were characterized by 3 features or more, whereas most premenopausal women (61.3%) had a healthy metabolic profile (0 features), and 6.9% were characterized by 3 or more features. Most postmenopausal women (54.3%) were characterized by 1 to 2 components of the metabolic syndrome, and 13% were characterized by 3 or more components. The proportion of participants characterized by the metabolic syndrome was lower in persons with SHBG values in the upper tertile compared with the lower tertile in both men and premenopausal women (17.7% vs 28.4% and 1.7% vs 14%, respectively). Logistic regression analyses showed that an SHBG level in the upper tertile was associated with a significant reduction in the probability of being characterized by the metabolic syndrome. Outcomes on logistic regression were not significant in postmenopausal women.

Conclusions.—Plasma SHBG levels may be a significant predictor of the metabolic syndrome in men and premenopausal women.

▶ The metabolic syndrome (abdominal obesity, inactivity, hypertension, hyperinsulinemia, glucose intolerance) is well established as a significant independent predictor of risk for cardiovascular disease. Since SHBG levels are known to correlate inversely with the individual parameters of the metabolic syndrome, the current authors undertook to see whether low SHBG levels could serve as a predictive biomarker for the syndrome as a whole, perhaps allowing new types of preventive intervention to be devised.

M. G. Bissell, MD, PhD, MPH

Soluble CD40 Ligand in Acute Coronary Syndromes
Heeschen C, for the CAPTURE Study Investigators (Univ of Frankfurt, Germany; et al)
N Engl J Med 348:1104-1111, 2003   23–3

Background.—It can be difficult to establish the correct diagnosis and initiate the appropriate treatment in patients with acute coronary syndromes who do not have ST-segment elevation. There is increasing evidence to suggest that CD40 ligand has an important role in the progression of coronary disease and in plaque destabilization. The predictive value of soluble CD40 ligand as a marker for clinical outcome was investigated, as well as the therapeutic effect of glycoprotein IIb/IIIa receptor inhibition in patients with acute coronary syndromes.

Methods.—Serum levels of soluble CD40 ligand were assayed in 1088 patients with acute coronary syndromes who had previously been enrolled in a randomized trial that compared abciximab with placebo before coronary angioplasty, and in 626 patients with acute chest pain.

Results.—The levels of soluble CD40 ligand were elevated in 221 of 1088 (40.6%) patients with acute coronary syndromes. Among the patients who received placebo, elevated soluble CD40 ligand levels were associated with a significantly increased risk of death or nonfatal myocardial infarction in 6 months of follow-up (Fig 3). The prognostic value of this marker was validated in the patients with chest pain. Among these patients, elevated soluble CD40 ligand levels identified those with acute coronary syndromes who were at high risk for death or nonfatal myocardial infarction. The increased risk in patients with elevated soluble CD40 ligand levels was significantly reduced by treatment with abciximab, whereas no treatment effect of abciximab was observed in patients with low levels of soluble CD40 ligand.

Conclusions.—Elevation of soluble CD40 ligand levels in patients with unstable coronary artery disease indicated an increased risk of cardiovascular events. Elevation of soluble CD40 ligand helps to identify a subgroup of persons at high risk who are likely to benefit from antiplatelet treatment with abciximab.

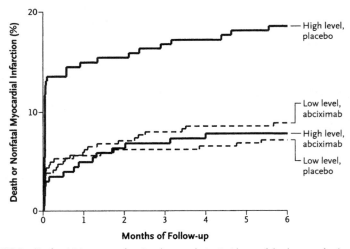

FIGURE 3.—Kaplan-Meier curves showing the cumulative incidence of death or nonfatal myocardial infarction during six months of follow-up, according to the base-line level of soluble CD40 ligand in the placebo group (544 patients) and the abciximab group (544 patients). High levels of soluble CD40 ligand were defined as levels greater than 5.0 μg per liter, and low levels as 5.0 μg per liter or less. (Courtesy of Heeschen C, for the CAPTURE Study Investigators: Soluble CD40 ligand in acute coronary syndromes. *N Engl J Med* 348:1104-1111, 2003. Copyright 2003 Massachusetts Medical Society.)

▶ With the acute coronary syndrome being the complex thing that it is patho-physiologically, with many stages, clinical variations, and degrees, there is definitely room for more biomarkers specific for various aspects. From this report, it appears that the circulating soluble ligand for CD40 from activated platelets is one of these.

M. G. Bissell, MD, PhD, MPH

Hemoglobin Glycosylation Index Is Not Related With Blood Glucose

Merino-Torres JF, Fajardo-Montañana C, Ferrer-Garcia JC, et al (Univ Hosp "La Fe," Valencia, Spain)
J Diabetes Complications 17:249-253, 2003   23–4

Introduction.—The accurate assessment of blood glucose control is paramount in preventing chronic complications in patients with diabetes mellitus. Glycosylation Index (HGI) quantifies the extent to which individuals demonstrate an HbA_{1c} greater or less than average for the population. The association between HGI and blood glucose was evaluated in 25 patients with type I diabetes.

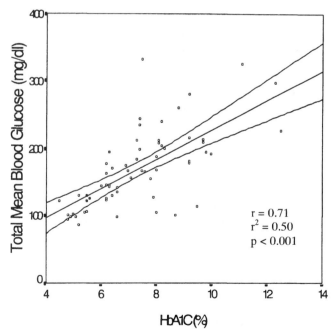

$$r = 0.71$$
$$r^2 = 0.50$$
$$p < 0.001$$

FIGURE 1.—Correlation of the total mean blood glucose with the HbA_{1c}. The regression line is indicated together with the 95% confidence interval. (Courtesy of Merino-Torres JF, Fajardo-Montañana C, Ferrer-Garcia JC, et al: Hemoglobin glycosylation index is not related with blood glucose. *J Diabetes Complications* 17:249-253, 2003.)

Methods.—All participants (12 males,13 females; mean age, 22.0 years) were instructed to self-monitor their glucose levels. The HbA_{1c} (determined by high-performance liquid chromatography [HPLC]) and self-monitored blood glucose levels were evaluated every 3 months. Patients were monitored for 3 to 9 months; 62 measurements of HbA_{1c} were included. The mean blood glucose (MBG) levels were calculated via self-monitored blood glucose records. A linear regression was determined between HbA_{1c} and MBG during the 60 days before sampling to ascertain HbA_{1c}. For each patient's MBG, a predicted HbA_{1c} was ascertained from the population regression equation. The HGI was then determined as HGI = observed HbA_{1c} − predicted HbA_{1c}. Blood glucose was evaluated within target range (WTR), below target range (BTR), and above target range (ATR) according to the European Diabetes Policy Group Consensus for type I diabetes.

Results.—A good linear regression between HbA_{1c} and MBG was seen ($r = .71$, $r^2 = .50$; $P < .001$) (Fig 1). No association was observed between HGI and the percentage of WTR, BTR, or ATR values. The percentage of self-monitored blood glucose ATR and BTR was the same for high glycosylators (HGI > 0 and ATR: mean, 56.2%; HGI > 0 and BTR: mean, 34.5%) as for low glycosylators (HGI < 0 and ATR: mean, 52.8%; HGI < 0 and BTR: mean, 25.1%).

Conclusion.—The HGI is determined by physiologic factors, along with blood glucose levels. A prospective investigation should be performed that would make it possible to determine whether HGI together with HbA_{1c} can predict the incidence and severity of chronic complications of diabetes.

▶ Although nonenzymatic glycosylation of proteins and other structures is known to be the basis for most of the long-term complications of diabetes mellitus, it is also known that there is considerable interindividual variation in the rate and degree to which glycosylation occurs. Not all patients with tightly controlled blood sugars avoid complications equally well. Perhaps, as these authors suggest, this new HGI will provide insight and better prognostic ability.

M. G. Bissell, MD, PhD, MPH,

Comparison of Intraoperative iPTH Assay (QPTH) Criteria in Guiding Parathyroidectomy: Which Criterion Is the Most Accurate?
Carneiro DM, Solorzano CC, Nader MC, et al (Univ of Miami, Fla)
Surgery 134:973-981, 2003   23–5

Introduction.—During the past decade, quick parathyroid hormone assays (QPTH) have been developed and have gained widespread use as intraoperative adjuncts during parathyroidectomy. The accuracy in predicting postoperative calcemia is associated with blood sample timing and the criteria applied. To improve specificity or to reduce the cost of QPTH, several criteria have been used to predict complete excision. A group of Miami surgeons have developed a new criterion for their predictions. The accuracy of the Miami criterion was compared with that of other published QPTH criteria in predicting operative outcome.

Methods.—Both QPTH and the Miami criterion (intact parathyroid hormone [iPTH] level decrease 50% or greater from the highest of either preincision or preexcision level at 10 minutes after gland excision) were used to predict postoperative calcium levels in 341 consecutive patients with sporadic primary hyperparathyroidism who were followed up for 6 or more months after the surgery or recognized as surgical failures. The intraoperative iPTH values of these patients were reexamined with the use of 5 published criteria to predict complete resection. The postoperative calcium levels were correlated with the criteria predictions.

Results.—The Miami criterion accurately predicted postoperative calcium levels in 329 (96.5%) of 341 patients; the 12 patients whose predictions were inaccurate included 3 false positives and 9 false negatives. Using other criteria, 2 of 3 false-positive results could have been prevented; the 3% incidence of false-negative predictions would then increase to between 6% and 24%, causing unneeded neck explorations to search for multiglandular disease.

Conclusion.—Surgeons attempting to increase QPTH specificity significantly reduce the accuracy and intraoperative usefulness of the assay. The Miami criterion has the greatest accuracy when compared with that of the other criteria.

▶ The availability of rapid intraoperative methods for parathyroid hormone has been accepted by many as a "chemical biopsy" supporting the surgeon's decision making in real time. But just how good a prognostic indicator the test is depends on the details of how it is used. Actually, this statement is as true of this assay than of any other. The current authors offer a head-to-head outcomes study of different iPTH interpretive criteria.

M. G. Bissell, MD, PhD, MPH

Cancer Antigen 125 Associated With Multiple Benign and Malignant Pathologies
Miralles C, Orea M, España P, et al (Hosp Universitario, Madrid)
Ann Surg Oncol 10:150-154, 2003   23–6

Background.—The tumor-associated cancer antigen (CA) 125 is a high molecular glycoprotein produced by normal cells of different tissues derived from the celomic epithelium. Increased levels of CA-125 have been found in several pathologic situations. This has been found to be useful for monitoring the course of epithelial ovarian cancer. The clinical utility of CA-125 for applications other than the follow-up of ovarian carcinoma has not been accepted, but many physicians nevertheless request the test in a variety of clinical situations, particularly as a potential marker of occult ovarian carcinoma when serosal structures are involved.

CA-125 testing is also requested frequently as a differential diagnosis in patients with pleural or peritoneal fluid. However, CA-125 is produced not only by the ovarian cancer cell but also by normal epithelia. The prevalence of CA-125 increases in a population of patients attending a general hospital was analyzed, and the possible clinical implications of increased CA-125 levels were explored.

Methods.—A total of 380 CA-125 assays were performed on 4 different days among randomly selected patients attending 1 hospital. Serum CA-125 was measured with a commercial enzyme immunoassay. Clinical records were reviewed for assessment of clinical parameters.

Results.—CA-125 was increased in 61 patients (16%). The pathologic processes in these patients were heart failure in 9 (14.7%), lung disease in 11 (18%), hepatic cirrhosis in 7 (11.4%), malignant tumors in 9 (14.7%), intra-abdominal nonhepatic disease in 6 (10%), previous surgery in 17 (27.8%), and miscellaneous in 2 (3%). Effusions were observed in 34 patients (55.7%).

Conclusion.—The findings provided confirmation of the variety of benign and malignant pathologic processes coursing with increased levels of CA-125. Cardiovascular and chronic liver disease were the most frequent diagnoses in patients with increased CA-125 levels. These results support the opinion that CA-125 lacks utility as a marker for malignancy. However, there may be a role for CA-125 in the follow-up of cardiovascular, hepatic, and tumoral diseases with serosal involvement.

▶ It should not surprise us to learn from this report that CA-125 is not specific for ovarian cancer. As with most serum tumor markers, the antigen actually proves to be associated with serosal tissue in a variety of locations. Like carcinoembryonic antigen and others, its linkage with carcinoma is coincidental. Thus, the wide spectrum of disease represented in this study helps account for the low predictive value as a screening test.

M. G. Bissell, MD, PhD, MPH

Seasonal Pseudohyperkalaemia
Sinclair D, Briston P, Young R, et al (Queen Alexandra Hosp, Portsmouth, England; Univ of Portsmouth, England)
J Clin Pathol 56:385-388, 2003   23–7

Background.—Factitious hyperkalemia has long complicated the estimation of serum potassium concentrations. A delay in centrifugation of blood samples is known to lead to an artificially high potassium concentration in the serum or plasma because potassium leaks from the blood cells and into the serum or plasma. Other important causes of factitious hyperkalemia are hemolysis, thrombocytosis, "leaky cell syndrome," other leukocytoses, and refrigeration of the whole blood sample before centrifugation.

However, other factors, such as fist clenching before venipuncture, also appear to influence potassium concentrations. The relationship between

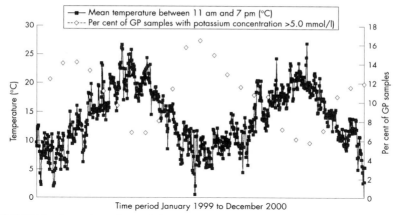

FIGURE 2.—Comparison of mean daily temperature between 11.00 and 19.00 hours and potassium concentrations of more than 5.0 mmol/L in general practitioner (*GP*) samples. (Courtesy of Sinclair D, Briston P, Young R, et al: Seasonal pseudohyperkalaemia. *J Clin Pathol* 56:385-388, 2003. With permission from the BMJ Publishing Group.)

ambient temperature and serum potassium concentrations in samples from primary care were investigated.

Methods.—Potassium concentrations were estimated in general practitioner and hospital ward samples in 1 hospital in the United Kingdom over a period of 2 years. The serum was obtained from gel separator samples. The number of general practice samples analyzed during each month ranged from 5093 to 8978, with a mean of 7068 samples per month.

Results.—The declining temperature during the winter months was associated with a rise in the mean daily serum potassium concentrations in samples from general practice; the inverse association was observed during the summer months (Fig 2). This effect was restricted to those samples obtained from general practice and was not observed in hospital ward samples.

Conclusion.—Exposure of samples to variations in ambient temperature during the transport of samples to the laboratory has a profound effect on the measured serum potassium concentrations.

▶ Here's a study documenting something that the operators of regional reference labs have long suspected: a potentially significant source of seasonal pre-analytic variation in test results. Specimens transported and temporarily stored under various environmental conditions not surprisingly appear to give rise to varying levels of specimen artifact, due in turn to varying levels of red cell fragility. Something to be aware of when analyzing results on shipped and transported specimens.

M. G. Bissell, MD, PhD, MPH

C-Reactive Protein and the Risk of Incident Colorectal Cancer

Erlinger TP, Platz EA, Rifai N, et al (Johns Hopkins Med Insts, Baltimore, Md; Johns Hopkins Bloomberg School of Public Health, Baltimore, Md; Harvard Med School, Boston; et al)
JAMA 291:585-590, 2004   23–8

Background.—It has been proposed that inflammation may increase the risk of cancer. Growing evidence from laboratory studies supports the role of inflammation in the pathogenesis of colorectal cancer, but data from epidemiologic studies are sparse. Inflammation could be of particular significance in the pathogenesis of colorectal cancers. C-reactive protein (CRP) is an acute-phase protein that is produced primarily in the liver in response to stimulation by interleukin 6. In recent studies, elevated levels of CRP have been shown to reliably predict cardiovascular events in several populations. The risk of incident colon and rectal cancer associated with elevated baseline plasma concentrations of CRP was investigated.

Methods.—A prospective, nested case-control study was conducted of a cohort of 22,887 adults 18 years of age or older. The patients were enrolled between May and October 1989 and followed up through December 2000. A total of 172 cases of colorectal cancer were identified through linkage with local and state cancer registries. Up to 2 controls (342 cases) were selected from the cohort for each case and matched by age, sex, race, and date of blood flow. The main outcome measures were the odds ratios of incident colon and rectal cancer.

Results.—The concentrations of plasma CRP were higher among all colorectal cancer patients combined than among control subjects (median CRP, 2.44 vs 1.94 mg/L). The highest CRP concentration was observed in persons in whom colon cancer subsequently developed compared with matched controls. Among the patients with rectal cancer, CRP concentrations were not significantly different from those of control subjects.

The risk of colon cancer was higher in persons in the highest versus the lowest quartile of CRP concentration. The corresponding association was stronger in nonsmokers. An increase of 1 standard deviation in log CRP (1.02 mg/L) was associated with an increased risk of colon cancer after adjustment for potential confounders and exclusion of cases occurring within 2 years of baseline or exclusion of those with late-stage colon cancer at the time of diagnosis.

Conclusion.—Plasma CRP concentrations are elevated in persons in whom colon cancer subsequently develops. These findings support the hypothesis that inflammation is a risk factor for the development of colon cancer in persons at average risk.

▶ We seem to be entering an era of increased appreciation for the role of inflammation in an ever-wider variety of conditions in which it was previously considered irrelevant. With this study, colorectal cancer enters the ranks of such conditions, and the interpretation of an elevated serum CRP has made one important condition more complex.

M. G. Bissell, MD, PhD, MPH

Novel Diagnostic Test for Acute Stroke
Lynch JR, Blessing R, White WD, et al (Duke Univ, Durham, NC)
Stroke 35:57-63, 2004   23–9

Background.—The diagnosis and management of stroke is significantly limited by the absence of a widely available and sensitive diagnostic test for acute cerebral ischemia. Absent such a test, the diagnosis of acute ischemic stroke in most facilities is made solely on the basis of clinical findings after intracranial hemorrhage or mass lesion is excluded by CT. The feasibility of developing a diagnostic panel of blood-borne biochemical markers of cerebral ischemia was investigated.

Methods.—Serial blood samples were obtained from 65 patients with suspected ischemic stroke and 157 control subjects seen in the emergency department of an academic medical center. Analyses were conducted of 26 blood-borne markers believed to play a role in the ischemic cascade, and a 3-variable logistic regression model was created to predict the clinical diagnosis of stroke, which was defined as persistent neurologic symptoms of cerebral ischemia of more than 24 hours' duration.

Results.—Of the 26 blood-borne markers evaluated, univariate logistic analysis showed that 4 were highly correlated with stroke: S100β, a marker of glial activation; matrix metalloproteinase-9 and vascular cell adhesion molecule (both markers of inflammation); and von Willebrand factor (a marker of thrombosis) (Fig 2). The logistic model developed for this study provided a sensitivity and specificity of 90% for prediction of stroke when the outcome level was set to a cutoff of $P = .1$.

Conclusion.—It appears that a panel of blood-borne biochemical markers may aid in the identification of patients with acute cerebral ischemia who could benefit from urgent care. A test such as this may also help in the identification of stroke patients in the prehospital setting so that they can be "fast-tracked" to an appropriately equipped facility.

▶ On every emergency room physician's list of "lab tests we wish we had available" 2 have always been prominent: a test for rule out congestive heart failure and a test for rule out stroke. With the dawn of the brain natriuretic peptide era, the first of these has become a reality. With the panel of 4 correlated analytes that is reported in this article, perhaps the second is now more of a concrete possibility than previously.

M. G. Bissell, MD, PhD, MPH

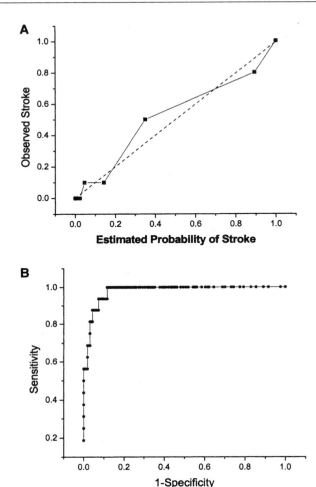

FIGURE 2.—**A,** Observed rates of stroke versus predicted rate of stroke for patients in whom blood was drawn within 6 hours of symptom onset on the basis of a logistic regression model using the variables von Willebrand factor, vascular cell adhesion molecule, and matrix metalloproteinase–9. Patients were divided into groups of 10 according to the probability of stroke as defined by this model. Actual stroke rate for each group is plotted versus average model prediction. *Dashed diagonal line* represents perfect calibration of the model predictions. **B,** receiver operating characteristic curve demonstrating sensitivity as a function of 1–specificity. This logistic model has a sensitivity and specificity of 90%. (Courtesy of Lynch JR, Blessing R, White WD, et al: Novel diagnostic test for acute stroke. *Stroke* 35:57-63, 2004. Reproduced by permission of *Stroke*. Copyright 2004 American Heart Association.)

C-Reactive Protein Concentration Distribution Among US Children and Young Adults: Findings From the National Health and Nutrition Examination Survey, 1999-2000

Ford ES, Giles WH, Myers GL, et al (Ctrs for Disease Control and Prevention, Atlanta, Ga; Harvard Med School, Boston)

Clin Chem 49:1353-1357, 2003   23–10

Background.—Inflammation is a component of many disease processes, and there has been a better appreciation of the contribution of inflammation to the pathophysiology of cardiovascular disease. There are many markers of inflammation, but C-reactive protein (CRP) concentrations are easily measured, providing an inexpensive and accurate marker of inflammation. The pathogenesis of cardiovascular disease often begins in childhood. The distribution of CRP concentrations among children and young adults in the United States, which until now has not been known, was investigated.

Methods.—Data were obtained from 3348 children and young adults in the United States, ages 3 to 19 years, who participated in the National Health and Nutrition Examination Survey, 1999 to 2000. These data were used to describe the distribution of CRP concentrations, based on results obtained with a high-sensitivity latex-enhanced turbidimetric assay.

Results.—The range of CRP concentrations was 0.1 to 90.8 mg/L, with concentrations increasing with age. Females aged 16 to 19 years had higher concentrations than males in this age range. Mexican Americans had the highest CRP concentrations among the major race or ethnic groups (Fig 1).

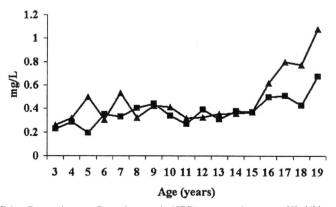

FIGURE 1.—Geometric mean C-reactive protein (CRP) concentration among US children and young adults after adjustment for race or ethnicity, body mass index percentile, and total cholesterol concentration, by sex and age. National Health and Nutrition Examination Survey, 1999 to 2000. *Squares* indicate males; *triangles*, females. CRP concentrations greater than 10 mg/L were excluded. (Courtesy of Ford ES, Giles WH, Myers GL, et al: C-reactive protein concentration distribution among US children and young adults: Findings from the National Health and Nutrition Examination Survey, 1999-2000. *Clin Chem* 49:1353-1357, 2003. ©2003 The American Association for Clinical Chemistry.)

Conclusion.—This study is the first to describe the CRP concentration distribution among children and young adults in the United States on the basis of results obtained with a high-sensitivity assay.

▶ New reference range data, particularly new reference range data on children, are always a valuable commodity to the laboratory medicine community. Here we have large-scale population-based reference intervals on the important new cardiac risk marker CRP in children and young adults. This fills a major gap in our armamentarium.

M. G. Bissell, MD, PhD, MPH

Automated Multicapillary Electrophoresis for Analysis of Human Serum Proteins
Gay-Bellile C, Bengoufa D, Houze P, et al (Hôpital St-Louis, Paris; Hotel Dieu, Nantes, France)
Clin Chem 49:1909-1915, 2003   23–11

Background.—The analysis of serum proteins by electrophoresis is routinely used for screening and monitoring not only B-cell malignancies but also immune and inflammatory responses. Capillary electrophoresis has emerged in the last decade as a powerful analytical tool. A new, automated multicapillary zone electrophoresis (CE) instrument—the Capillarys instrument—for analysis of human serum protein was evaluated.

Methods.—The Capillarys β1-β2+ reagent set was used to separate proteins at 7 kV for 4 minutes in 15.5 cm × 25 µm fused-silica capillaries (8 capillaries) at 35.5°C in a pH 10 buffer with online detection at 200 nm. Serum samples with different electrophoretic patterns (265 samples) or potential interference (69 samples) were analyzed and compared with agarose gel electrophoresis.

Results.—CVs were less than 3.5% for albumin, less than 11% for α_1-globulin, less than 4.1% for α_2-globulin, less than 7.4% for β-globulin, and less than 5.8% for γ-globulin (3 control levels). The measured throughput was 60 samples per hour. For 116 patients without paraprotein, the median differences between CE and agarose gel electrophoresis were −5.4 g/L for albumin, 4.0 g/L for α_1-globulin, 0.7 g/L for α_2-globulin, 0.6 g/L for β-globulin, and −0.1 g/L for γ-globulin (not significant).

A majority of samples had at least oneγ-migrating peak detected by CE (135 vs 130 samples), but fewer were quantified (84 vs 91 samples) because of γ- to β-migration shifts. There was a 1.2 g/L median difference between CE and agarose gel electrophoresis for γ-migrating paraprotein quantification. Several ultraviolet-absorbing substances (lipid emulsion, hemoglobin) or molecules (contrast agent, gelatin-based plasma substitute) induced CE artifacts.

Conclusion.—The Capillarys instrument is a reliable multicapillary zone electrophoresis instrument for serum protein analysis. The advantages of full automation are combined in this system with high analytical performance and throughput.

▶ Serum protein electrophoresis is generally a more broadly utilized technique in Europe than in the United States, and so it is not surprising that new methods for high-volume work in this area seem to have been implemented there more readily. The first multicapillary electrophoresis method was the Beckman Paragon CZE2000 system released in 1994, but it was far from universally adopted. Here the authors evaluate a new European-produced instrument.

M. G. Bissell, MD, PhD, MPH

Subject Index

A

Acanthocyturia
in differentiating diabetic nephropathy from glomerulonephritis, 380
Accessory nipples
clear cells of Toker in, 100
Acquired immunodeficiency syndrome (AIDS)
(*see also* Human immunodeficiency virus)
classification of transmission risk, 374
Acute coronary syndrome
soluble CD40 ligand levels in, 409
Acute lymphoblastic leukemia/lymphoblastic lymphoma
vs. lymphocyte-rich thymoma, flow cytometry in diagnosis of, 286
Acute megakaryoblastic leukemia (AML)
novel karyotype in, 385
Acute myeloid leukemia (AML)
detection of *FLT3* gene mutations by multiplex polymerase chain reaction and capillary electrophoresis assay, 324
gene expression profiling to identify prognostic subclasses, 322
Acute promyelocytic leukemia (APL)
gene expression profiling during all-*trans* retinoic acid–induced cell differentiation in, 378
Acute respiratory distress syndrome (ARDS)
open-lung biopsy in, 121
Adenocarcinoma
endometrial
vs. endocervical adenocarcinoma, 171
myoinvasive, unusual epithelial and stroma changes in, 182
vs. ovarian endometrioid tumors of low malignant potential, 168
prostate (*see also* Prostate cancer)
interphase fluorescence in situ hybridization in prostate needle biopsy specimens, 189
quantitative GSTP1 methylation and detection in sextant biopsies, 194
pulmonary, adenomatous hyperplasia as precursor, 107
salivary gland, KIT expression in, 232
sinonasal, 237
Adenoid cystic carcinoma
KIT expression in, 229, 232
Adenomas
monomorphic, KIT expression in, 232
serrated, colorectal, 40

Adenomatous hyperplasia
as precursor for bronchioloalveolar cancer, 107
Adrenal gland
cortical vs. medullary tumors, 212
African Americans
hereditary prostate cancer in, 196
AGUS (*see* Atypical glandular cells of undetermined significance)
AIDS (*see* Acquired immunodeficiency syndrome)
AITL (*see* Angioimmunoblastic T-cell lymphoma [AITL])
ALK protein
in evaluation of lymphoma, 287
ALL/LBL (*see* Acute lymphoblastic leukemia/lymphoblastic lymphoma)
All-*trans* retinoic acid (ATRA)–induced cell differentiation
in acute promyelocytic leukemia, gene expression profiling during, 378
Allelic imbalance
plasma DNA, as tumor-specific marker in lung cancer, 325
α_1-antitrypsin (α_1-AT) deficiency
genomic DNA extraction from small amounts of serum for detection of, 396
Aluminum
apoptosis in neurons and exposure to, 245
Alzheimer's disease
neuronal depletion of calcium-dependent proteins in the dentate gyrus in, 256
AML (*see* Acute megakaryoblastic leukemia; Acute myeloid leukemia)
Amniotic infection syndrome
nosology and reproducibility of placental reaction patterns, 313
Anaplastic large cell lymphoma
vs. lymphomatoid papulosis, 91
Angiogenesis
survivin-dependent, in ischemic brain tissue, 258
Angioimmunoblastic T-cell lymphoma (AITL)
CD10 expression in extranodal dissemination, 284
Anthrax
inhalational, accuracy of screening after a bioterrorist attack, 368
Antibiotic resistance
of gram-negative pathogens, patient- and institution-specific variables and, 373

Author Index